# Allied Health
## *Practice Issues and Trends in the New Millennium*

# Allied Health
## *Practice Issues and Trends in the New Millennium*

Pedro J. Lecca, PhD
Peggy A. Valentine, EdD
Kevin J. Lyons, PhD
Editors

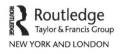

Routledge
Taylor & Francis Group
NEW YORK AND LONDON

First Published by
The Haworth Press, Inc., 10 Alice Street, Binghamton, NY 13904-1580.

Transferred to Digital Printing 2009 by Routledge
270 Madison Ave, New York NY 10016
2 Park Square, Milton Park, Abingdon, Oxon, OX14 4RN

Cover design by Jennifer M. Gaska.

**Library of Congress Cataloging-in-Publication Data**

Allied health : practice issues and trends in the new millennium / [edited by] Pedro J. Lecca, Peggy A. Valentine, Kevin J. Lyons.
    p. cm.
Includes bibliographical references and index.
    ISBN 0-7890-1846-2 (hardcover : alk. paper)—ISBN 0-7890-1847-0 (softcover : alk. paper)
1. Allied health personnel.
    [DNLM: 1. Allied Health Personnel—trends—United States. 2. Allied Health Personnel—education—United States. 3. Delivery of Health Care—trends—United States. 4. Health Policy—United States. 5. Professional Competence—United States. W 21.5 A4355 2003] I. Lecca, Pedro J., 1936-. II. Valentine, Peggy A. III. Lyons, Kevin J.

R697.A4 A438 2003
610.69'0973—dc21

2002014718

# CONTENTS

**About the Edtiors**                                                    xi

**Contributors**                                                         xiii

**Preface**                                                              xv

**Chapter 1. Historical Overview: Evolution of the Allied
Health Professions**                                                     1
> *Harry E. Douglas III*

Introduction                                                             1
The Changing Medical Paradigm                                            2
Toward a Definition of Allied Health                                     3
The Evolving U.S. Health Care System                                     6
The Evolving Role of Education and Standards
    for the Allied Health Professions                13
A New Majority in the Health Professions                                 16
Toward Recognition of the Allied Health Professions                      19
Summary                                                                  26

**Chapter 2. Role of the Federal Government in Allied
Health Education**                                                       31
> *Norman L. Clark*

The Nebraska Story: A Case Study                                         31
The Federal Government and Health Professions Education                  32
Program Examples                                                         41
Conclusion                                                               42

**Chapter 3. Primary Health Care**                                       45
> *Howard Straker*
> *Marvin Barnard*

Introduction                                                             45
Case Study                                                               45
Primary Care Definition                                                  46
Major Specialties That Interact with Primary Care                        53

Who Practices Primary Care? 55
Controversies and Conceptual/Systemic Flaws 58
Summary and Future Considerations 59

**Chapter 4. Rehabilitative and Restorative Therapies** **61**
*John Echternach*

History of the Development of Rehabilitative
    and Restorative Therapies 64
How Teams Work Together 72
The Role of Research 73

**Chapter 5. Health Care Management** **75**
*Joan M. Kiel*

Health Management Defined 75
Health Care Management Organizational Structure 79
Health Care Management Functions 82
Meeting the Challenge 98

**Chapter 6. Chemical and Dietary Therapies** **101**
*Barbara F. Harland*

Case Study of Testimonials of Efficacy of Certain
    Therapies 101
Complementary and Alternative Medicine 102
Dietary Supplements 104
Facts About Food 110
Summary 116

**Chapter 7. Diagnostic Services** **119**
*Veronica A. Clarke-Tasker*
*Marguerite E. Neita*
*Marvin Barnard*

Multidisciplinary Health Care Team 119
Case Study 120
Factors in Selecting Laboratory Tests 121
Laboratory and Other Diagnostic Procedures 125

**Chapter 8. Psychosocial Interaction and Its Therapeutic Impact on Patients' Physical and Mental Health: Implications for Health Care Providers**     **137**

*K. Habib Khan*

Introduction     137
Technical Competence versus People Skills     138
Definition of Health     140
Psychosocial Therapies     140
Expectations from a Successful Health Care Provider     146
Health Workers and Stress     147
How to Handle Stress     148
Health Workers As Care Providers, Leaders, and Managers     151

**Chapter 9. Interdisciplinary and Community-Based Health Care**     **155**

*Ivan Quervalu*

Interdisciplinary Behavioral Approaches     156
Behavioral Services in Hospitals     156
The Case of Jason     157
Depression in Primary Care     160
Community Health Services     162
Complementary and Alternative Medicine Treatments     165

**Chapter 10. Demographic and Health Trends in the Twenty-First Century**     **171**

*Richard E. Oliver*
*Stephen L. Wilson*

Aging Population     173
Racial and Ethnic Diversity     177
Poverty and Underserved Populations     179
Changes in the Family Structure     180
Demographic Changes and the Allied Health Professions     182

**Chapter 11. New Directions for Accreditation of Allied Health Education Programs**     **187**

*John E. Trufant*

Part I: Overview of Accreditation     188
Part II: Accreditation in Allied Health     193

Part III: Issues in Allied Health Education                    197
Part IV: New Directions                                        201
Conclusion                                                     211

**Chapter 12. Allied Health Education in a Global Community**                                                  **215**
    *Cheryl T. Samuels*

Introduction                                                   215
Overview of Race and Origin of the U.S. Population             216
Cultural Competence in a Global Community                      218
Trends Shaping Use of Complementary and Alternative
   Approaches                                   220
Implications for Education and Practice                        222
Summary                                                        231

**Chapter 13. Genomics, Proteomics, and Allied Health**        **235**
    *Thomas W. Elwood*

Introduction                                                   235
Overview                                                       236
Role of Genetics in Health Care                                239
Ethical, Legal, and Social Issues                              242
Pharmacogenomics                                               244
Conclusion                                                     247

**Chapter 14. Interprofessional Collaborative Alliances**      **249**
    *Lorna Hayward*
    *Rosanna DeMarco*
    *M. Marcia Lynch*

Introduction                                                   249
Definition of Terms                                            250
Need for Collaboration                                         251
Case Example                                                   253
Barriers Related to Interprofessional Work                     255
Interprofessional Alliance Model                               259
Case Example: Interprofessional Alliance Model                 263
Summary                                                        268

**Chapter 15. Impact of Technology on Allied Health Education**     **271**

> *Elzar Camper Jr.*
> *Amani M. Nuru-Jeter*
> *Carole I. Smith*

Case Study     271
Familiarity with Technology     273
Preservice Technology Preparation of Allied Health
    Practitioners     275
Core Curriculum and Technology Course     276
Connecting Preservice Theory and In-Service Practice     277
Determining and Applying Content     280
Internet and Searching     282
Policy     285
Technology and Online Education     287
Trends in Adult Learning and Postsecondary Education     290
Health Promotion     291
Summary     294
Recommendations     294

**Chapter 16. Allied Health and Public Policy: Making Change Happen**     **299**

> *Thomas W. Elwood*

Separation of Powers     300
Ergonomics     302
Discussion     308
Other Determinants in Making Public Policy     310
Interest Groups     312
Conclusion     315

**Chapter 17. Gaps in Knowledge and Research Needs**     **319**

> *Kevin J. Lyons*

Introduction     319
Case Study     320
Importance of Research to the Allied Health Professions     322
Types of Research Being Conducted by Allied Health
    Professionals     324
Strategies for Becoming Professional     325
Conclusion     331

**Chapter 18. Preparing Future Allied Health Leaders**    **333**
   *Gail A. Nielsen*

Case Study: What Would the Leader Do?    333
Why Allied Health Professionals Should Prepare
   for the Future    336
Observations from the Front Line    340
Coalition for Allied Health Leadership (CAHL)    343
Recommendations for Students of Allied Health    348
Summary    349

**Chapter 19. Employment Opportunities in Allied Health**    **353**
   *Peggy Valentine*
   *Pedro J. Lecca*

Introduction    353
Preparing for Careers in a High-Tech Age    353
Where Are the Jobs?    355
Maximizing the Undergraduate Educational Experiences
   for Future Employment    359
Maximizing the Graduate Educational Experiences
   for Future Employment    360
Summary    361

**Conclusion and Recommendations**    **363**

**Appendix. Allied Health Organizations and Affiliates**    **369**

**Index**    **385**

# ABOUT THE EDITORS

**Pedro J. Lecca, PhD, RRh, LMSW,** is Professor and Dean of the College of Pharmacy, Nursing, and Allied Health Sciences at Howard University in Washington, DC. Dr. Lecca has received many honors, including an American Council on Higher Education Fellowship and two UTA awards: Outstanding Faculty Representative and Outstanding Faculty Senate President. He has been an examiner for the Malcolm Baldrige Award since 1998. Dr. Lecca has also been recognized by many community organizations for his volunteer work. He is a recipient of the Paul Harris Fellow Award from Rotary International. Dr. Lecca has served as Commissioner of Planning and Zoning for the City of Arlington, Texas, and served on the boards of over 10 community organizations. He is a participant in national and local Hispanic organizations, including the Educational Organization for United Latin Americans (EOFULA), ASPIRA of America, LULAC of Arlington, the Arlington Hispanic Advisory Council, and the Tarrant County Hispanic Clearinghouse. Dr. Lecca has written research grants totaling over $100 million and has written or contributed to over twenty books, including *Cultural Competency in Health and Human Service* and *Interdisciplinary Team Practice.*

**Peggy A. Valentine, EdD, PA-C, RN,** is Associate Dean and Associate Professor for the Division of Allied Health Sciences and a member of the graduate faculty at Howard University. She has published numerous articles on AIDS, minority health issues, and health care for the homeless. She is the recipient of many grants and subcontracts, and presently serves as Principal Investigator for the Establishing a Complementary Health Care Curriculum for Allied Students project, funded by the Ford Foundation. She is also Principal Investigator for the University Technical Assistance Project for HIV Prevention in Malawi, Africa, funded by the Centers for Disease Control and Prevention. Dr. Valentine is listed in *Who's Who of American Women* and was honored as Educator of the Year by the American Academy of Physician Assistants. She serves as Chairman of the Board for My Brother's Keeper and is a board member of the United Negro College Fund's Project HOPE. Dr. Lecca is the immediate Past President of the National Society of Allied Health.

**Kevin J. Lyons, PhD,** is Associate Dean in the College of Health Professions and the College of Graduate Studies, and Director of the Center for Collaborative Research at Thomas Jefferson University. Dr. Lyons has served in the Institute of Medicine of the National Academy of Sciences' Committee on Health Services Research (Training and Workforce Issues) and has written a white paper for the National Commission on Allied Health as well as numerous other publications. He is Editor of the *Journal of Allied Health,* the scholarly journal of the Association of Schools of Allied Health Professions (ASAHP). He is a recipient of the J. Warren Perry Distinguished Author Award and is a Fellow of ASAHP.

# CONTRIBUTORS

**Marvin Barnard, MD,** is Chairman of the Physician Assistant Department at Howard University, Washington, DC.

**Elzar Camper Jr., EdD,** is Professor in the Department of Media, Communication and Technology, East Stroudsburg University, East Stroudsburg, Pennsylvania.

**Norman L. Clark, DDS, MPH, JD,** is a Captain (Retired) in the United States Public Health Service, Reedville, Virginia.

**Veronica A. Clarke-Tasker, PhD, RN, MBA,** is Assistant Professor in the Division of Nursing, Howard University, Washington, DC.

**Rosanna DeMarco, PhD, RN, ACRN,** is Assistant Professor, Bouve College of Health Sciences, School of Nursing, Northeastern University, Boston, Massachusetts.

**Harry E. Douglas III, DPA, MPA,** is Executive Vice President of Charles R. Drew University of Medicine and Science, Los Angeles, California.

**John Echternach, EdD,** is Professor and Eminent Scholar in the School of Physical Therapy, Old Dominion University, Norfolk, Virginia.

**Thomas W. Elwood, DrPH,** is Executive Director of the Association of Schools of Allied Health Professions, Washington, DC.

**Barbara F. Harland, PhD,** is Professor, Department of Nutritional Sciences, College of Pharmacy, Nursing and Allied Health Sciences at Howard University, Washington, DC.

**Lorna Hayward, EdD,** is Assistant Professor, Bouve College of Health Sciences, School of Health Professions, Department of Physical Therapy, Northeastern University, Boston, Massachusetts.

**K. Habib Khan, PhD,** is Associate Professor in the Health Management Program, Division of Allied Health Sciences, Howard University, Washington, DC.

**Joan M. Kiel, PhD,** is Chairman of the Health Management Systems Department, Duquesne University, Pittsburgh, Pennsylvania.

**M. Marcia Lynch, DNSc, RN,** is Associate Professor, Bouve College of Health Sciences, School of Nursing, Northeastern University, Boston, Massachusetts.

**Marguerite E. Neita, PhD,** is Associate Professor in the Department of Clinical Laboratory Science, Howard University, Washington, DC.

**Gail A. Nielsen, BSHCA,** is Patient Safety Administrator, Iowa Health System, Des Moines, Iowa.

**Amani M. Nuru-Jeter, MPH,** is PhD Candidate and Research Associate in the Department of Health Policy and Management, Bloomberg School of Public Health, The Johns Hopkins University, Baltimore, Maryland.

**Richard E. Oliver, PhD,** is Dean of the School of Health Professions, University of Missouri, Columbus, Missouri.

**Ivan Quervalu, PhD,** is Director of the Office of Training, Development and Grants in the Department of Mental Health, Mental Retardation and Alcoholism Services, New York, New York.

**Cheryl T. Samuels, PhD,** is Dean of the College of Health Sciences, Old Dominion University, Norfolk, Virginia.

**Carole I. Smith, MS,** is Executive Director of the Mayor's Telecommunications Policy Advisory Commission, Executive Director of the Workforce 2000 Advisory Council, President of Carole I. Smith and Associates, and Cofounder and CEO of DigitalSistas.net, Philadelphia, Pennsylvania.

**Howard Straker, MPH,** is Assistant Professor in the Physician Assistant Program at George Washington University, Washington, DC.

**John E. Trufant, EdD,** is Dean and Vice President of the College of Health Sciences, Rush University, Chicago, Illinois.

**Stephen L. Wilson, PhD,** is Director of the School of Allied Health Professions and Associate Dean of the College of Medicine and Public Health, Ohio State University, Columbus, Ohio.

# Preface

The field of allied health continues to be the fastest growing employment sector in the United States, and by 2005, approximately 4 million new jobs will be added. Many of these new jobs will be in the disciplines of advancement of technologies and allied health practice, with home health care in the greatest demand.

When combined, allied health professionals comprise 60 percent of the health care workforce, the largest and most diverse pool of health workers in the United States. There are estimates of 140 to 200 distinct allied health occupations in the nation, representing approximately 2 to 3 million individuals.

Allied health professionals are trained individuals who share responsibility for the delivery of health care services or related services. They compliment, supplement, or support the functions of physicians, dentists, and other health professionals in the delivery of health care, thus playing a critical role in health care delivery. The National Commission on Allied Health in 1995 reported that allied health providers have tremendous potential for addressing issues of health care cost, quality, and access within the health care system. They provide disease detection, prevention, dietary, health promotion, rehabilitation, and health management services, and work in all levels of health care delivery.

Allied health professions are widely accepted for the critical and flexible services they provide. Given changing demographics, increasing longevity of the population, and a shift from health to high-tech careers, new computer technology, drug information, and health insurance options, the role of allied health professionals will undoubtedly expand. It will be challenging for the allied health educational system to keep up with the major changes impacting the health care system.

The health care system has undergone a remarkable transformation over the past decade. More than two decades ago, the expansion of health maintenance organizations (HMOs), through Kaiser in the West, and health insurance plans in the East, helped fuel the need for interdisciplinary cooperation and advances in manpower needs. HMOs provide a wide range of health services at low cost through expanded utilization of nonphysicians, thus reducing the cost of health care. Managed care plans now enroll more than 80 million Americans. Today, some critics complain about the rapid growth of insurance companies and programs targeted for the public, while some government officials say they have not expanded enough.

As the managed care system seeks to provide efficient and effective care for the nation, it has impacted allied health practice. The quality of health care has often been sacrificed for efficiency in delivering care at a reduced price. We believe the health care system must be redesigned to ensure that care is safe, effective, efficient, equitable, and tailored to each individual's specific needs. This can be achieved by using the knowledge and skills of all the allied health professionals.

New immigrants have also affected the health care system. It is interesting to note the U.S. population has increased significantly with new immigrants from South and Central America, Asia, and Africa. This population is younger, and will become the majority population in the next two decades. Today's children offer a preview of the nation's future citizens, workers, and parents.

An aging population has further impacted the health care delivery system as more people face questions about long-term care and insurance for themselves or family members. Through new drugs and technology, the elderly are living longer and healthier lives. The number of "old elderly" (eighty-five plus) is expected to rise 75 percent in the next two decades. In Washington, DC, for example, persons over the age of sixty comprised 17.8 percent of the total population, with those over the age of seventy-five being the fastest growing segment of the population. More than 25 percent of these individuals reside in nursing homes or community residence facilities staffed by a cadre of health care providers including allied health.

The economy, population, demographics, technology, and health care system will continue to expand in the twenty-first century. With this expansion, the general public will have greater access to health care information and therefore a demand for improved services. These and other changes have resulted in an expansion of allied health programs.

A number of reasons are cited for the expansion of allied health programs. The primary reason is the multidisciplinary approach taken during the past two decades for delivering health care services, which led to an expansion of providers. As mentioned earlier, managed care, a growing elderly population, and an increased need for rehabilitation services have also contributed to this expansion.

For the past few years, many of the allied health professions have expanded their educational programs, and advocated for more interdisciplinary approaches to practice, as concerns about the health and well-being of children and adolescents who live in poverty have grown. Many groups in the United States fall outside the economic and medical mainstreams, particularly the millions of low-income individuals with limited or no health insurance. It is critical that allied health professionals join public and private policymakers and educators in improving access to health care for all people.

Allied health professionals are in a key position to significantly contribute to the health care of this country. We know more about cancer prevention, detection, and treatment than ever before—yet not all segments of the population have benefited to the fullest extent possible from these advances. There are many reason for this, e.g., manpower shortages, cost, out-reach, and lack of access to adequate care. The Institute of Medicine's 1999 report, "The Unequal Burden of Cancer: An Assessment of NIH Research and Programs for Ethnic Minorities and the Medically Underserved," documents the gaps existing in this area and why the whole health care team is needed to make a difference.

Despite the expanded roles of allied health professionals, there continues to be a national shortage of some key disciplines. For example, a shortage of physician assistants in 1995 led to a doubling in the number of educational programs. Enrollment in physical therapy and occupational therapy programs declined in the late 1990s, resulting in a severe shortage of these professionals in the early 2000s. Certain diseases such as HIV/AIDS have led to the need for more home health providers. Coupled with advances in research, these changes will drive the demand for more allied health professionals. An example of this is human genome mapping which will revolutionize disease diagnosis and treatment. At the same time, the convergence of genomics, structural biology, and informatics, coupled with related changes in the research environment, is transforming biomedical research and the entire health care environment. All aspects of how health practitioners deliver health care will be affected. These trends create a series of problems in managing a public-private interface that does not yet have a well-articulated set of rules to match the new science. Protecting the privacy of personal health information while enabling improvements in clinical care and research has been intensely debated and is still far from being resolved.

Allied health professionals will be involved in these and other debates on protecting the privacy of health-related information. Allied health practice will be one of the most important policy issues of the next few years. Providing answers to the complex health questions facing today's society requires an integrated approach that melds multiple disciplines.

Chapter 1

# Historical Overview: Evolution of the Allied Health Professions

Harry E. Douglas III

## *INTRODUCTION*

Modern medicine, considered by many to be the foundation for the allied health professions, is rooted in ancient traditions of healing. Indeed, some aspects of those traditions are relevant and complementary to modern medical practice. The allied health professions are included in the ancient traditions of the healing arts. This is an important point because the general populace has shown deep reverence for the esoteric and special skills for healers of all types since the early dawn of humanity. Contemporary society continues to revere the health worker, including the allied health professional. While there has always been a central figure who ministered to the physical, mental, spiritual, and social conditions of people, such as the medicine man of shamanistic folk tradition, the physician in primitive society was physician, priest, magician, and philosopher in one person. In addition, other healing types were concerned with what was perceived to be the spiritual and emotional causation of illness. In the ancient world, it was commonly accepted that a function of religion was to heal disease.[1] Magicians and others were called upon to handle the mystical dimensions of life, e.g., ancestral spirits, evil spirits, and witchcraft. They were traditional folk healers who were familiar with the mental and psychological needs of individuals and communities. Such health providers could, in a real sense, be construed as a community working within the community. As such, each provider played a defined role within a system of community service that addressed the needs of the whole person.

Thus, to fully appreciate and understand the evolution of allied health professions one must study the evolution of the healing arts within the context of society while recognizing that the allied health sciences have always been an essential partner in the delivery of health and mental health services around the world.

## THE CHANGING MEDICAL PARADIGM

The medical paradigm has undergone considerable change since its early beginnings. The most significant of these has been the manner in which the health care profession, especially in the Western approach to medicine, viewed the patient and ultimately organized the delivery system to respond to patient needs.

### The Early Approach to Medicine

The early formative stages of medicine evolved around the concept of holistic health. Ancient medicine integrated mind-body medicine and was rooted in a social and religious matrix of a culturally defined people within a definite belief system.[2] Most societies had their shamans, magicians, and witch doctors who possessed psychological influence over individuals and the communal health belief system. Family and community were the basis for social healing. On the other hand, many cases of illness never reached a physician or professed healer. Such maladies were often treated by the sick person or by relatives. Early communities were organized according to tribal traditions of protection, social support, pooling of resources, expertise, and family. Each community had its elders (leaders), but more important, they had village social organizers who ensured that rituals and cultural events ministered to the social health of the community. Each of these, and other approaches, were the focus of early practice of individual and community health.

While the aforementioned approaches were not necessarily integrative or cross-disciplinary in approach, nonetheless, the health services consumer was insulated by a complex web of alternative and complementary services bound by a culturally defined community and belief system. In addition to the physician, this complement included, but was not limited to, folk healers, magicians, masters of the occult sciences, pharmacists, druggists, psychologists, neighborhood activists, and religious leaders, each of whom offered their services to the ill.

The concept of a culturally defined belief system is rooted in a number of traditional health systems. For instance, traditional healers in southern Africa treat illnesses mainly with plant products and some animal products and use spiritual resources to augment the healing process.[3] In the system, the traditional healer is concerned with relieving suffering, controlling symptoms and restoring physical functioning, and social and psychological connection. In Asia, traditional Chinese medicine is a healing art that includes both acupuncture and herbology as major components of therapy.[4] Other dimensions of traditional Chinese therapy include exercise and nutrition. Both are concrete examples of the healing arts ministering to the health of the whole person within a culturally defined system.

### *Toward a Modern (Western) Approach to Medicine*

Over the years, Western concepts of medicine, which "rest on the axiom of Cartesian dualism or the separation of mind and body,"[5] have evolved and wholly displaced the ancient view. Only recently have we returned to the concept that health is a function of the physical, spiritual, mental, and social aspects of life. However, to minister to the physiological, psychological, social, and spiritual aspect of a person and/or community at the same time is an extremely difficult and time-consuming task. Through a process of professionalism, reductionism, and specialization, twentieth-century Western medicine evolved into a fragmented system of health care that distinguishes physical health from the mental, social, and spiritual aspects of health. In this paradigm, allied health personnel emerged as one of a number of individual support and complementary healers in a specialized and compartmentalized health care system. This is the tacit operational model for the allied health profession.

## TOWARD A DEFINITION OF ALLIED HEALTH

As a singular profession, allied health has struggled to define itself for a number of years. There have been numerous attempts to define allied health and to categorize the health workers who should be included in a universal definition. In 1980, the National Commission on Allied Health Education defined the field as ". . . all Health personnel working towards the common goal of providing the best possible service in patient care and health promotion."[6] A shortcoming of this definition, as cited in a 1989 Institute of Medicine report, was that it does not define boundaries for groups of health care providers, nor does it describe commonalities of task or education that identify the fields to be included.[7] In effect, this definition leaves it to each occupational area to decide for itself whether or not it would be listed under the allied health umbrella.

The U.S. Department of Health and Human Services' 1995 "Report of the National Commission on Allied Health" defined allied health professional as written in the Health Professions Education Extension Amendments of 1992, section 701 of the Public Health Service Act:

> A health professional (other than a registered nurse or physician assistant) who has received a certificate, an associate's degree, a bachelor's degree, a master's degree, a doctoral degree, or post baccalaureate training in a science relating to health care, who shares in the responsibility for the delivery of health care services or related services, including (1) services relating to the identification, evaluation and prevention of disease and disorder, (2) dietary and nutrition services, (3) health promotion services, (4) rehabilitation services, or (5) health systems management service, and who has not received a degree of doctor of medicine, a degree of doctor of osteopathy, a degree of doctor of veterinary medicine or equivalent degree, a degree of doctor of optometry or equivalent degree, a degree of podiatric medicine or equivalent degree, a degree of doctor of pharmacy or equivalent degree, a graduate degree in public health or equivalent degree, degree of doctor of chiropractic or equivalent degree, a degree in health administration or equivalent degree, a doctoral degree in clinical psychology or equivalent degree or a degree in social work or equivalent degree.[8]

This definition excludes those allied health fields that have specific federal legislation for programmatic funding. The physician assistant occupation is widely acknowledged as falling under the allied health umbrella; however, it is specifically excluded from this definition because it has a federal line item for funding. Other occupations may or may not regard themselves as allied health but are nonetheless included in Health and Human Services' definition. The lack of a consensus on how to define allied health contributes to the confusion about which fields fall under the Allied Health rubric.[9] An approach to staking out the boundaries of allied health is offered by Schloman.[10] She brings together four definitions and organizes them into a typology that can aid people to decide what allied health is. The following are Schloman's four definitional areas:

- *Broadly defined* (U.S. Division of Allied Health Manpower, 1969) "All those professional, technical, and supportive workers in the field of patient care, community health, public health, environmental health and related research who engage in activities that support, complement, or supplement the professional of administrators and practitioners."
- *Vaguely defined* (American Medical Association [AMA], 1995) "A large cluster of health-related personnel who fulfill necessary roles in

the health care system, including assisting, facilitating, and complementing the work of physicians and other health care specialists."

- *What it is not* (Pew Advisory Panel for Allied Health, 1992) "Allied Health includes all health related disciplines with the exception of nursing and the MODDVOPP disciplines . . . medicine, osteopathy, dentistry, veterinary medicine, optometry, pharmacy and podiatry."
- *Avoiding the issue* (Institute of Medicine, 1989) "The benefits of making the term Allied Health more precise are less clear than the benefits of continued evolution."

One approach to defining the field not mentioned in the literature is that the term allied health refers to all health workers as caregivers who are allied with the patient.* Many health personnel and health professional organizations neglect or fail to consider this critically engaging, socially meaningful, and philosophically compelling point. In their 1977 report *Health Personnel: Meeting the Explosive Demand for Medical Care,* Goldstein and Horowitz noted:

> This report will use the terms Allied Health or health personnel or occupation with no intention of slighting or disparaging any occupation or group. Our interest is to include all those persons in the industry who relate directly to the patient—"laying hands-on." The terms allied health or health profession are intended to cover the whole range of health workers from physician and physician extenders (such as pediatric nurse practitioners and graduate registered nurses with four or five years of formal schooling after secondary school) to entry-level nurse's aide or assistant (NA) and the laboratory assistant who may have less than a high school education plus on-the-job training, in-service education or both.[11]

As we review the evolution of the allied health professions, it is clear that the definition of allied health is not universally accepted today. For the most part, this state of affairs is an outgrowth of the intense professionalization of medicine, the fragmentation of health care to manageable parts, and overspecialization of the health care workforce. These issues, coupled with the need to maintain a professional hierarchy within the U.S. health care sys-

---

* In a number of professions meetings sponsored by the American Association of Schools of Allied Health and the National Society of Allied Health from 1972 to present, the relationship of health personnel has been referred to not as a pecking order in terms of education and professional hierarchy, but rather in terms of each health professions' relationship with the patient. In this view, all health care providers should be considered allied with the patient.

tem, one that is dominated by the physician and focuses on the patient, produces an extremely trying context for allied health and contributes to its current identity crisis. The following section reviews a few of the social epochs contributing to the identity crisis.

## THE EVOLVING U.S. HEALTH CARE SYSTEM

The history of organized medicine in the United States is generally acknowledged to begin with the founding of the American Medical Association (AMA) in 1847. The first invitation to an AMA organizational meeting stated that a national convention would be conducive to elevating the standard of medical education in the United States. However, it was not until many years later that improvement was achieved in medical education.[12] Many of the economic, social, political, and technological factors that contributed to the rapid development of medical education and the physician community similarly contributed to the evolution of the allied health community. The most compelling of these was the Shattuck Report.

### The Shattuck Report (1850)

The Report of the Sanitary Commission of Massachusetts (1850), commonly referred to as the Shattuck Report because it was authored by Lemuel Shattuck, is one of the most important works ever published in the field of public health. Shattuck's report marks the beginning of the rationalization of the U.S. health care system. It established the basis for defining and differentiating the role of several important concepts that help define the U.S. health system and health worker roles. The report is significant for several reasons, including (1) its documentation of the history of public health efforts and (2) its focus on health from a holistic perspective. Specifically, the report discussed the following concepts:

- *Industrial Police*—The laws and regulations concerning the occupations of people. This concept is similar to the present-day field of occupational health.
- *Sanitary Police*—The laws and regulations for the prevention of disease and promotion of health. This was an extraordinary finding in light of several Surgeon General's reports on health promotion and disease prevention published in the past twenty years.

- *Medical Police*—The laws and regulations for the practice of medicine. It established the basis for medical education and public health service.[13]

The Shattuck report also provided the rationale for government involvement beyond the role of policy planners to include a new role as a limited care provider.

At this stage of U.S. history, it was a revolutionary concept for government to become involved in the delivery of health services. Health care was primarily a private matter and people were expected to take care of themselves by obtaining the services of private physicians, nurses, and other health providers, and by purchasing medications from "mom and pop" drugstores, and by personally paying for these services. Society's social values were tied to a laissez-faire approach, namely, individuals and communities were left to define and defend for themselves. The government's role at the federal, state, or local level was, for the most part, nonexistent. For those who could not afford to pay for medical services, their recourse was charitable care from voluntary organizations. The Shattuck Report indicated that some community health issues were so significant that local government was compelled to provide service as a matter of public policy. In furtherance of the public policy concern, Shattuck's report recommended training health workers who could provide service in a broadly defined system of public health:

> The great objectives of sanitary science are to teach the causes of disease, how to remove or avoid these causes, how to prevent disease, how to live without being sick, how to increase the vital force and how to avoid premature decay.[14]

Thus, the Shattuck Report had a strong influence on rationalizing the U.S. health care system. It established a framework for defining various types of health workers, e.g., occupational health workers, preventive health, public health, and medical healers, and expanded the landscape to include a limited role for government in the provision of health care services. Finally, it promoted the idea of educating health workers according to principles of public health.

### Flexner Report (1910)—Moving Beyond a Guild System

In 1910, the Flexner Report established the foundation for formal medical education in the United States. By inference and practice, it became the prototype for all health education programs. Furthermore, the Flexner Report was the beginning of relating state licensure to the accreditation of education programs. The report provided a detailed analysis of medical education, i.e., a state-of-the-art work, and concluded with recommendations for major change. The report characterized medical education as (1) being a supplement to the apprenticeship system and (2) a rote education process based on commercialism. At the time, medical education was essentially an on-the-job training program. It was recommended that medical education be grounded in the basic sciences, have a clinical component based on specific standards, and assist the student in developing problem-solving skills. Moreover, the report cast the medical profession as a collective body that has major social responsibilities that transcend medicine:

> The medical profession is a social organ, created not for the purpose of gratifying the inclinations or preference of certain individuals but as a means of promoting health, physical vigor, and happiness, and the economic independence and efficiency immediately connected with these factors.[15]

The report (1) outlined a new model for physician education, (2) recommended minimal standards for medical school accreditation, and (3) proposed uniform criteria for student selection at medical schools. The rationale for Flexner's recommendation was grounded in the belief that states have an affirmative duty to certify doctors and the quality of schools providing their education:

> The state boards are the instruments through which the reconstruction of medical education will be largely effected. The law that protects the public interest against the unfit doctor should in fairness protect the student against an unfit school.[16]

Hindsight suggests the Flexner Report may have been given more importance than it deserved. The report was published at a time when the AMA was pursuing medical education reform. Shortly after the turn of the century, the AMA was reorganized to include creation of a council on medical education. The council was a major driving force behind voluntary accreditation in the United States. The Flexner Report provided public recognition for the needed changes, however, the report would not have been as influential were it not for the groundwork laid by the medical eduction council in terms of initiating movement for reform of medical education and establishing the model for accreditation.[17] Nonetheless the Flexner Report is widely considered the most influential factor in transforming the U.S. medical education system into a system whose accomplishments and contributions are today the envy of the world. The resultant medical school education model has emerged as the prototype for allied health and other health professions.

## *The Emerging Partnership Between the AMA and the Allied Health Professions*

The Great Depression of the 1930s was the impetus for social change and movement toward equality within a number of political and economic environments, including health care. It was a time when many new relationships were formed between the AMA and various allied health professions. The AMA formalized its role in accrediting allied health professions in the mid-1930s, when it began developing minimal education standards for occupational therapists (1935), and medical technologists and physical therapists (1936). The AMA increased its involvement with allied health until the 1990s.* The following statement summarizes the AMA's rationale for its involvement in the accreditation of allied health education:

> The AMA recognizes that it has great responsibility and that it must be actively aware of, and related to, all the allied fields for one extremely important reason: that all of the allied health workers find their focus, indeed their reason for existence, in the care of the patient; and where the care of the patient is concerned, the physician ultimately has legal, moral and ethical responsibility. As the major professional organization for physicians, the AMA feels this responsibility keenly and believes that it must increasingly be involved in coordination, guidance and direction of the multiple, increasingly fragmented components of the health care team, through which the care of the patient is provided.[18]

While not all allied health fields became partners under the AMA's umbrella accreditation body, many of the major groups did. It was a self-described system designed to provide education standards and a level of professionalism for allied health professions education programs. In furtherance of its legal, moral, and ethical responsibility, the AMA adopted a 1960s report by the Committee to Study the Relationships of Medicine with Allied Health Professions and Services by its House of Delegates. The report announced

---

*The AMA discontinued its role of allied health accreditation in 1993. Allied health professions are now accredited by the Commission on Accreditation of Allied Health Education Programs (CAAHEP) or have independent recognition with the U.S. Department of Education.

the medical profession had a responsibility to serve as a unifying body in assisting other vitally important, technical allied health groups in recruitment, education, and professional growth.[19] This was the organizing foundation on which the long-term partnership between allied health professions and the AMA was established.

## The War Years—World War II and Beyond

During World War II millions of Americans were exposed to new levels of health care because of their service in the military. This exposure resulted in higher levels of medical expectation which would later prove difficult to lower. A national employer-paid health insurance policy was an additional direct consequence of the war effort. These two events contributed to increased construction of hospitals and rapid proliferation of various specialty medical and allied health education programs.

### Hospital Construction

In 1946, Congress passed the Hospital Survey and Construction Act (Hill-Burton), which was responsible for developing construction programs for public and other nonprofit hospitals and facilities. The legislation's intent was to make funds available to every state to create an adequate number of hospital beds and to ensure teaching hospitals were available in every major community. This initiative was also a major force increasing hospital construction following the war, and was a wellspring for the increasing need for all types of health personnel. As the number of available beds serving the postwar population increased, so did the need for more health workers.

### Proliferation of Specialty Medical and Allied Health Education Programs

There were only a few doctors who became specialists in the medical field before World War II. Following the war, the federal government insisted on upgrading specialty training and downgrading general practitioners![20] This policy change increased the demand for specialty residency positions held by physicians who had served in the war. The increased growth in interns and residents on staff at most hospitals was, for the first time, more than the number of third- and fourth-year students enrolled in medical school.[21] The growth of graduate medical education not only transformed medical education but also transformed and defined the allied health professions.

Allied health professions experienced rapid growth following World War II. The need for additional allied health personnel has traditionally been explained by the economic theory of joint demand. The joint demand theory posits that if a need exists for health manpower at the highest occupational level (MDs), then a corresponding need exists at other levels within the hierarchy of the health manpower system. Because of the field's close relationship with the AMA, this theory was applied to the allied health professions following World War II. The Graduate Medical Education National Advisory Committee (GMENAC), established in the 1970s by the secretary of the Department of Health, Education, and Welfare (DHEW), now the Department of Health and Human Services (DHHS), published the first report to break with the joint demand theory in 1980. The report concluded that more non-physician providers (e.g., physician assistants, nurse practitioners, and nurse midwives) would be needed in the 1990s, even though a surplus was projected for physicians (refer to *A New Majority in the Health Profession* for details on the growth of the allied health profession). Even though there was a surplus projected for physicians, the demand for allied health workers continued beyond the war years. Now, the demand for allied health manpower is projected independently of physician requirements and is no longer driven by the economic theory of joint demand.

New hospital-based education programs also began to emerge in the years following World War II. An example of one such allied health field is respiratory therapy. The first professional association to represent respiratory therapists was founded in Chicago in 1947. Now known as the American Association for Respiratory Care (AARC), the organization's purpose was to advance the science, technology, ethics, and art of respiratory therapy (formerly known as inhalation therapy).[22] Collier and Youtsey chronicle the profession's birth as a need for hospital orderlies to transport oxygen tanks to patients' rooms. The orderly became known as a "tank jockey."[23] Eventually, service expanded, orderlies were assigned more complicated tasks, and their role evolved into an allied health specialty. The therapist today is considered a highly specialized profession involving sophisticated life-support systems. It is a critically important patient service.

Here we see how the rapid expansion of hospitals following the war resulted in the need for improved patient services and the need to control health care costs by using allied health professionals. These phenomena created at least two results: (1) It established a close professional bond between a new allied health field (respiratory therapist) and the physician, and (2) further fragmented the specialized health care delivery system. On a more positive note, the physician has been freed to focus attention on patient management issues with the introduction and evolving role of this allied health function.

## The Social Experiments of the 1960s

In the 1960s, the U.S. government began a series of noble experiments to expand and extend health care insurance coverage and increase the health manpower supply. First, the government became involved in personal health service assistance programs. In 1965, the Medicare program was created to provide health care services for persons age sixty-five years and older and to disabled persons of any age. That same year, Medicaid was also enacted into law as a shared state/federal program to enable the poor, including those defined as medically indigent, to receive health care. These two programs dramatically increased the utilization patterns and demand for health care in the United States. Those who did not have health insurance in the past were now eligible to participate in a national health insurance program. Legions of Americans were brought into the private health care system, resulting in greater utilization of medical services than ever before.[24]

In 1964, Congress passed the Economic Opportunity Act, which included funding for a job corps program. The program provided youths ages sixteen to twenty-one with education, vocational training, and work-training programs in which they could obtain useful paid experience. In their book *New Careers for the Poor,* Pearl and Reissman indicated the broad field of health services was an area where potential for employment was great. They further indicated that almost every aspect of health services could be enlarged or improved by using the new career concept.[25] The notion of a para-professional or sub-professional became very popular, especially in the health industry. It was the authors' premise that workers could provide useful and purposeful service at an unskilled level while participating in a training program to upgrade their skills to a more professional level. The authors also indicated that:

> The unique quality of the new career proposal might be best emphasized by consideration of the present inability of a registered nurse (allied health profession) to obtain credit for training and skill toward becoming a medical doctor. It is proposed that ultimately such a course would be available. The nurse-to-doctor sequence, while probably more fraught with difficulty than most, would indicate the nature of resistance to be encountered and overcome before the new career concept can become a reality.[26]

An incentive to devise and develop new careers in the health fields was provided by the federal government. The U. S. Department of Health, Education and Welfare (now Health and Human Services) established the Office of New Careers to support the new career concept. The office provided funding for a number of projects to encourage the development of new career opportunities.

The concept of new careers became extremely popular in the health care industry. The pedagogical principle of a career ladder and lattice became household words. The idea of an entry level employee, such as a laundry worker, food service helper, social worker-aide, laboratory assistant, dietary aide, etc., moving up and across the professional hierarchy into an allied health profession and beyond was no longer a novel concept but an operational reality.* It was considered a way to (1) increase the numbers of health workers to support the professional to carry out her/his duties, (2) create meaningful upward mobile jobs for entry level employees and other low skilled workers, and (3) meet the demands of rising expectations for health care in inner-city and medically underserved communities. In the allied health community, the new career concept was not well received. The term sub- or paraprofessional had negative connotations, suggesting that allied health workers were less than professional, when in fact, the allied health field consists of health workers who are professionals of the highest standards. Notwithstanding concerns about the new careers movement, it was a major social force in promoting and defining the allied health field.

## THE EVOLVING ROLE OF EDUCATION AND STANDARDS FOR THE ALLIED HEALTH PROFESSIONS

During the twentieth century, the education of allied health professionals evolved from a guild system, to hospital-based, to a college model. In the early part of the century, most health professions modeled their education on a guild system. Specifically, a doctor or some other type of practitioner would recruit an individual to serve for a period of apprenticeship under their tutelage. Upon completion of training, the apprentice would be allowed to hang out a shingle advertising themself as a fully competent practitioner. There were neither uniform standards for training nor methods for certifying the competence of these guild system trainees. A number of the health professions, including physicians, contain vestiges of the guild/

*This author was once the director of a program at Los Angeles County General Hospital funded by the Department of Labor to introduce new career opportunities for entry-level employees and Native Americans. The program was considered highly effective. He also created radiological technologist, nuclear medical technician, and physician assistant training programs for community residents in South Central Los Angeles prior to the opening of the Martin Luther King Jr. Hospital in 1970-1972.

apprenticeship system as part of their training today. Although resident training programs for MDs are more organized and grounded in specific educational theories, learning outcomes, and defined competencies, they are nonetheless a more sophisticated model of an earlier practice. Many of the allied health professions have an apprenticeship component. For example, the orthotic and prosthetic education programs require residency before certification. Occupational therapists, physical therapists, radiologist technicians, physician assistants, medical social workers, medical records technicians, medical assistants, etc., each have an experiential component of varying degrees.

The early guild model of rote learning was transformed to its current model based on the work of the AMA's Committee on Medical Education as well as the recommendations of the Flexner Report. Several changes were most evident for the allied health field including (1) that education/training programs became more formal and for the most part evolved into hospital-based training programs and (2) the fields began to develop standards for accrediting allied health programs.

Radiological technology is an example of how one allied health field evolved from a guild system into a formal hospital-based training program, and how standards were established for providing such programs. Like most health fields in the early twentieth century, many x-ray technicians were trained informally via the guild system. However, as both the complexity of radiographic equipment and the volume of radiological procedures being performed by radiologists continued to grow, the need became apparent for a new class of technical workers to assist radiologists with much of their routine work. There was no formal training system for x-ray technician—training usually was an apprenticeship of sorts, with the radiologist training an individual—frequently a nurse or other staff member—to be the x-ray technician. Ed C. Jerman was considered the first to formally instruct x-ray students. In the early 1920s he established the first educational department in the x-ray industry, and was considered the first to establish an orderly radiographic procedure by defining radiographic qualities, and identifying and arranging the factors that contribute to those qualities.[27] (The impetus for hospital-based training programs was a direct result of World War I. War veterans and military authorities were pressing for better levels of services for returning military personnel.) Jerman is also considered a major influence for creating the American Registry of X-ray Technicians in 1922. Hence, he influenced both the educational model and procedure for certifying the competence of these new practitioners. Ultimately, the profession affiliated with the AMA's Council of Medical Education for purposes of establishing standards for approved programs and procedures for accrediting educational and training programs.

It was not long, however, before hospital-based training programs began to phase out and transition to a collegiate format. This transformation occurred for several reasons: (1) Medicare and Medicaid and various other insurance carriers discontinued the practice of permitting hospitals to write off training costs as a part of patient care, and (2) the pressures from accreditation and certification requirements forced the training programs to affiliate with academic institutions. The following is a brief explanation of the role and function of accreditation and certification.

*Accreditation*

The U.S. accreditation system is unique to our system of government. While accreditation is a voluntary, non-governmental system, it has been organized with the express purpose of maintaining an external peer review process to ensure maintenance of pre-determined levels of academic standards. The goal of accreditation is to ensure that educational programs meet acceptable levels of quality. The allied health field has accreditation systems in place to monitor and verify standards. There are two basic types of educational accreditation, namely, institutional, and specialized (or programmatic). Institutional accreditation applies to an entire institution and is conducted by a regional or national accrediting agency. Its purpose is to determine if the overall institution (1) has established goals, (2) is performing in a purposeful manner in pursuit of its stated goals, and (3) is maintaining academic quality according to regional standards. Specialized or programmatic accreditation applies to programs, departments, or schools that are part of an institution. For example, a medical school and each of its academic departments in a university would receive programmatic accreditation. Additionally, each of the university's allied health programs would receive some form of programmatic accreditation. However, the sponsoring university would receive regional or institutional accreditation. Both types of accreditation are essential for monitoring and maintaining academic quality. The following chart delineates some functions of accreditation.

1. Verifying that an institution or program meets established standards
2. Assisting prospective students in identifying acceptable institutions
3. Assisting institutions in determining the acceptability of transfer credits
4. Helping to identify institutions and programs for investment of public and private funds
5. Protecting an institution against harmful internal and external pressures

6. Creating goals for self-improvement of weaker programs and stimulating a general raising of standards among education institutions
7. Involving the faculty and staff comprehensively in institutional evaluation and planning
8. Establishing criteria for professional certification and licensure and for upgrading courses offering such preparation
9. Providing one of several considerations used as a basis for determining eligibility for federal assistance[28]

## *Certification*

In addition to accreditation, the health professions have a certification system. Certification is the process by which a nongovernmental agency or association grants recognition to an individual who has met certain predetermined qualifications specified by that agency or association. The primary goal of certification is to prevent unqualified persons from entering the profession and to publicly certify the standards of those who are qualified. The allied health professions model was patterned on the certification system developed by the AMA. Established in 1917, The American Board of Ophthalmology became the first American medical specialty board and was the prototype for certifying all health fields. The model requires a specific amount and kind of formal education preparation and experience, or some combination of the two, in order to sit for a certifying examination. It is also generally stipulated that the educational and clinical portion of the academic preparation and clinical experience must be received in an appropriately accredited education program and accredited health facility.

The gradual changes in payment methods for hospital-based educational programs, and demands of both programmatic and institutional accreditation, coupled with the new professional standards required by professional associations/societies, were contributing forces that helped change the allied health education/training model. The basic educational model for the allied health professions is today primarily collegiate, e.g., programs are offered in junior/community colleges, senior colleges, and universities. For allied health practitioners to become certified in a specific occupational area they must have successfully completed an accredited education program.

## A NEW MAJORITY IN THE HEALTH PROFESSIONS

The allied health professions have evolved into the single largest body of workers employed in our nation's health care delivery system. It is estimated that approximately 60 percent of the health care workforce is allied health personnel.[29] However, this has not always been the case. As late as 1910, there were essentially three members of the formal health care team, namely, the physician, the nurse, and the aide.[30] Presently, the figure is estimated between fifty and 600 individual health care occupations. The National Commission on Allied Health indicated "employment in Allied Health is projected to increase by 43 percent, nearly twice as fast as the average for all occupations over the 1992-2005 period."[31] Supporting this projection is a recent Bureau of Labor Statistics occupational outlook report indicating that allied health is one of the fastest growing occupational groups (Table 1.1). The report further revealed:

- Health services is one of the largest industries in the country with about 11.3 million jobs.
- Twelve occupations projected to grow fastest are concentrated in health services.[32]

The genesis of this significant increase in demand for new types and categories of allied health professions is driven by the need to keep pace with rapid social, economic, and political changes coupled with advances in technology and specialized use of technology in health care. Indeed, available technology has grown from almost zero at the time the Shattuck Report was published to a condition of such variety that the health care system has been virtually overwhelmed and captured by the technology it has created. However, a significant social lag prevents immediate use of new technologies in the treatment of patients as well as rapid development of new categories of health care workers.

Notwithstanding the delays caused by social lag, the history of the healing arts is replete with stories about the emergence of new and innovative types of health professionals. For example, therapeutic touch, which has its origin in antiquity, is now part of a number of health professions including nursing, sports medicine, exercise physiology, physical therapy, and occupational therapy. Each of the health professions having direct patient care responsibility is in one way or another involved in therapeutic touch, whether they realize it or not. Likewise, herbal medicine is also part of this early tradition. In 400 B.C., Hippocrates, the father of medicine, is reported to have said to his students, "Let thy food be thy medicine and thy medicine be thy food." Because foods were often used as cosmetics or as medicine in early civilization, could it be that the nutrition healers were some of the first allied health practitioners? Modern medicine now recognizes the dietitian's role as a critical function in the health care system.

TABLE 1.1. Employment in Allied Health in Health Services, 1998, and Projected Change, 1998-2008 (Employment in Thousands)

| Selected Occupations | 1998 Employment | | 1998-2008 Projected Percent Change |
|---|---|---|---|
| | Number | Percent | |
| Social Workers | 157 | 1.5 | 47.4 |
| Physical Therapists | 109 | 1.0 | 34.5 |
| Respiratory Therapists | 84 | 0.8 | 43.0 |
| Physician Assistants | 60 | 0.6 | 52.0 |
| Occupational Therapists | 49 | 0.5 | 30.3 |
| Computer Systems Analysts, Engineers, and Scientists | 41 | 0.4 | 62.3 |
| Speech-Language Pathologists and Audiologists | 39 | 0.4 | 37.3 |
| Dietitians and Nutritionists | 29 | 0.3 | 20.1 |
| Medical Assistants | 246 | 2.3 | 58.8 |
| Dental Assistants | 222 | 2.1 | 43.4 |
| Physical Therapy Assistants and Aides | 79 | 0.7 | 44.7 |
| Pharmacy Assistants | 34 | 0.3 | 11.6 |
| Clinical Laboratory Technologists and Technicians | 277 | 2.6 | 17.4 |
| Radiologic Technologists and Technicians | 160 | 1.5 | 19.8 |
| Dental Hygienists | 140 | 1.3 | 41.3 |
| Medical Records and Health Information Technicians | 81 | 0.8 | 48.2 |
| Emergency Medical Technicians | 35 | 0.3 | 37.6 |
| Health Services Managers | 175 | 1.6 | 36.1 |

*Source:* Adapted from Bureau of Labor Statistics, *Career Guide to Industries,* <stats.bls.gov/oco/cg>, September 2001.

It is also important to note that when new and innovative types of health professions emerge, their development closely parallels changing environmental, economic, technological, and social conditions of the prevailing health requirements of the day. Currently, an emerging new field is telemedicine. Several positions have been proposed for telemedicine technicians. In a few years, there will be accreditation standards for education programs and certifying examinations for entry into this young occupational area.

As the scientific community discovers new methods and acquires more knowledge, technology will continue to play an important role in defining the need for personnel in the health care field. However, health workers must be trained in the appropriate use of technology. This means educational programs must keep abreast of changing technology. The allied health field is mandated to ensure that technology used to treat and diagnose disease is used appropriately and must produce positive clinical patient outcomes. These increasing education requirements have contributed to a social lag that has slowed the production of new workers coming into the field. However, it has not reduced the demand for new allied health manpower. On the contrary, it has intensified the demand. It is anticipated that the need for more allied health workers will exist well beyond the 2005 projections described by the National Commission on Allied Health.

## TOWARD RECOGNITION OF THE ALLIED HEALTH PROFESSIONS

A number of studies have been commissioned and legislative initiatives undertaken to inform the public of the roles, importance of the field, manpower requirements, and future of allied health. This section chronicles the most germane of these reports and legislation to clarify the evolving role of the allied health professions.

### The Allied Health Personnel Training Act of 1966

The Allied Health Personnel Training Act of 1966 was a landmark federal law. It was enacted to provide federal grants to assist in the construction of new facilities for training allied health professionals. However, it provided much more, to include federal recognition of the emerging importance of allied health professions. In the 1960s, the concern was access to health care and the lack of personnel to provide services. Also, a significant increase occurred in the number of educational training programs that were offered in technical schools, junior and senior colleges, and universities. The act was also designed to provide federal funds to increase the number of allied health schools in the United States. It was also the first federal recognition of allied health as a key health manpower field. Before the training act, recognition was limited to state and local levels of government, and through professional association. It is important to note the Association of Schools of Allied Health Professions (ASAHP) was formed in 1967 and emerged as a natural constituent for the Bureau of Health Manpower Education, the federal agency administering the Allied Health Personnel Training Act.

## Health Training Improvement Act of 1970

In 1970, Congress enacted the Health Training Improvement Act which extended and expanded the programs outlined in the Allied Health Personnel Training Act of 1966. Programs authorized by the training improvement act included the following:

1. Construction grants for teaching facilities
2. Formula grants to improve and to strengthen allied health curricula at allied health training centers
3. Special improvement grants to provide, maintain, and improve specialized training function at allied health training centers
4. Grants for planning or developing new allied health programs
5. Grants for developing, demonstrating, or evaluating new or improved teaching methods or curricula
6. Advanced traineeships that would prepare teachers, administrators, supervisors, and nonresearch specialists
7. Scholarships, loans, and work-study programs for allied health students

The emphasis of this legislation was to (1) increase the quality of allied health education training programs, (2) coordinate educational efforts in the allied health field, (3) upgrade teacher competence and develop new teaching methods, (4) strengthen the curriculum to include core courses, and (5) make various forms of financial assistance available to students. The training improvement act marked the beginning of a new direction for allied health education, supported and strengthened the education and training of allied health within a collegiate model. Further, the act began to define the field as distinguished from the new career concept.

## The Study of Accreditation of Selected Health Education Programs (SASHEP), 1971

The previously cited Health Training Empowerment Act of 1970 required a special licensure report. The secretary of health, education and welfare was required to prepare a report identifying the major problems associated with licensure, certification, and other qualifications for practice of health personnel as well as recommend steps to be taken to solve them.

The secretary's report contained a number of recommendations, including a two-year moratorium on any legislation that would establish new categories of health personnel. The proposed delay would allow time for deliberating issues about the tasks and functions of new health care occupations.[33]

Given the serious implications inherent in the secretary's report, the Advisory Committee of Education for the Allied Health Professions and Services of the American Medical Association proposed a study on accreditation. The Study of Accreditation of Selected Health Education Programs (SASHEP) was sponsored by the AMA's Council on Medical Education, the Association of Schools of Allied Health professions and the National Commission on Accrediting. The study was financed by a grant from the commonwealth funds.[34] The report was far reaching and addressed the difficult regulatory tasks of accreditation, certification, licensure, and registration. The report established the foundation on which future processes and procedures for allied health education, accreditation, and certification have been modeled. The two-part report is considered foundational in terms of understanding the history and current state of accreditation, licensure, certification, and registration for all health professions.

### *The National Commission of Allied Health (1980): The Future of Allied Health Education*

Supported by a grant from the W.K. Kellogg Foundation, the American Society of Allied Health Professionals conducted a study that focused on alliances that need to be built within the allied health field and called for a more collaborative approach to providing health services. The society's National Commission on Allied Health made the following recommendations:

1. Strengthening alliances in services and education. The objective was to bind together the various groups of health practitioners. There should be more collaboration within the allied health field and with other health professions.
2. Determine appropriate content and level of education. The commission believed more emphasis should be placed on team building, core curricula development, multi-skills development, teacher training, and leadership development to help improve the situation.
3. Improvement of clinical education. The connection between classroom instruction and clinical practice requires closer articulation. The commission recommended that clinical instruction be developed to move beyond the guild system model for all programs.

4. Building a capacity for leadership and innovation. The commission recognized that allied health professionals must assume a greater role in defining their profession. To do so they must engage in more scholarly activity. Success in this area should increase the capacity for leadership and generate more innovation.
5. Supplying adequate funding for allied health education. This area has been a persistent theme for allied health beginning with the Allied Health Personnel Training Act of 1966.

This study was the first of a number of reports that recognized the need to increase the number of minority group members in allied health occupations, especially African American and Latinos.

### The Allied Health Services: Avoiding Crises (1989)

In 1989, the Institute of Medicine (IOM) sponsored a study to explore policies on the role of allied health personnel in health care delivery. The report was prompted by the Health Manpower Training Act of 1985. This study was the first major independent examination of the allied health field. Congressional mandate required the study commission to:

1. assess the role of allied health personnel in health care delivery;
2. identify projected needs, availability, and requirements of various types of health care delivery systems for each type of allied health worker;
3. investigate current practices for licensing, credentialing, and accrediting allied health personnel;
4. assess changes to allied health educational programs and curricula and the delivery of services by allied health personnel that are necessary to meet the needs and requirements identified in paragraph (2); and
5. assess the role of federal, state, and local governments, educational institutions, and health care facilities in meeting the needs and requirements identified in paragraph (2).

In 1989 the results of the study were published by the Institute of Medicine in a book titled *Allied Health Services: Avoiding Crises*. Although the study covered many recommendations identified in earlier reports, the recommendations listed in this report were given greater recognition because of the IOM's prestige. The most significant recommendations were:

1. more graduate programs should be developed;
2. more allied health personnel will be needed to handle the problems of an aging population, and that the various curricula will need to address this concern for all allied health personnel;
3. students should be sought in less traditional applicant pools, including minorities, older students, career changers, those already employed in health care, men (who are underrepresented), and individuals with handicapping conditions; and
4. federal and state governments as well as foundations should make funding available for special activities such as faculty development, faculty exchangers, research, and policy studies.

The report concluded by recommending a novel approach to implement its recommendations. It stated that the committee was cognizant no one entity in the public or private sector has the power or responsibility to determine whether allied health education and practice will adequately respond to the challenges of changing patterns of illness and care requirements.[35] The solution was for collaborative action to occur. "None of the committee's recommendations is self-implementing. Each requires a principal party to convince others to join in their efforts or to accede to alterations in traditional ways of operating, whether in educating students, delivering services or supporting professional interests."[36] Clearly, the commission recognized that without a mandate and an identified party to implement recommendations nothing would happen. Therefore it was the commission's belief that relevant constituent groups could voluntarily take charge and implement its recommendations.

### The Pew Health Professions Commission

The Pew Health Professions Commission has been in existence since 1990. The commission's mission is to systematically study the health professions. The allied health professions have always been an integral part of the commission's work. In 1993 the commission released a report titled *Health Professions Education for the Future: Schools in Service to the Nations.*[37] The report was ground breaking for all health professions, especially allied health. It strongly argued that health workers of the future would require a radically different set of skills, values, and attitudes to minister to the health needs of society. To achieve this, the commission recommended specific strategies for allied health educators and schools:

Strategy 1: Explore models for unifying parts of the allied health professions in clinical service and education.
Strategy 2: Encourage continuous validation of clinical practice in allied health.
Strategy 3: Improve linkages among allied health practitioners and within allied health education.
Strategy 4: Develop, test, and evaluate new ways of utilizing allied health workers in the health care systems.
Strategy 5: Enact institutional accreditation for allied health programs.
Strategy 6: Broaden efforts to enhance minority representation in allied health.[38]

In 1995, the commission released *Reforming Health Care Workforce Regulation: Policy Consideration for the 21st Century.*[39] The report provided ten recommendations concerning the regulations and composition of the health professions. Many of the commission's recommendations were considered revolutionary. Indeed, the report recommended that states take the lead role in changing the process for regulating the health professions, to include adopting entry-to-practice standards for each profession. Perhaps the most radical idea was the report's recommendation, which proposed that states should base practice acts on demonstrated initial and continued competence. This process would permit different professions to share overlapping scopes of practice. "States should explore pathways to allow all professionals to provide services to the full extent of their current knowledge, training, experience, and skills."[40] In some respects, this recommendation revisited the new careers concept espoused in the 1960s by Pearl and Reissman. The recommendation suggested that we not narrowly define and limit scope of the prevailing state practice acts. It proposed breaking-down barriers that contribute to our fragmented health care delivery system, namely, professionalism, reductionism and specialization, especially as they relate to practice acts for the allied health professionals. In this regard, the report addressed a number of the issues defined in previous reports. What was new was the recommendation to use government and regulatory agencies to restructure the practice domain of health workers.

### National Commission on Allied Health (1995)

Established by the Health Professions Extension Amendments of 1991, the National Commission on Allied Health undertook a comprehensive review of the issues, problems, and potential solutions pertaining to the education, supply, and distribution of allied health personnel in the United States.

The review resulted in the commission publishing *The Report of the National Commission on Allied Health* which examines allied health issues following four major themes: (1) workplace relationships, (2) education, (3) research, and (4) data.[41] The report indicated that although allied health providers are the largest and most diverse constituency within the health care workforce and have enormous potential for addressing questions of cost, quality, and access to care, serious issues are defined within the previous four themes that prevent their engagement in these issues. The problem of fragmentation, which is compounded by health professions resistance to change, lack of practice pattern uniformity caused by state licensure laws and practice regulation, inflexible curricula, accreditation standards, licensure requirements, degree requirements, and disciplinary boundaries prevent allied health educational institutions from responding to a rapidly changing workforce.[42] The report further indicates that there is an inadequate supply of allied health professionals trained as health services researchers and that limited resources have restricted development and dissemination of data pertaining to allied health personnel.

The allied health report is the most comprehensive ever produced by the federal government. It states that allied health is a major educational, research, and service resource that has not realized its maximum potential. The report attributes this lack of unrealized potential to poor collaboration and cooperation between and among the allied health professions and major stakeholders. Unfortunately the report is grounded in a statement that encourages all entities providing allied health education to voluntarily achieve the recommendations of the commission. Given the nature of our fragmented health care system, which is compounded by the health professions' resistance to change, lack of practice pattern uniformity caused by state licensure laws and practice regulations, inflexible curricula, accreditation standards, licensure requirements, degree requirements, and disciplinary boundaries, one could not expect much in terms of achieving the report's recommendations.

Since the mid-1960s, the allied health field has made considerable progress in terms of informing the public about its roles, importance of the field, manpower requirements, and future of the profession. Themes that emerged from these various reports and legislative initiatives include:

- The requirement for more allied health workers will continue for years to come.
- The field will continue to strengthen academic preparation for entry into the profession, including creation of more graduate programs.

- Students will be sought in less traditional applicant pools, e.g., minorities, older students, career changers, and individuals with handicapping conditions.
- Improving teacher competence both in the classroom and in clinical practicum will be stressed.
- Infusion of new resources in support of academic programs continues to be a high priority issue.
- Continual collaboration and coordination within the allied health profession and between other health fields is essential.
- Finally, the skills, values, and attitudes recommended by the first Pew report are a twenty-first century mandate for all health professionals.

## *SUMMARY*

Since the dawn of humankind, allied health practitioners have played a role in the healing arts. Indeed, even though the medical paradigm has undergone considerable change since its early beginnings, allied health professionals have evolved into major providers of health services in the United States. They are today the single largest body of workers employed in our nation's health care industry. Some estimates suggest as much as 60 percent of the health care workforce are allied health personnel. Furthermore, these numbers are predicted to grow. Historically, there were a number of forces that contributed to the increased demand for allied health workers. Those forces, especially technology, continue to be present today. The Graduate Medical Education National Advisory Committee (GMENAC) report of 1980 was the first study to discount the joint demand theory as a method for projecting allied health manpower needs. Currently, allied health manpower is projected independently of physician requirements and no longer driven by the economic theory of joint demand. Although these workers represent a new majority in the health workforce, allied health is suffering from an identity crisis and is struggling to define itself. Thus, the various definitions of allied health are neither universally accepted nor understood.

The modern concept of allied health emerged because of the profession's close relationship with the organizing history of the AMA. The Shattuck and Flexner reports provide the foundation and framework for the practice and education of all health professions, and hence, are the prototype for allied health. In the 1930s, the AMA and Allied Health began a partnership of collaborating to improve the standards of educational programs by establishing accreditation processes and procedures. This arrangement continued until the 1990s, when the AMA discontinued accreditation of allied health programs. The field organized to create the Commission on Accreditation of Allied Health Education Programs (CAAHEP) as the new umbrella organization to coordinate the accreditation of allied health programs. A number of programs chose to seek independent recognition with the U.S. Department of Education. As with most health professions, allied health has evolved from a guild system of education and training into a highly specialized collegiate model of professional education. The field controls entry into the profession through certification examinations.

Since the mid-1960s, the allied health field has been actively engaged in promoting special studies and legislative initiatives to inform the public of its role, importance, manpower requirements, and future. These studies and legislative initiatives have strengthened the profession and, more important, have helped redefine not only allied health, but all health professions. Indeed, the Pew Commission's recommendation that health workers of the future need radically different skills, values, and attitudes was the impetus for changing health professions education in the U.S. It is now clear the collective voice of allied health has not maximized its influence in the health policy and educational arenas. However, the historical evolution of allied health suggests that within the early part of the twenty-first century the new majority of health workers will have a clearer view of themselves and begin to establish their identity. Moreover, it is essential that allied health projects a more dominant position in the policy arena if it truly desires to establish a recognizable identity. Hence, it is paramount that allied health reformulates the relationship between itself and health establishments in its role as the highly professional new majority.

## REFERENCE NOTES

1. Gary B. Ferngren, Early Christianity As a Religion of Healing, *Bulletin of the History of Medicine* 66 (Baltimore, MD: John Hopkins University Press, 1992), p. 1.

2. Peter Morrell, Integrative Medicine Is Not New, *BMJ* 322(7279): 168 (BMJ.com, January 20, 2001).

3. Mariana G. Hewson, Traditional Healers in Southern Africa, *Annals of Internal Medicine* 128(12), part 1, 1998.

4. Margaret W. Beal, Acupuncture and Related Treatment Modalities, Part 1: Theoretical Backgrounds, *Journal of Nurse-Midwifery* 37(4), 1992.

5. Hewson, Traditional Healers in Southern Africa, p. 1029.

6. Institute of Medicine, *Allied Health Services: Avoiding Crises* (Washington, DC: National Academy Press, 1989), p. 15.

7. Ibid., pp. 15-16.

8. U.S. Department of Health and Human Services, *The Report of the National Commission on Allied Health* (Rockville, MD: USDHHS, 1995) p. 25.

9. *Allied Health Services: Avoiding Crises,* p. 15.

10. Barbara F. Schloman, Staking Out the Boundaries: Mapping the Literature of Allied Health, paper presented to the Medical Library Association, Seattle, WA, May 25, 1997.

11. Harold Goldstein and Morris A. Horowitz, *Health Personnel: Meeting the Explosive Demand for Medical Care* (Germantown, MD: Aspen Systems Corp., 1977) pp. 9-10.

12. William K. Selden, "Historical Introduction to Accreditation of Health Educational Program," Study of Accreditation of Selected Health Education Programs (SASHEP), Part One: Working Papers, 1971, p. A-1.

13. Lemuel Shattuck, *Report of the Sanitary Commission of Massachusetts, 1850* (Cambridge, MA: Harvard University Press, 1948) p. 16.

14. Ibid.

15. Abraham Flexner, *The Flexner Report on Medical Education in the United States and Canada* (Washington, DC: Science and Health Publications, Inc., 1910) p. 42.

16. Ibid., p. 167

17. Selden, The SASHEP Report, p. A-4.

18. Jerry W. Miller, "Structure of Accreditation of Health Education Program," SASHEP Report Part One, p. B-5.

19. Ibid., p. B-6.

20. Kenneth M. Ludnerer, *Time to Heal: American Medical Education from the Turn of the Century to the Era of Managed Care* (New York: Oxford University Press, 1999) pp. 181-182.

21. Ibid., pp. 183-184.

22. Stephen H. Collier and John W. Youtsey, "Development, Issues and Education in Respiratory Care," *Review of Allied Health Education 3* edited by Joseph Honburg (Lexington, KY: University Press of Kentucky, 1979) p. 100.

23. Ibid., pp. 100-101.

24. Ludnerer, *Time to Heal,* p. 223.

25. Arthur Pearl and Frank Reissman, *New careers for the Poor: The Non-Professional in Human Services* (New York: The Free Press, 1965) pp. 12-13.

26. Ibid., pp. 14-15.

27. Richard Terrass, The Life of Ed C. Jerman: A Historical Perspective, *Radiologic Technology* 661(5), 1995.

28. Adapted from Overview of Accreditation, U.S. Office of Postsecondary Education, <www.ed.gov/offices/OPE/accreditation/index.html>, January 2001.

29. *The Report of the National Commission on Allied Health,* 1995, p. 25.

30. Harold M. Goldstein and Morris A. Horowitz, *Health Personnel: Meeting the Explosive Demand for Medical Care* (Germantown, MD: Aspen Systems Corp., 1977) p. 10.

31. *The Report of the National Commission on Allied Health,* 1995, p. 111.

32. Bureau of Labor Statistics *Career Guide to Industries,* <stats.bls.gov/oco/cg>, September 2001.

33. *Allied Health Services: Avoiding Crises,* p. 240.

34. SASHEP, p. G-1.

35. *Allied Health Services: Avoiding Crises,* p. 14.

36. Ibid.

37. *Health Professions Education for the Future: Schools in Service to the Nation,* The Pew Health Professions Commission Report, San Francisco, CA, UCSF Center for the Health Professions, 1993.

38. Adapted from the Pew Health Professions Commission Report.

39. *Reforming Health Care Workforce Regulations: Policy Considerations for the 21st Century,* The Pew Health Professions Commission Report, San Francisco, CA, UCSF Center for the Health Professions, 1995.

40. Ibid.

41. *The Report of the National Commission on Allied Health,* 1995.

42. Ibid., p. 81.

Chapter 2

# Role of the Federal Government in Allied Health Education

Norman L. Clark

## THE NEBRASKA STORY: A CASE STUDY

One winter day, a young mother named Jane was sitting at her kitchen table drinking coffee and looking out the window at the snow covered fields of her North Platte, Nebraska, ranch. Jane was dreaming about her life and how she would like to continue her education. She had always wanted to pursue a career in one of the allied health professions, particularly in the medical laboratory field. Jane's sister, a medical technologist at a major hospital in Omaha, had often talked about the medical technology profession and the satisfaction of being an allied health professional. Jane loves working with patients and has volunteered at a small, rural hospital for several years. She feels an overwhelming need to do more for patients, but that would require additional training. As a mother of two and a supporting wife for her rancher husband, the possibility of getting that training seems remote. Jane could spend some time each day in training while the children are at school and her husband is working. Although her family would support this, Jane lives miles away from any academic institution that could provide the training she needs for a career in allied health. In addition, her family responsibilities preclude her from leaving home for any extended period of time.

Jane recognizes the local hospital has a desperate need for trained allied health professionals. This need is especially true for medical technologists in urban and rural areas. Jane has noted the shortage has delayed hospital personnel from receiving critical laboratory results and compromised the quality of health care. Attracting and retaining qualified professionals in rural Nebraska is a continuing challenge.

*31*

Enter the federal government! As one of its major focus areas, the government has sought to improve access to affordable quality health care, especially in medically underserved and rural communities. Federal grants are made available to encourage such focused initiatives.

Luckily for Jane, the University of Nebraska's Medical Center in Omaha has responded to the government's call to develop innovative models for improving access to health care in rural areas. The university established a training model called the Rural Health Education Network (RHEN) which was designed to train and increase the number of medical laboratory personnel at health care facilities in rural Nebraska. RHEN established medical technology programs in several rural Nebraska communities, including North Platte, to provide more accessible education to both traditional and nontraditional students who wished to remain in their home communities but required either formal professional education or retraining.

A nontraditional student, Jane learned about the university's new program through her local hospital. What an opportunity! Now she could realize her dreams! With her family's support, Jane enrolled in the program. She successfully completed her training and is currently employed as a medical technologist at the local hospital and outpatient clinic in North Platte.

Another RHEN graduate and father of four, Jerry from Gering, Nebraska, became a medical technologist by completing an educational program in his home community. After completing the program, he began working at a small rural hospital near his home. Prior to hiring Jerry the hospital had been trying to recruit medical technologists for more than two years.

The federal government's support of the RHEN project has also proven successful in retaining allied health professionals in rural areas. Ninety-seven percent of the project's graduates are now employed in rural hospitals and clinics in their own communities throughout Nebraska. The Nebraska story is only one of many that has been made possible by the support of the federal government. Not only have many students been trained as allied health professionals, but also access to quality health care in rural and underserved communities has improved significantly throughout America because of federal support.

## THE FEDERAL GOVERNMENT
## AND HEALTH PROFESSIONS EDUCATION

Let us look in more detail at the legislative and executive branches of the federal government and their involvement in health professions education.

## Legislative Branch

Federal agencies, such as the Health and Resources Administration, the Food and Drug Administration, the Centers for Disease Control, the National Institutes of Health, and others, are part of the executive branch of government. Such agencies administer the laws passed by the legislative branch or Congress. A brief review of Congress's role in the health professions education process is in order.

Congress hears from many different constituents almost daily about the severe problems found in hospitals and other health care delivery settings throughout the nation. They hear about personnel shortages and insufficient staff. They hear about educational institutions with insufficient funds to support education programs, faculty shortages, and inadequate numbers of students, particularly minority students, to serve vulnerable populations. They also hear about the continuing challenge to recruit and retain personnel in rural and medically underserved communities, such as noted for rural Nebraska.

Congress has duly noted these problems and determined that federal support of health professions education is critical. Federal support may be the primary or only resource for improving access to quality, cost-effective health care, especially in rural and medically underserved areas. Many times care may not be provided by the private sector to such communities.

### Congressional Members

How does Congress make the determination to support health professions education? Members of Congress may first make a determination individually. Usually this occurs when a shortage of health professionals is noted by members of Congress as a problem for the area they represent. For example, our office was recently contacted by a senator's office about the shortage of radiographers in the senator's state. This call was prompted by constituents' (both hospitals and patients) complaints that mammography-screening programs could not continue throughout the state due to the shortage of radiographers. Pressure from constituents to an elected official will most likely result in some positive action. In this example, legislation was introduced by the senator to increase funding for the Allied Health Grant Program.

### Lobbying

Another way members of Congress learn about the need for health professions education is through the lobbying efforts of interest groups such as professional associations and societies, academic institutions, state and local community groups, individual constituents, and other interested parties. Such groups provide Congress with data and other appropriate information about the need for training health professionals. Lobbying efforts become particularly important and useful as new health professions educational legislation is introduced. Lobbying becomes critical during annual appropriation deliberations by the budget committees of both the House and Senate. Health professions educational programs are discretionary and must compete for limited budget resources.

*Mandated Reports*

Congress also mandates reports when specific information is needed for decision making. A mandate typically requires studies be conducted by an appropriate federal agency. For example, the Health Resources and Services Administration's Bureau of Health Professions administers various health professions educational programs for physicians, dentists, nurses, and the allied health professions. If a report is mandated to determine supply and demand for certain types of professionals, the bureau would be the lead for such a study.

Let us look at two specific cases for mandated reports. The first is a mandated report that required the Health Resources and Services Administration to examine issues related to the allied health workforce. To accomplish this task, the 102nd Congress authorized Section 301 of the Health Professions Education Extension Amendments (PL 102-408) to establish the National Commission on Allied Health within the Bureau of Health Professions. Commission members were selected and approved by the secretary of health and human services. The commission then conducted a comprehensive review of the issues, problems, and potential solutions pertaining to education, supply, and distribution of allied health professionals throughout the United States. The bureau was responsible for publishing the final report that was distributed to Congress and the secretary of health and human services.

A second example of a mandated report is the recently completed Pharmacist Workforce Study. This report to Congress responded to mounting concerns regarding a possible shortage of licensed pharmacists in the United States. By law the final report was also distributed by the bureau to the appropriate Senate and House committees for their review. Such reports are used by Congress as they consider new legislative authorities for health professions educational programs during budget reauthorizations.

Generally, lobbyist and Congressionally mandated reports point out that federal support is needed for health professions education. Among the reasons they may include is that federal support allows the creation of new types of work environments that emphasize quality of care, access, flexibility, and cultural diversity. The federal government is also in a position to encourage collaboration among all health professions' communities of interest, including academia, practice, employers, and policymakers, to better address questions of cost, quality, and access to care in the health care system. The government can also encourage health professionals to take advantage of career development programs.

*Legislation*

After Congress has identified a need, they may pass a law or statute to address that need. The statutory authority, or laws passed by Congress and signed by the president, provides the basis for programs that are administered by federal agencies. In our case, Public Law 105-392, the Health Professions Education Partnership Act of 1998 is the current legislative authority for the allied health program. Section 755 of the law details the training of professionals within the allied health program. The program is administered by the Health Resources and Services Administration, Bureau of Health Professions.

Legislation typically takes a prescribed path through Congress: Normally, a member of Congress introduces a bill after receiving information and data from lobbyists, public constituents, academic institutions, and other groups who may be interested in seeing certain legislation passed. For example, there may be a need to improve access to quality health care in medically underserved areas in America. Certain data or results of studies completed by federal agencies on the subject may be requested, or Congress may mandate a report to provide certain information that is not currently available from other sources.

After the bill is drafted, it is referred to a committee and, in turn, to a subcommittee. The subcommittee holds hearings on the bill to obtain additional information and pertinent data from interested groups. The subcommittee then amends the bill and sends it back to the full committee. The full committee may amend the bill further before issuing a report. The bill is now ready for floor action where it may be debated and further amended. If it passes, the bill is sent to the other congressional chamber (either House or Senate, depending on where the bill originated) where it undergoes the same process. If, as is frequently the case, each chamber works simultaneously on the same or similar legislation and both chambers pass their versions of a bill, any differences can be reconciled by agreeing to or modifying the amendments of the other chamber or by sending the measure to a conference committee. The conference committee tries to arrive at language acceptable to both bodies. Once this is done, the legislation is sent to the president for signature.

After the president signs the bill, federal staff begin drafting program materials and regulations necessary to implement and administer programs authorized by the new law. The parameters for these program materials are determined by congressional intent as defined by the law and House and Senate reports.

## Congressional Set-Asides

Congress may pass a law that requires funds be provided to a particular training institution or institutions to accomplish certain things. This is rare, however, occurring only twice in the past decade for the Allied Health Grant Program. Usually, Congressional mandates or "set-asides" are the result of lobbing efforts by interest groups from a member's home district. Set-aside may last for several years with a predetermined sum of money for each year.

One example of a set-aside program for allied health, the Allied Health Occupations Training for Impoverished Citizens in Illinois, included specific language from the House Appropriations Committee to fund an allied health professions training program for impoverished citizens in the Chicago area. Three community colleges were named specifically to provide this training, with funds to be administered by the Illinois Community College Board. It should be noted that set-aside grants are treated the same as any other grant and must meet the same program reports and requirements.

## Executive Branch

### Regulations

Once a federal agency receives a new law, the administrative process begins. Regulations are basic documents for implementing legislation. Once federal staff drafts a regulatory document, it is reviewed and undergoes a clearance process through the appropriate federal agency and department. In the case of allied health, this would be the Health Resources and Services Administration's Department of Health and Human Services. Once approved, regulations are published in the daily *Federal Register.* Congress established the *Register* to inform the public of new rules and regulations.

There are three basic stages of regulatory development that should be discussed. The first is the Notice of Proposed Rulemaking, a document that proposes a specific change in the Code of Federal Regulations (CFR) either by suggesting an amendment to an existing regulation or by proposing a new regulation. The CFR is a compendium of all effective regulations promulgated by the federal government. It is revised and published annually by the Office of the Federal Register.

The second regulatory document is the Interim Final Rule. This document has the legal authority of a final rule and is codified in the CFR. The Interim Final Rule generally solicits public comment and promises a reissuance of regulations based on a consideration of comments received. This document is generally used so agencies can respond to emergency situations.

After public comment on the Interim Final Rule, the Final Rule is promulgated. This document has the force of law and is codified in the CFR. It is effective until revoked.

Another action document called a General Notice is most useful when a federal agency wants to make certain information available to the public. This document has been very useful to the Bureau of Health Professions when publishing information about grant programs and cooperative agreements for the public.

Regulations can become burdensome and are not used as much today as in the past for most of the Bureau of Health Professions' grant programs. Instead, information about the allied health grant program is now published in the Health Resources and Services Administration's *HRSA Preview*. The *Preview* lists competitive grant offerings for each fiscal year and is considered to be more user friendly than regulations. Information in the *Preview* continues to be available in the *Federal Register* as well as on the Internet. However, regulations continue to be used as an administrative tool for many programs within the executive branch of the federal government.

*Program Materials*

To facilitate the process of awarding grants to eligible entities, the Health Resources and Services Administration uses program materials that include all the information needed to complete an application. Program materials found in the application kit include specific information and requirements unique for completing a grant for a specific program, such as allied health, nursing, or medicine. For example, program specific information includes the purpose of a particular grant program, eligibility requirements, funding factors (which we will describe in more detail later), special initiatives, and review criteria that will be used by peer reviewers in making funding decisions. The remaining part of the application consists of uniform information that applies to all grant programs. Uniform information includes forms for completing a detailed budget, biographical sketches, as well as general information such as page restrictions and other general submission requirements.

Why is program specific information so critical to successful grant writing? A grant application may include innovative ideas or unique educational models to accomplish a statutory purpose of a grant program and get excellent reviews, but if it does not meet each of the specific program or uniform requirements, or address the funding factors described in the following, the chance of receiving an award is unlikely.

*Funding Factors*

Addressing funding factors is critical to the successful review of a grant application. Funding factors are either statutory or administrative. Statutory funding factors are placed in the legislative language by Congress; administrative funding factors by a federal agency. The purpose of funding factors is to provide ways of adjusting or improving grant application scores that address certain issues or problems such as access or diversity as mentioned.

Three different kinds of funding factors are available to grant programs. They include funding preference, funding priority, and special consideration. The most common are funding preferences and priorities described in the following text.

A funding preference may be statutory, such as the following example for the allied health program. Funding preferences are either met or not met. No scores attach to a preferences but meeting them is critical to receiving a funding award. An example of a funding preference (statutory) for the Allied Health Grant Program is as follows:

> A funding preference shall be given to applicants who have a high rate of placing graduates in practice settings having the principal focus of serving residents of medically underserved communities. High rate refers to a minimum of 20 percent of graduates in an academic year who spend at least 50 percent of their work time in clinical practice in the specified settings.

On the other hand, a funding priority is the actual favorable adjustment of aggregate review scores when applications meet specified criteria. This can be critical for applicants who are competing for a funding award. An example of an administrative funding priority for the Allied Health Grant Program follows:

> A funding priority will be given to qualified applicants who provide community-based training experiences designed to improve access to health care services in underserved areas.

Funding factors are useful tools when the federal government, either Congress or an administrative agency, wants to target a specific issue or problem. Although the previous are specific examples for improving access to health care in rural and underserved communities for the allied health program, such funding factors are used by most grant programs to address specific issues or problems.

*Legislative Purpose*

All legislatively based programs that provide for grants and/or contracts have authorizing and appropriation legislative language in their charter. The authorizing language tells federal agencies what can be done within the framework of the grant program, while appropriations language provides the budget authority.

As mentioned earlier, the Health Professions Education Extension Amendments of 1992 is the current authorization for the Allied Health Grant Program. This act authorizes grants to eligible entities to meet the costs associated with expanding or establishing programs to increase the number of individuals trained in allied health professions. This fits within the act's mission of improving access to quality health care. The authorizing language then gives nine different legislative purposes that further define this general language. The following are two examples of the nine legislative purposes for allied health:

> The establishment of community-based allied health training programs that link academic centers to rural clinical settings.

> The expanding or establishing of clinical training sites for allied health professionals in medically underserved or rural communities in order to increase the number of individuals trained.

Applicants must address at least one of the nine different legislative purposes listed for the allied health program to be eligible for an award. This is usually done in an innovative way that can serve as a model for other eligible entities with similar goals. The previous examples have been used by many applicants to develop models that embrace the concept of distance learning and to provide rural area practitioners and organizations with high quality distance learning programs. Examples of such distance-based training models developed by grant support will be described later.

*Eligibility*

Eligible entities for most of the Bureau of Health Professions' training grant programs are health professions schools, academic health centers, and state or local governments. To provide the programs some flexibility for special cases that may arise, most eligibility requirements also include a clause for "other appropriate public or private nonprofit entities."

*Definition of Allied Health Professionals*

Each training grant program must specify the disciplines eligible for training under their grant authority. For training disciplines such as nurses, dentists or physicians, eligibility is clear. For the allied health disciplines, eligibility is not as clear since these disciplines are the largest and most diverse constituency within the health care workforce. Therefore, the definition for allied health professionals used by the bureau is broad:

- Health professionals who have received a certificate, an associate's degree, a bachelor's degree, a master's degree, a doctoral degree, or post baccalaureate training, in a science relating to health care.
- Health professionals who share in the responsibility for the delivery of health care services or related services, including:
    —services relating to the identification, evaluation, and prevention of diseases and disorders
    —nutrition and dietetic services
    —health promotion services
    —rehabilitation services
    —health systems management services

Such a broad definition may include allied health disciplines ranging from those that receive on the job training to disciplines trained at the doctoral level.

*Application Process*

Potential applicants who meet eligibility criteria and want to apply for grant funding may do so by using the World Wide Web. World Wide Web addresses are published in the *HRSA Preview* mentioned earlier, as well as specific program "fact sheets" that are available as hard copies. Such addresses will provide access to the grant program's home page. For example, the allied health program's home page includes the program's description, purpose, eligibility, and availability of allied health project abstracts.

The Bureau of Health Professions uses Adobe Acrobat to publish grant documents. Such documents include all the program specific information and application materials needed to complete an application. These materials also include review criteria peer reviewers use to evaluate applications. These materials are usually available in July of each year and the deadline for submission is typically January or February.

If additional programmatic information is needed, the project officer can be contacted directly. Questions regarding grant policies and business management issues are directed to grants management at the Bureau of Health Professions. Also, for applicants who are unable to access application materials electronically, a hard copy can be provided by the agency's application center.

## PROGRAM EXAMPLES

As noted under the section on legislative purposes, access to quality health care is a critical part of the Allied Health Grant Program. Two of the nine statutory purposes are directed at improving access through the development of community-based learning programs. The Health Resources and Services Administration also has as one of its core missions the enhancement and expansion of access of care to medically underserved areas. Many applicants have therefore embraced the concept of distance learning as a community-based experience using the newest technologies to improve access to care in rural and underserved areas—such as the program in Nebraska.

Approximately forty allied health grantees have developed innovative community-based training programs since 1990 to train students to practice in underserved areas. Many of these programs are using Web- and Internet-based systems, Interactive Television, Compressed Video, and Audio using fiber optics to support their distance-based training programs. The use of such multipurpose communication technologies to prepare students for practice in rural and underserved communities has been very rewarding.

Let us look at a few examples of allied health programs using various technologies to develop new types of educational experiences for rural and underserved distance education programs.

One such example is the Center for Creative Instruction and the School of Allied Health at the Medical College of Ohio where they have created interactive educational software for their distance education programs. The software includes video and audio clips that allow students to "see and hear" what persons with compromised sight and hearing see and hear. Another example is a University of Texas Medical Branch's Health Information System Simulation (HISS) project, which simulates patient cases. Interacting via computers with the simulated patient, other students, and faculty, students in the project learn to collaborate with colleagues in other disciplines while mastering skills in diagnosis and treatment planning. A component of the HISS called the Electronic Patient Record includes patient histories, physicals, laboratory results, photographs, and diagnostic tests. By incorporating social, economic, locational, and medical information, students can achieve increased awareness of the needs of underserved populations.

In the case study presented earlier in this chapter, the multipurpose communication techniques made available for Jane by the RHEN program allowed her to take major courses online, maintain up-to-date skills after graduation, and meet continuing education requirements.

The federal government has supported other distance-based learning programs where new technologies are being used to deliver educational material to learners at distant sites. These programs address the isolation barriers of many underserved and rural areas, as well as the lack of human resources and face-to-face collaboration.

One federally supported grant was used to develop an electronic classroom geared toward improving access, quality, and delivery of health care through multilevel, innovative training programs at Southwest Texas State University. Using problem-based learning, the university developed an innovative Web-based course that presents interactive curricula in a modular form. The course was developed by a multistate, multi-institutional faculty team representing several different allied health professions, nursing, medicine, and social work. Such a classroom can provide health care students with the opportunity to digest and reflect course material at leisure, while consulting and incorporating outside resource materials as needed.

The electronic classroom is only one of many evolving distance education modalities that receive federal support. Certainly, no single technological solution will work for all programs or all communities. Each location is unique, and systems designed to address access problems must be tailored to meet the particular needs and culture of each community, both rural and underserved.

## CONCLUSION

As noted earlier, new technologies for distance education programs have been developed with federal support to help mitigate problems posed by geographic distance and the lack of human resources in rural and underserved areas. However, it is important to remember that one important role the federal government has in allied health education in general is to provide support and leadership to eligible training institutions in the development of various types of allied health training programs. The Allied Health Grant Program has provided support for various training models for more than forty different allied health professions. These trained professionals have provided quality health care services to major hospitals, outpatient clinics, independent and private practices, and the federal government, including the Indian Health Service, Federal Bureau of Prevention, and U.S. military. Federal support promotes affordable and accessible quality health care services in the twenty-first century for underserved communities.

Chapter 3

# Primary Health Care

Howard Straker
Marvin Barnard

## INTRODUCTION

The term "primary care" is gaining popularity in health care discussions, yet, what is meant by the term varies from setting to setting. This ambiguity can be the source of miscommunication and misunderstanding between clinician and patient. The lack of clarity is compounded by a changing health care situation. This chapter will provide a definition and discuss key elements, characteristics, and functions of primary health care. This chapter will also discuss attributes of primary care practices and the clinicians who provide such care. Controversial features, overlapping concepts, and future directions of primary care will also be explored.

## CASE STUDY

S.J.W. is a thirty-nine-year-old female who presented to the emergency room with a chief complaint of increased shortness of breath and wheezing for five to six hours. She has a history of asthma typically controlled by an inhalant. However, she recently relocated to the area and her medications have run out. S.J.W. was cleaning her apartment when she began to cough sporadically and experience tightness in her chest. Her psychosocial history was positive for post-traumatic stress disorder following a robbery assault one year ago for which she was prescribed an antidepressant. She does not smoke or drink, but has a positive family history for asthma, coronary heart disease, and cancer.

S.J.W.'s physical examination was remarkable for an elevated blood pressure (160/120) and pulse (120), as well as labored breathing with a rapid rate of twenty-six breaths per minute. She is five feet five inches tall,

165 pounds, and in moderate distress. Her chest exam revealed a two-centimeter lump in her left breast, and her lungs exhibited expiratory wheezing on both sides.

Diagnostic studies were significant for mild EKG changes only.

She responded well over several hours in the emergency room to multiple nebulization treatments, intravenous hydration, and oxygen therapy.

Consultations with internal medicine (asthma), cardiology (cardiovascular disease), surgery (breast mass), and psychiatry (post-traumatic stress disorder) were made with subsequent clinic referrals for follow-up in the next few weeks. An obstetrics and gynecology (OB/GYN) referral was added upon patient request to perform an overdue follow-up for a borderline Pap smear.

S.J.W. was given prescriptions and told to return to the ER if the condition recurred. She was not aware of the health coverage and benefits provided by her new job at time of discharge. On her way out, S.J.W. was heard asking, "Who is my doctor?"

This case study highlights the need for primary care. S.J.W. was seen in the emergency room for an attack that probably could have been avoided with proper primary care attention. Her visit uncovered additional possible health concerns such as obesity, high blood pressure, a breast mass, and history of mental health problems. Had S.J.W. been previously placed in primary care she would have been prescribed asthma medications, and would have received appropriate medical services for her other problems. More important, she would know who her doctor is!

In reality, S.J.W.'s "doctor" is many people. As with the rest of health care, primary care is made possible by the contributions of multiple professionals and workers. Physician assistants (PA), nurse practitioners (NP), clinical chemists, medical technologists, nutritionists, radiology technicians, physical therapists, occupational therapists, health educators, as well as physicians each have roles in primary care.

### *PRIMARY CARE DEFINITION*

In 1996, the Institute of Medicine's Committee on the Future of Primary Care adapted the following definition of primary care:

> Primary care is the provision of integrated, accessible health care services by clinicians who are accountable for addressing a large majority of personal health care needs, developing a sustained partnership

with patients, and practicing in the context of family and community. (Donaldson et al., 1996, p. 31)

This definition focuses on primary care as a type of health care service that is broad and versatile enough to address most of the daily health care needs of the population. It emphasizes a continuous relationship between the clinician and the patient. It also implies the American primary care delivery system is comprehensive enough to address many individual health needs with an awareness of family and community.

The primary care practice is the central focus around which the medical system is organized. It is the point of entry in the medical care system and is designed to meet most health care needs and services. In the primary care practice the patient has a personal clinician, allowing for a continuity of care. The clinician establishes a relationship with the patient and follows the patient over the years. A record is kept of care the patient receives and coverage is provided for the times that the personal clinician is unavailable.

The primary care practice is responsible for coordinating additional patient care beyond the capabilities of the practice. If a patient requires services beyond primary care, then he or she is referred to the appropriate medical practice. Although patients may be referred to a medical specialty, they are still patients of and are seen by the primary care practice. At times a back-and-forth relationship may occur with the patient being sent to a practice area outside of primary care for specialized treatment, but returning to the primary care practice to receive ongoing health services.

## *Continuity*

One element of primary care is continuity. Primary care is an ongoing process that is the dominating and central part of a person's medical care, involving an ongoing patient/clinician relationship over time, and provides a flow and cohesion of information throughout the medical care process.

The primary care practitioner/patient relationship may continue for years. It can go from birth to the grave with the patient having the same clinician. Most medical visits patients make over their lifetime are usually to a primary care practice. In this unique relationship, the clinician's knowledge of the patient's medical, psychological, and social situations grows with each encounter; therefore, the patient does not have to start over at the beginning at each visit. This also helps the clinician approach and treat the patient in a holistic manner. The patient goes to the primary care clinician during episodes of illness or injury, for ongoing management of chronic disease, as well as preventive services such as physical examinations and routine screenings. If patients are healthy, they may only require a routine annual visit to their primary care clinician. If there is an exacerbation of chronic disease or an episode of acute illness, then clinician encounters should be more frequent. Primary care is the major provider for medical care over time.

Primary care also provides continuity of information by maintaining ongoing medical records and information about the patient. When the practice coordinates additional services, it transfers necessary information to other practices and services, and maintains communications and records resulting from the referral. For example, if a patient is referred to an orthopedic practice, the primary care practice forwards relevant medical history and test results such as X rays. The primary care practice then receives reports back from the orthopedic practice about findings, test results, treatments, and suggestions for further treatment. This information is placed in the primary care practice records to maintain a comprehensive and continuous patient history.

### Levels of Care

The medical care delivery system is organized into several levels: primary, secondary, and tertiary. Primary care is the "first contact" of health care service provided to the population. It is a system of basic yet extensive medical care including periodic physical examinations, routine medical examinations, and treatments for common illnesses. Primary care also includes preventive services such as immunization for infectious diseases and screenings for chronic diseases, continuing care for chronic problems, as well as mental and physical health concerns. It encompasses referrals for more specialized care and advisement for various diagnostic and treatment options. Primary care is performed in an ambulatory setting, be it an office of a solo practitioner, an office of a group practice, a neighborhood clinic, a health maintenance organization (HMO), or a hospital outpatient office.

Secondary care is usually acute medical care for an episode of illness or injury. Many times it involves more complex or elaborate diagnostic work or treatment services than provided for in a primary care setting. It includes routine hospitalizations and most specialty care. Emergency care, specialty care, outpatient clinics, and inpatient stays in community hospitals or medical centers encompass secondary care. In addition to physicians, physician assistants, and nurse practitioners, many other health professionals participate in secondary care. Clinical chemists, administrators, radiation technologists, physical therapists, and occupational therapists are just a few of these professionals.

Tertiary care is advanced specialty care. It involves complicated and technical services for diagnosis and treatment. These services are usually provided by specialty hospitals and medical centers having the technical equipment and expertise for the care of complicated or advanced illness and injury. Many health professionals and health care workers work at this level of care.

## *First Contact*

Many times primary care is described as "first contact" medicine. It is said to be the point of entry for the patient into the health care system. The patient chooses or is assigned to a primary care clinician. Although primary care provides preventive services, many times a patient's first contact with the medical system comes when there is a problem. Many patients' insurance plans require them to choose a primary care clinician upon first entering the plan. If a patient waits too long to choose a primary care provider the insurance plan assigns one. Ideally this is how patients enter the medical care system, but sometimes they enter via self-referrals to a specialist or through the emergency department, such as S.J.W. in our case study.

Embedded in the first contact function of primary care is the function of *gatekeeper.* The primary care clinician has the knowledge and ability to decide when a patient needs services beyond the practice. As the main provider of medical care, the primary care clinician provides as much diagnostic work and treatment possible to minimize unnecessary trips to emergency departments or specialists, and to avoid unnecessary complications or duplication of activities.

## *Integration of Services and Comprehensive Care*

The Institute of Medicine's primary care definition also emphasizes integration of services and comprehensive care. Primary care has three main areas of focus: preventive care, acute care, and chronic care. Integration of these areas into individual patient care provides for comprehensive service.

Preventive care has the goal of reducing mortality and morbidity. It concentrates on diseases and injuries that can be prevented with periodic screenings, immunizations, education, and behavioral modifications. Primary care clinicians incorporate these functions into their practice, sometimes directing patients to other health professionals to provide these services. For example, a patient might be sent to a nurse for immunization, or a female smoker with early signs of heart disease might be sent to a health educator for a smoking cessation program, and to a nutritionist to reduce chances of having a heart attack.

Acute care is provided on an episodic basis. As patients experience an episode of discomfort, illness, or injury, they present themselves to the primary care clinician. Hopefully they seek care early in their illness. The clinician provides a diagnosis and treatment for this problem. Sometimes this may require several visits over a relatively short period of time. The majority of primary care visits are for acute care services. Some overlap may occur between primary and secondary acute care services. Many times patients go to the emergency department for an acute problem that could be treated in a primary care setting.

Chronic care is provided for diseases that are ongoing and usually do not have a cure. In these cases primary care clinicians manage the disease, i.e., they provide care that includes treatment to slow down the disease process, minimize symptoms or damage to the body, and/or optimize activities of daily living. Patients might periodically see a specialist, but care is coordinated and managed by their primary care clinician. Management of many chronic diseases requires specialization of other health professionals such as physical therapists, occupational therapists, radiation therapists, and nutritionists.

Primary care provides patients with preventive services, and acute and chronic care on a continual basis regardless of organ system. It is comprehensive, integrating diagnosis, treatment, disease management, and patient advisement. When required, primary care also coordinates other services related to patient care.

Primary care is the core of medical care. It facilitates transition between various clinicians and types of care. This coordinated transition provides for a flow of information and services to the patient's benefit. Figure 3.1 highlights the central role primary care plays in the medical system. Primary care links with the secondary care specialties like a two-way street. If a patient needs specialty care services, the primary care practice coordinates or refers the patient to that service. If a patient enters the medical care system from outside of the primary care practice, e.g., specialty care, then the patient should be referred to a primary care clinician for long-term follow-up care.

The branches of medicine that are considered primary care include family medicine, internal medicine, general medicine, and pediatrics. Although OB/GYN is considered primary care by some organizations and agencies, it was not included in the categorization of primary care because of its focus on the reproductive system. This controversy will be discussed later.

The patient enters the medical system by establishing contact with one of the primary care practices. Family medicine and general medicine provide

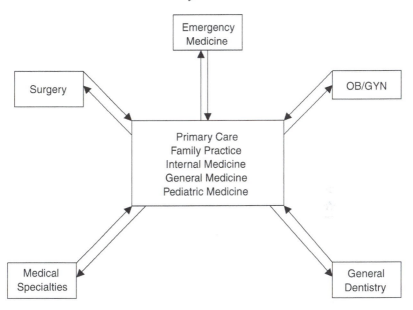

FIGURE 3.1. Primary Care Components Flowchart

care for anyone at any age. Internal medicine takes care of adults and pediatrics provides care for children. Patients are followed by the primary care practice until they are referred to a specialist or another level of care. Patients continue to be followed by the primary care practice even if they need to remain at another level of care for an extended period (e.g., hospitalization).

Family medicine provides care for every member of the family regardless of the organ system of involvement, age, or sex. Emphasis is placed on the family as a unit. Family medicine provides general medical care that includes pediatrics, internal medicine, OB/GYN, and surgery. They can also provide men's and women's medical care, and may perform procedures and therapies such as minor and simple surgeries, and birthing. Doctors (doctor of medicine, MD, or doctor of osteopathy, DO) who have completed a graduate medical training program in family medicine practice family medicine. Physician assistants and family nurse practitioners (nurse practitioners with a training emphasis in family care) may also practice family medicine.

Internal medicine provides general care for adult men and women, with emphasis on treating diseases of the internal organs in a nonsurgical fashion (though internalists can perform minor surgical procedures and provide basic gynecological care. Internal medicine is practiced by doctors (MD or

DO) who have completed a graduate medical training program in internal medicine, as well as physician assistants, and adult nurse practitioners (nurse practitioners with a training emphasis in adult care).

Pediatrics involves health care for children from birth through the end of adolescence. Pediatricians also treat diseases of children in a nonsurgical fashion, although they can perform minor surgical procedures and basic gynecological care. Doctors (MD or DO) who have completed a pediatrics graduate medical training program, physician assistants, and pediatric and family nurse practitioners can practice pediatrics.

General medicine encompasses general knowledge from other branches of medicine. Unlike the previously mentioned primary care practices, physicians practicing general medicine usually have completed only one year of graduate medical training. The number of general practitioners has been decreasing over the years. In the 1930s, 87 percent of physicians in private practice were general practitioners. By 1994, general practitioners accounted for less than 18 percent (Donaldson et al., 1996). Physician assistants and nurse practitioners can also practice general medicine.

OB/GYN is the branch of medicine that provides care for women. Obstetrics deals with childbirth from pregnancy through the postpartum period while gynecology deals with the female reproductive system, including the breasts. OB/GYN includes treatments such as surgery and medication. Care for adolescent and young women can be included in the OB/GYN practice. OB/GYN is practiced by doctors (MD or DO) who have completed a graduate medical training program in this field; physician assistants, nurse-midwives, and women, family, and adult nurse practitioners. In addition, primary care practices such as family or internal medicine can also provide basic obstetrical and gynecological care.

As mentioned earlier, some controversy exists among various organizations and agencies whether OB/GYN should be included in primary care. For example, the Institute of Medicine does not recognize OB/GYN, but the Federal Bureau of Primary Health Care does. By the Institute Of Medicine's definition, OB/GYN is too focused on the reproductive system to address most patients' personal health care needs and thus is generally not considered to be primary care. Some argue that OB/GYN should be considered a primary care practice since many women use it as their first point of contact and basic gynecological care is a major primary care function for health care of women. In addition, all OB/GYN clinicians received some primary care training before specializing in women's medicine. Some women even have nonreproductive problems addressed by their gynecological clinician. Although the discipline of OB/GYN was not included in the diagram of primary care (Figure 3.1), what is more important is whether OB/GYN clinicians are performing the functions of primary care, i.e., providing continuous, comprehensive care with coordination of health care services.

Women seen by OB/GYN clinicians are usually referred by a primary care clinician or by an emergency medicine practitioner. Women go to the OB/GYN practice for routine care such as Pap smears, pregnancy, or specialized care such as infertility treatment. Many women enter the medical system by referring themselves to gynecologists for their annual gynecological examination. Gynecologists should then refer patients to a primary care practice for overall care. Women may also be referred to the OB/GYN after being seen by the emergency department. Subsequently, OB/GYN should then refer her to a primary care practice for overall care.

## MAJOR SPECIALTIES THAT INTERACT WITH PRIMARY CARE

Mental health is the branch of medicine that provides care for mental and social functioning. A range of problems and disorders affect mental functioning, including depression, schizophrenia, alcohol use, drug use, bulimia, and anxiety. Several types of clinicians provide mental health care. Psychiatrists are doctors (MD or DO) who have completed a graduate medical training program in psychiatry. Physician assistants and nurse practitioners can also provide mental health care. These three types of clinicians can prescribe medications for mental and physical health. Other mental health clinicians include psychologists, social workers, therapists, and advance practice nurses.

Patients may refer themselves to mental health clinicians, although primary care can help identify mental problems. Many physical disorders seen by primary care clinicians can be treated in primary care with mental health consultation, while others must be referred to mental health. If patients enter the medical system via mental health channels they should be eventually be referred to primary care for overall health care.

Dentistry provides care for teeth and the oral cavity. It is practiced by dentists (doctor of dental medicine, DMD, or doctor of dental science, DDS), who have completed graduate schools in dentistry. Dentistry has several areas. General or primary care dentistry provides comprehensive overall dental care including routine prevention, diagnosis, and treatment for diseases of the teeth and gums. Specialized areas of dentistry such as orthodontics deal with the alignment of teeth and periodontics deals with the gums and other supporting structures of the teeth. In addition, dental assistants and dental hygienists also assist the dental practice.

Patients can refer themselves to the dentist or be referred by a primary care clinician. Primary care clinicians will refer patients to dentistry for routine preventive care or for treatment of oral cavity problems the primary care clinician has detected. Primary care clinicians can provide supporting treatment for acute dental problems such as pain management and infection control, but they will refer patients to dentistry for definitive care. Emergency medicine can also refer patients to dentistry. Dentists should refer patients to primary care clinicians for overall care if the patient is not in the medical care system. Dentists may refer patients to primary care for routine care or treatment of diseases they may detect.

Emergency medicine specializes in the treatment of patients with acute episodes of injury and disease, particularly life threatening problems. The role of emergency medicine is to provide definitive care when possible, otherwise its role is to stabilize patients enough to send them to definitive care such as the operating room or hospitalization. Patients can even be sent home (in the case of chronic problems) to follow up in the future with an outpatient clinician. Emergency medicine requires broad knowledge that includes pediatrics, internal medicine, OB/GYN, surgery, and critical care. Most of emergency medicine is practiced in hospital emergency departments. It can also be practiced in urgent care clinics. It is practiced by doctors (MD or DO) who have completed a graduate medical training program in emergency medicine, as well as physician assistants, and nurse practitioners.

Patients may bring themselves to the emergency department or they may be referred by another clinician. If patients enter the medical system through an emergency department visit then they should be referred to primary care practice or to a specialist upon discharge. The majority of emergency department visits are for primary care type problems and are not life threatening. For example, a child sustains a laceration and is brought by their parents to a pediatrician who decides the child needs extensive suturing. After cleansing and bandaging the wound the pediatrician refers the child immediately to the emergency department, where the child is sutured and referred back to the pediatrician.

Surgery provides care for disease and injury through operations and physical manipulation, regardless of age or gender. Areas of specialization in surgery are organized by organ systems and are practiced by doctors (MD or DO) who have completed a graduate medical training program in surgery and who are considered surgeons. Physician assistants and nurse practitioners can provide surgical care, but only physicians can initiate an operation.

Patients are usually referred to surgery by other clinicians, including primary care clinicians. If a patient has been referred by a specialist or is self-referred then the surgical practice should refer the patient to primary care for general medical care.

Medical specialties are branches of internal medicine that focus on a specific organ system. Physicians who are specialized have additional training beyond internal medicine. Nurse practitioners and physician assistants who practice in the medical subspecialties have either received additional formal training or informal training by working in that practice setting.

Patients are usually referred to medical specialists by the primary care clinicians or the emergency medicine clinicians. Patients may also refer themselves. Specialists will then refer patients to a primary care practice if they are not affiliated with one. If the problem requires continued intervention by a specialist, then the patient can be referred back to primary care between specialty care visits.

Hospitalization occurs when patients have a problem that requires diagnostic study or treatment that must take place in the hospital. Patients can only be admitted to a hospital through referral from a clinician. The hospital grants privileges or authority to the clinician to provide care within the hospital. The emergency department also has the authority to admit patients to the hospital, though they do not provide inpatient care. Patients are referred back to the primary care practice for overall care upon discharge from the hospital. Regardless of the problem, primary care should be involved in the care process even if it is only through referral or to be kept informed. This process ensures a flow of proper information, maximizes everyone's time, avoids duplication of services, and prevents contradictory events such as medication interactions.

## WHO PRACTICES PRIMARY CARE?

Primary care clinicians are responsible for addressing the majority of personal health care needs. This means clinicians must have knowledge of most of the body's organ systems. A primary care clinician can see a patient for a headache, muscle strain, and even heart disease. They are generalists. Most medical specialists are focused on a specific organ system such as the heart (cardiology), nervous system (neurology), or muscle and bones (orthopedics). Thus primary care clinicians come from the following areas of medicine: family practice, internal medicine, general medicine, and pediatrics. OB/GYN is too focused on the reproductive system to address most patients' personal health care needs and thus is generally not considered to be primary care.

## Primary Care Clinicians

Physicians have graduated from an allopathic or osteopathic medical school. Graduates of allopathic schools are called medical doctors (MD), while graduates of osteopathic schools are called doctors of osteopathy (DO). After medical school physicians receive graduate medical training through a hospital residency for an average of three years. Family practice, internal medicine, and pediatric residencies train the physician primary care workforce.

Physician assistants (PA) are clinicians who have received two or more years of professional training to perform duties traditionally assigned to physicians including evaluating, diagnosing, treating illness and injuries, monitoring, prescribing medication, counseling, and referral. Physician assistants work with the supervision of a physician. The majority of physician assistant graduates have been trained at primary care physician assistant programs.

Nurse practitioners are advanced practice nurses. They are nurses with advanced graduate education in specialty areas such as family practice, pediatrics, or adult and women's medicine. They are trained to perform medical histories and physical examinations, order and interpret diagnostic tests, diagnose and treat illness and injuries, conduct patient health maintenance, and provide prevention counseling. They may also prescribe medications.

## The Role of the Primary Care Clinician

Primary care clinicians are usually physicians, physician assistants, or nurse practitioners. Clinicians are chosen by or assigned to patients. When a patient sees the clinician for a medical concern, the clinician addresses the concern regardless of the problem. If the problem requires more extensive or specialized care, the clinician arranges that care. The patient may be referred to an emergency department, a specialist, or may even be hospitalized. The clinicians should conduct follow ups with patients after emergency department or specialist visits, as well as during and after hospital stays.

One role of primary care and its clinicians is the coordination of patient medical services, while another is that of "gatekeeper" for the medical system. Most of the time these roles overlap. As the first or primary contact, primary care clinicians direct patients to appropriate care and services. This includes arranging various tests to diagnose a problem, referring patients to other clinicians, and managing the recommendations of other clinicians.

This helps ensure a level of quality care for patients. Clinicians refer patients to specialists when the situation requires another level of expertise, such as referring a patient to the dermatologist for an advanced skin problem, or to a social worker to help arrange home nursing service. Without coordination and oversight, it is possible for a patient to see several specialists who each address one specific problem and offer therapies that might be contradictory. For example, Mr. Jones is an elderly man who was taking several medications for hypertension, diabetes, and arthritis. Each set of medications was prescribed by a different specialist. Mr. Jones' antihypertension medication was contraindicated for a patient with diabetes. If Mr. Jones had been cared for by a primary care clinician, he would have returned to that clinician soon after his visit to the specialist who prescribed his antihypertension medication. The specialist would have communicated with Mr. Jones' primary care clinician and Mr. Jones would have been placed on different medication.

The primary care clinician's coordination of diagnostic and treatment options and gatekeeper functions can minimize the cost of medical care. Medical care costs increase with the use of specialists and high technology. Patients should not be referred to specialists or specialized tests for functions that can be performed by primary care clinicians. Managed care organizations see this as an important factor in controlling costs.

## *Other Contributors to the Primary Care Team*

Quality primary care is actually made possible by a team of clinicians. Some clinicians come from disciplines that perform primary care functions such as pediatrics, internal medicine, and family medicine. Other clinicians contribute to primary care. General dentists, podiatrists, and optometrists are examples of clinicians who perform primary care functions, but do not fit the definition of a primary care clinician because they do not address the majority of their patients' personal health care needs. Some specialists perform primary care functions with some of their patients, such as the cardiologist who refers his or her patient to the dentist and provides the patient with pneumococcal immunizations. These clinicians generally do not fit the definition of primary care clinician.

## *The Primary Care Practice*

The primary care practice is composed of all the professions and functions involved in the primary care clinical setting. Some practices are small and have only one clinician and one or two other staff members. Other practices are quite large, with fifty or more employees. The number and type of professionals involved depends on the size of the practice. The primary care clinician may be a physician assistant, nurse practitioner, or a physician. A medical assistant may be the first person in the office to come in contact with patients by registering them. A nurse may take vital signs and do an initial assessment. The nurse may also provide a treatment such as an injection, a breathing treatment, or may dress a wound after the patient has been evaluated by the clinician. A clinical chemist or medical technologist might take and analyze blood, urine, or other body specimens for diagnostic purposes. A radiology technician may take a roentgenogram (X ray) ordered by the clinician. A physical therapist may provide some therapeutic modalities for the patient. A nutritionist may provide dietary counseling. A health educator may offer classes to help the patient manage a disease or to promote wellness. An office or clinic manager coordinates office functions. Each of these professions and more can participate in the primary care practice.

## CONTROVERSIES AND CONCEPTUAL/SYSTEMIC FLAWS

Controversies and conceptual flaws abound when we think of primary care medicine. This is mainly due to the *scope of practice overlap* ("fuzzy medicine"), *perspective variations* in defining the primary care specialties (e.g., OB/GYN), and the *large numbers of health care personnel* whose roles may be poorly defined. In addition, rapidly growing areas such as geriatrics and midwifery are challenging prevailing boundaries and blurring the lines of primary care medicine. The lines continue to blur and shift with the incorporation of health promotional initiatives into primary care practices. This targets a state of wellness that does not focus on the absence of disease alone.

Key phrases such as first contact, coordination, comprehensiveness, continuity, accessibility, and accountability in health maintenance and management tend to define primary care. However, must *all* these elements be present to establish definition? As in other fields of medical statistical classification, can a portion of those elements be present to designate primary care status? If so, how much and in what combination? It is no wonder that so much confusion exists; addressing these questions would be a strong first step toward properly defining primary health care.

## *SUMMARY AND FUTURE CONSIDERATIONS*

Much work remains to be done. Continuous education of patients, clinical practitioners, and administrative personnel is critical for minimizing chronic problems. It must be emphasized that the patient is the only *person* who undergoes *all* diagnostic and therapeutic interventions, and therefore must be empowered to make key decisions. Pivotally, patients must secure a *central point of reference* in their health care. A primary care clinician's role is to be the chief facilitator of the health care delivery process. It is imperative to inform each patient of his or her options and associated risks in order to select the best choice. It would appear that all clinical practitioners are linked in the primary care network. Many perform some or all of the duties that are readily accepted as primary care. A consideration involving a three-pronged approach for each patient encounter may aid in distinguishing the function and degree of primary care elements for the clinical practitioner. As individual providers simply resolve to understand the following: (1) What were the circumstances that brought the patient to me? (2) What are the specific interventions that I should perform? (3) Where does the patient go for follow-up and/or referral? This approach should help the clinical practitioner discern the extent of primary care versus episodic care involvement.

Administrative personnel embrace cost effective measures that are linked to patient outcome and satisfaction. Patient feedback instruments such as surveys, polls, comments, etc., should act as barometers for the health care delivery network and reflect its core value. A fundamental response involves active listening and enhanced communication between patient and health care providers. Clarity in process/procedural flow and patient directed options will help maintain focus on the big picture. A colleague once stated, "We can get the sand out of our eyes, if we take our heads out of the sand."

In closing, discussions that attempt to quantify the criteria that tend to define primary care medicine and address a patient's biological, behavioral, and social needs are recommended. Subsequently, the number or portion of the criteria that establishes primary care status needs to be determined. Input from key segments including patient consumer groups, clinical practitioners from multiple specialties, HMO personnel, and governmental health agencies would be highly beneficial. This is just a small step, but at least it is a step toward answering or rephrasing S.J.W.'s question: "Who is my doctor?"

## BIBLIOGRAPHY

American Academy of Family Physicians (2000). Retrieved from the World Wide Web: <http://www.aafp.org/x6988.xml>.

American Academy of Nurse Practitioners (n.d.). Retrieved from the World Wide Web: <http://www.aanp.org>.

American Academy of Physician Assistants (n.d.). Retrieved from the World Wide Web: <http://www.aapa.org/employer.html>.

American College of Nurse Practitioners (n.d.). Retrieved from the World Wide Web: <http://www.nurse.org/acnp/facts/whatis.shtml>.

American College of Nurse-Midwifes (n.d.). Retrieved from the World Wide Web: <http://www.midwife.org/prof/display.cfm?id=137>.

American Medical Association (n.d.). Retrieved from the World Wide Web: <http://www.ama-assn.org/apps/pf_online/pf_online?f_n=browse&doc=policyfiles/HOD/H-200.969.HTM>.

Bureau of Primary Health Care (n.d.). Appendix A to Part 5—Criteria for Designation of Areas Having Shortages of Primary Medical Care Professional(s). Retrieved from the World Wide Web: <http://bphc.hrsa.gov:80/dsd/hpsa_fr2.html>.

Donaldson, M.S., Yordy, K.D., Lohr, K.N., and Vanselow, N.E. (Eds.) (1996). *Primary Care: America's Health in a New Era*. Washington, DC: National Academy Press.

Jones, P.E. and Cawley, J.F. (1994). "Physician Assistant and Health Reform: Clinical Capabilities, Practice Activities and Potential Roles." *Journal of the American Medical Association*, 271:1266-1272.

McKenzie, J.F., Pinger, R.R. and Kotechi, J.E. (1999). "The Structure of the U.S. Health Care System." *An Introduction to Community Health, Web Enhanced* (Third edition), pp. 428-432. Boston: Jones and Bartlett.

Stevens, R.A. (2000). Professional Competence and Board Certification. Paper presented to the American Board of Medical Specialties. Retrieved from the World Wide Web: <http://www.abms.org/downloads/conferences/stevens%20paper.doc>.

U.S. Department of Health and Human Services, Health Resources and Services Administration. (July, 2000). Community Health Status Report: Data Sources, Definitions, and Notes. Retrieved from the World Wide Web: <http://www.communityhealth.hrsa.gov:80/documents/CHSI-CompanionView.pdf>.

William, S.J. (1993). "Ambulatory Health Care Services." *Introduction to Health Services* (Fourth edition), pp. 108-134. Albany: Delmar.

Chapter 4

# Rehabilitative and Restorative Therapies

John Echternach

The focus of this chapter is to explore briefly the health professions and health occupations that might be involved with a patient's rehabilitative and restorative care. This section will begin with a brief case report.

The patient is a sixty-year-old woman named Mary who went to the emergency room of the local medical center complaining of left-side weakness and dizziness. The initial impression was that she had labyrinthitis, which would account for her dizziness. Because of the persistence of the problem, the physician admitted her to the hospital and obtained a magnetic resonance image (MRI) which showed that the patient was developing a right-sided infarct. The diagnosis was that the patient had had a cerebral vascular accident (CVA).

Over the next few hours, the patient developed left hemiparesis. The patient remained in the hospital for two weeks when she was admitted to a rehabilitation unit. Her time in the hospital was spent stabilizing her condition and she began to receive physical therapy services during this time. The physical therapy services consisted primarily of maintaining range of motion and having the patient sit and stand for brief periods of time.

The patient's previous history included a diagnosis of hypertension. The patient smoked two packs of cigarettes per day at the time of admission. The patient also had hyperlipidemia.

Upon admission to the rehabilitation unit, the patient was evaluated by personnel in the departments of physical therapy, occupational therapy, speech pathology, clinical psychology, dietetics, and physiatry. It was noted that the patient had weakness on the left side of her body and had very little function of her left arm. The patient could initiate flexion and extension at the hip, however, extension was very poor. The patient essentially was a hemiplegic with weakness in the upper extremity that was far more severe than the weakness in the lower extremity. It was noted that the patient's hypertension was poorly controlled and her resting blood pressure was 160/100 with a resting pulse of 84. Prior to the patient's current illness, she had co-owned a dry cleaning store and had worked long hours supervising two other employees.

The team that evaluated the patient, in discussion with the patient, determined the following goals: (1) the patient would walk independently with the use of an assist, (2) the patient would be independent in dressing and self-care, (3) the patient would have community ambulation ability. Each of the service teams that saw the patient set particular goals for their aspect of patient care. Nursing would work on being sure the patient developed continence with both bowel and bladder. Occupational therapy would work on the patient's abilities to conduct personal hygiene, including toileting and being able to use a tub and shower with minimal assistance. Physical therapy would be concerned primarily with independence in transfers. Initially, transfers were directed at getting the patient into a wheelchair and later ambulating with a walker. Psychological services determined they would work with the patient concerning the psychological liability that occurs after a CVA. The dietetic service would work toward weight reduction since the patient weighed 227 pounds. Their goal was for the patient to lose nearly fifty pounds under supervision. Both occupational therapy and the physical therapy service would work with the patient's husband and help him understand his responsibilities in terms of supervising the patient's ambulation and other self-care activities after discharge. Occupational therapy personnel also had the goal of helping the patient develop a kitchen in which she could function and continue to prepare family meals. The patient spent approximately three weeks in the rehabilitation unit.

At that time, the patient was being prepared to be discharged to her home. A home inspection was done by the physical therapist and occupational therapist. They noted that the patient's house had three entrance steps, with a banister for assistance. There were no inside stairs. At this point, the patient could walk 150 feet with a walker and could walk a shorter distance using a cane. The patient did a better job of going up stairs than coming down them. The patient had begun to regain some fine motor control in her upper extremity but still used her left arm primarily as a "helper extremity" for her right arm. Occupational therapy personnel assessed the kitchen arrangements and felt the patient could function in the kitchen with a few minor modifications. At the time of discharge from the rehabilitation unit, it was also determined that the patient should be followed for an additional six weeks as an outpatient with physical therapy and occupational therapy. The psychological services staff felt the patient's cognitive abilities at this time were within the normal range. The patient continued to work with the dietetic service at losing weight and has had some success. The patient also stopped smoking during the time she was in the hospital and continued cessation while she was in the rehabilitation unit. The patient stated she did not intend to resume smoking. When she was discharged from the rehabilitation unit, the patient stated her goal was to eventually return to work. The various team members felt this was a realistic goal for the future, after the patient had completed outpatient services.

Since the patient had left-sided weakness and right-sided CVA, there was not much in the way of speech impairment. Even though speech services personnel had evaluated the patient, they did not feel that they had an important role to play with this patient. However, if the patient's stroke had resulted in a left CVA and right-sided weakness, speech services would have been an integral part of the patient's care because the patient would have had some form of aphasia as a result of the stroke. Fortunately, the patient did not need speech services, but it was important to note that speech services did evaluate the patient for potential problems.

The dictionary defines rehabilitation as the process of treatment and education that helps disabled individuals to obtain maximum function, a sense of well-being, and a personally satisfying level of independence. Rehabilitation may be necessary for any disease or injury that causes mental or physical impairment serious enough to result in functional limitations or disability. The term restoration refers to the act of returning something to a previous state.

In regard to rehabilitative and restorative services, there is a tendency to think of them primarily as the professions or occupations that are most noted for working in these areas. Most of those professions were part of the team that saw the patient in the case study. This chapter will focus on three of these groups: occupational therapy, physical therapy, and speech and language therapies. This is not to exclude other groups from the concept of rehabilitation. The dictionary's definition makes the case that rehabilitation can be performed by any health care practitioner who is dealing with someone with disabilities serious enough to require a team approach. The team approach is an important concept in the idea of modern health care regardless of whether it is considered a rehabilitative environment or other environment. Rarely does an individual with a serious disease or injury receive care from only one individual. The idea of a team providing services for individuals is one that is becoming more and more important. Therefore, the concept of team work among rehabilitative health care practitioners is also becoming increasingly important. The concept of rehabilitation seems to refer more frequently to functional limitations and disabilities than does the concept of acute care. Acute care is the process of either saving lives or helping patients recover from an illness that does not result in serious residual functional limitations or disability. An example of this might be a patient who has pneumonia and is acutely ill while having the disease but is treated with an antibiotic in the acute care environment and recovers within a relatively short time without residual problems. The acute care environment provides care for nearly every patient who becomes a rehabilitation patient by providing life-saving services early in the course of the disease or injury, and therefore contributes in very important ways to the overall rehabilitation of the individual. Health care represents a continuum of care from acute illness through long-term chronic illness with various health care practitioners making their contribution along the way. Rehabilitative and restorative health care practitioners contribute by dealing with serious long-term functional limitations and disabilities.

The overall purpose of rehabilitation is to simply decrease functional limitations, increase a person's functional abilities to their highest level, and decrease the person's level of disability as much as possible. The Nagi model or the World Health Organization model for health care provides a fairly good framework for understanding the concept of rehabilitation as part of the continuum of care. The illustrations provided will show that this continuum of care focuses primarily on understanding what the persons' impairments are, trying to improve their ability to function while decreasing functional limitations, and ultimately having a patient whose disabilities are as minimized as possible.

## HISTORY OF THE DEVELOPMENT OF REHABILITATIVE AND RESTORATIVE THERAPIES

This section will briefly describe how each of the rehabilitative and restorative therapy groups developed, beginning with physical therapy.

The history of physical therapy in the United States can be traced to the outbreaks of poliomyelitis in the late 1890s and early 1900s, when physicians realized patients would benefit from supervised exercise programs. Generally speaking, these programs were conducted by women who were physical educators and, as time went by, became a more specialized practice. In terms of regulation, the first recognition of physical therapy as a separate field came in 1915 when a licensure law was passed in Pennsylvania. World War I was the impetus for the development of the profession, when women were employed by the U.S. Army to aid in the care and rehabilitation of injured servicemen. These women received training and were called reconstruction aides. In 1921, a veteran reconstruction aide named Mary McMillan organized a meeting of reconstruction aides in New York City. The group formed a professional organization that ultimately became the American Physical Therapy Association (APTA).

One of the early goals of this association was to develop educational standards for the field of physical therapy. Development of the profession was slow during the 1920s and 1930s, particularly during the Great Depression. The next burst of growth came during World War II, when the military commissioned women with appropriate levels of education to function as physical therapy officers. Following the war, the profession continued to grow and this growth is reflected both in the kinds of education physical therapists receive as well as the variety of environments in which physical therapists function. The APTA developed a detailed definition of physical therapy for the purpose of licensure and licensure has now been achieved in all states. The APTA's definition of model practice protects both the title of physical therapist as well as the practice of physical therapy. The APTA has also developed a philosophical statement on physical therapy which is a more general definition for informing the public what physical therapists do.

The education of physical therapists has evolved over time from one which started in the 1920s as essentially on-the-job training in a hospital physical therapy department to the development of physical therapy educational programs at universities. Originally, many of these university educational programs were postbaccalaureate certificate programs. Gradually bachelors degree programs were developed and in the 1950s and 1960s a few programs were developed that led to a master's degree as the entry level degree for physical therapy. In 1979 the APTA's house of delegates stated that physical therapy education after 1990 should lead to a postbaccalaureate degree. The goal was not met by 1990, but as of 2002 all physical therapy educational programs are postbaccalaureate in nature. Many of these programs lead to physical therapy degrees titled master of physical therapy (MPT) or master of science in physical therapy (MSPT). More recently there has been a call for doctor of physical therapy degree (DPT) as the entry level degree. This concept is growing rapidly and the APTA has developed a vision statement which states that by 2020 physical therapy will be provided by physical therapists who are DPTs.

For many years, the number of physical therapists supplied by physical therapy educational programs fell far short of the number of physical therapists needed. However, when the federal government curtailed Medicare payments in 1997, many therapists lost their jobs due to decreased demand for services. This resulted in an excess of physical therapy professionals. Since then, the number of applicants to physical therapy educational programs has decreased and recent developments have led to the recovery of physical therapists to near full employment. The most recent figures provided by the APTA state that only about 1 percent of physical therapists who are seeking employment are not currently employed. Recent graduates usually find employment relatively soon after graduation. It is estimated that the number of applicants to physical therapy educational programs will soon rise.

Currently, the educational pathway for becoming a physical therapist follows one of three patterns. The first pattern involves choosing a bachelor's degree with certain prerequisite courses, followed by a two-year master's degree program. Following completion of this two-year program, graduates would receive an MPT degree. The second pattern involves three or four years of education at the undergraduate level (often leading to a bachelor's degree) followed by application to a DPT program. After thirty-five to thirty-six months (or nearly three calendar years), graduates would achieve a DPT degree. The third pattern is a combination of these two patterns in which students complete three years of college and then enter a three-year professional program in which the fourth year of the six-year program is a transitional year from an undergraduate to a professional degree program.

All physical therapy educational programs in the United States are accredited by the Commission on Accreditation of Physical Therapy Education (CAPTE). Licensure is dependant upon graduation from an accredited program.

Another historical development in physical therapy, which is occurring gradually over time, is the change in how much access physical therapists have to patients. Originally, all physical therapy patients were referred by physicians, dentists, or osteopathic physicians. Over time, physical therapists have gained more autonomy in their professional practice and more access to patients without referral from other practitioners. This access now extends to thirty-seven states in which physical therapists can both evaluate and treat patients under defined circumstances without a referral from another practitioner. In an additional nine states (making a total of forty-six states), physical therapists can evaluate patients without a referral for the purposes of screening, health promotion, and disease prevention. In these nine states where physical therapists may not treat patients without a referral, patients at least have the benefit of physical therapists being the point of entry into the health care system since they can be referred by physical therapists to appropriate health care practitioners if a problem is discovered.

Within the field of physical therapy other individuals assist physical therapists in the provision of services. Since the 1960s, physical therapist assistants are educated at the community college level. These individuals attend community colleges and receive an associate in applied science (AAS) degree in physical therapy. These individuals work under the direct supervision of physical therapists and are an important asset to the profession by strengthening the services provided to patients through teamwork. In addition, many physical therapy practices also employ physical therapy aides. These individuals are trained to perform certain tasks that free physical therapists and physical therapist assistants to perform more complex tasks required in patient care.

As with physical therapy, occupational therapy developed in the late nineteenth and early twentieth centuries. However, the philosophical background that led to the development of occupational therapy was much different than physical therapy. In physical therapy, the emphasis was primarily on the physical rehabilitation of individuals, while in occupational therapy the early thought process and philosophy was based on the concept that those who were mentally ill deserved the appropriate treatment to be administered to them with both kindness and consideration.

At the turn of the century, when chronic illness was increasing and industrial accidents were becoming a part of life in modern society, a physician named Herbert Hall proposed the concept of adapting the arts and crafts movement as a treatment method. Two other individuals are often credited with having an important role in the development of occupational therapy. A psychiatrist named William Rush Dunton Jr. is credited with developing some of the early occupational therapy programs, particularly as they developed in specialized institutions and hospitals. A social worker named Eleanor Clark Slagle is also credited with being the founder of occupational therapy as a profession for her work in the early 1900s, particularly in developing a workshop for the chronically unemployed. Slagle also organized the first professional school for occupational therapy practitioners.

In 1917, a small group of individuals, including those mentioned previously, met in Clifton Springs, New York, and incorporated the group called the National Society for the Promotion of Occupational Therapy. Occupational therapy showed a great deal of growth during World War I, as did physical therapy. Following World War I, occupational therapy grew slowly, inhibited in some ways by the Great Depression. Occupational therapy services during World War II were recognized by the military and there was more widespread use of occupational therapists as part of rehabilitation teams.

Following World War II, occupational therapy continued to grow in stature and numbers. As with most health professions, concern arose during the early years about the educational programs provided for occupational therapists. An outgrowth of this concern was the development of a required registration examination in 1945. In the 1960s, the American Occupational Therapy Association (AOTA) sought regulation from state licensing agencies to regulate the practice of occupational therapy, however licensure was not pursued vigorously until the late 1980s. Occupational therapists are now licensed in most states.

Entry level education for occupational therapists has paralleled that of physical therapy in many ways. In the beginning, many occupational therapists were trained on the job and supervised by other occupational therapists. Later, a certificate in occupational therapy was created as a postbaccalaureate program requiring one to two years of study. Current occupational therapists are required to have one of the following qualifications: bachelor's degree in occupational therapy, BS with a postgraduate certificate, an entry-level master's degree (MSOT), or a recently developed clinical entry-level doctor of occupational therapy (OTD). Many educational programs provide a combinational bachelor's and master's degree approach, with professional qualification at the end of five or six years.

The American Occupational Therapy Association (AOTA) is the nationally recognized professional association for occupational therapists and occupational therapist assistants. The AOTA has more than 50,000 members. The AOTA is responsible for accrediting occupational therapy educational programs through the Accredition Council for Occupational Therapy Education (ACOTE). Occupational therapists also have a group of individuals who assist them in their practice called Certified Occupational Therapy Assistants (COTA). Currently, COTAs are required to be graduates of an accredited two-year degree program and have completed appropriate supervised field work for certification. Originally, COTAs were individuals who were essentially trained on the job in a formal program. However, since 1965 COTAs have been required to be graduates of a community college program.

In addition to COTAs, occupational therapists also use occupational therapy aides defined as those trained to perform specific tasks under the supervision of either the occupational therapist or the COTA. However, the occupational therapist retains responsibility for acts performed by this individual.

The occupational therapy profession has relied heavily on the importance of individuals in the field passing a certification exam, and the occupational therapist must pass a national certifying examination after completion of their education. This is also true for COTAs, who must pass a national certification examination after completing their educational requirements. All fifty states, including the District of Columbia and Puerto Rico, regulate the practice of occupational therapy; however, not all of these states require licensure. Some states require registration of the certification as evidence that individuals are capable of practicing occupational therapy.

Occupational therapy has always been particularly attractive to women; only a small percentage are men. The number of occupational therapists with entry-level postbaccalaureate degrees is increasing and now approaches 40 percent. Occupational therapy as a profession has continued to expand employment opportunities for occupational therapists. Occupational therapists work in nearly every health care setting imaginable, from private practices and school systems, to long-term care facilities such as nursing homes and rehabilitation centers. Occupational therapy has followed the example of many other health professions by developing areas of specialization and ways for occupational therapists to develop certifications in various specialties either through the American Occupational Therapy Association or other organizations. Even as the profession has expanded into new areas and taken on additional roles, it has maintained that occupational therapy is based on the unique philosophy that treatment by occupational therapists should be based on purposeful activities that tend to improve or increase the independence of the clients they work with.

While maintaining its unique boundaries, occupational therapy is also a highly collaborative profession whose members work comfortably with other health professionals. Occupational therapists have traditionally been very comfortable working with physical therapists, speech therapists, and others in rehabilitative and restorative professions. Occupational therapists frequently work with individuals who have physical disabilities, with individuals who have psychological or emotional difficulties. as well as individuals with developmental problems. Occupational therapists are frequent visitors to patients' homes as part of the home health care system, and contribute to health promotion and disease prevention.

Occupational therapists often are involved in adapting equipment or ordinary household objects for patients' use and, as computerized technology has gained its place, occupational therapists have also begun adapting computer-aided equipment. Generally speaking, employment opportunities for occupational therapists have remained high. Although occupational therapists were affected by the actions that restricted Medicare payments in 1997, employment opportunities for both occupational therapists and COTAs are looking healthy again now that the ceiling on Medicare payments has been adjusted.

The third group this section will direct attention to are those professionals who work in speech/language pathology. In many instances, patients who have neurological difficulties resulting from disease or trauma will have problems with speech and communication that are part of the problem that must be rehabilitated. Action is then required to improve the patient's function following an incident. Speech language pathologists are involved in the examination, evaluation, and treatment or intervention with patients who have speech or language problems resulting from any number of conditions. They may also be involved in counseling patients and their families about these disorders and assisting them with coping with stress and some of the resulting problems and misunderstandings that accompany difficulties in communication.

Speech language pathology and audiology have always been closely associated, but in the United States they evolved into two separate professional groups. Both of these professions share a common interest, which is improving communication. The focus of this section will be on speech language pathologists since problems in audiology often affect a different population and for different reasons than those patients who are seen by rehabilitative and restorative services teams.

Individuals working with speech problems in the United States began to appear in the early 1900s and were primarily associated with public schools. The history of speech language pathology and audiology can be approached from several different angles. One approach would be the obvious observation that speech and hearing are primary human functions and therefore have received attention throughout history. However, this attention was not necessarily scientific. In the early nineteenth century, nonscientific methods were developed for treating patients with hearing and speech problems that were based on recurring common problems. As time went on, and the mechanisms of speech and hearing were better understood, more scientific methodology was introduced and the professions of speech language pathology and audiology were created. In the early states of their development, it was difficult to separate the two professions. As time passed, they eventually became distinct disciplines, each with their own educational and qualificational standards. Many writers have suggested that even though there is a separation in the professional qualifications for these two groups, each must understand the other to a high degree because of the overlapping knowledge and abilities required to understand speech and hearing problems.

Interest in speech language problems in the late nineteenth and early twentieth centuries led to the training of individuals who were responsible for treating school-age children with speech disorders. By the early 1900s schools were employing these individuals in the United States and Europe. By 1913 there were treatment centers for persons with communicational disorders established at many universities in the United States, with Columbia University, University of Pennsylvania, and the University of Wisconsin leading the way. During World War I, hospitals were established for treating brain-injured soldiers, including aphasics. This was the first large-scale attempt to rehabilitate individuals with aphasia.

By 1920, speech correction services were offered at public schools in a number of American cities, and there were both international and national groups forming who were expressing concerns about education and qualifications of those individuals who were practicing in this field. In 1925 the American Academy of Speech Correction, currently known as The American Speech Language/Hearing Association (ASHA), was formed. The ASHA is the national association for U.S. speech language pathologists and audiologists. In 1936, the first issue of *The Journal of Speech Disorders* was published. Increased interest in childhood speech disorders during the 1930s resulted in more money being provided to school systems for children's programs. World War II also saw the establishment of special programs for brain-injured soldiers, which were continued at many veteran's hospitals after the war.

Audiology became a separate profession after World War II, mostly due to the growth of treatment programs established by veteran's hospitals for hearing-impaired veterans. In the period following World War II there was considerable growth in both professions. The remainder of this section will concentrate on speech language pathologists since they are most commonly associated with rehabilitative efforts combining physical therapists, occupational therapists, and others in a restorative and rehabilitative environment.

Today, speech language pathologists are required to have master's degrees. Although there are undergraduate or preprofessional programs in speech language pathology, these programs simply prepare one to be admitted to a graduate program that leads to a master's degree. Speech language pathologists are licensed by most states and these states specify that a master's degree or graduate degree is the minimum for receipt of a license. In addition, many employers require the speech language therapist to be credentialed by the ASHA. Since 1962, the minimum requirements for membership in the ASHA have been a master's degree and the ASHA's certificate of clinical competence (CCC). The CCC is currently the standard for entry into the practice of speech language pathology.

The ASHA has a role in the accreditation of educational programs for speech language pathologists. The accrediting organization is the Council on Academic Accreditation (CAA) which accredits speech language pathologist programs and acts a component of the ASHA. The number of educational programs in speech language pathology has grown and currently there are 240 or more master's degree programs in communication sciences and disorders in the United States that are accredited by the CAA. There has been no move among speech language pathologists to adopt a required entry-level doctoral degree. However, this has happened in the companion profession of audiology, where the doctor of audiology degree (AuD) has become the most desirable graduate degree for qualification as an audiologist. Many speech language pathologists have attended graduate school and earned degrees at the doctoral level (primarily PhD or EdD).

As in other health professions, a move occurred toward specialization within speech language pathology and the ASHA set up a mechanism for recognizing various specialties. Speech language pathologists work in a wide variety of settings, from school systems to long-term rehabilitation settings to private practices, and in all environments teamwork with other health care professionals is an important aspect of their work. Speech language pathologists are also involved in home health care, which has been a growing area for all the professions discussed in this chapter.

Speech language pathologists believe there is a bright future for their field despite the temporary decrease in services, particularly financing services, when the Medicare administration enacted the prospective payment system and created competition between physical therapists, occupational therapists, and speech language pathologists for funds for treatment of individual patients. This problem at present has been rectified, however, as all three professions continue to be concerned about financing health care for individuals who need their services, particularly when an aging population requires increased services from these three professions.

## HOW TEAMS WORK TOGETHER

The case study presented earlier and the description of the professions in this chapter have emphasized the importance of teamwork, not only between these professions but with other health professions in the rehabilitative and restorative care of individuals. All three professions are not only comfortable with and used to the idea of teamwork, they understand the importance of teamwork in rehabilitating individuals with serious disabilities. It is obvious that in today's health care environment, where patients have complex problems requiring complex answers, no one health profession can provide all the answers for the care of one patient. The concept of teamwork crosses all boundaries in health care and the three groups discussed in this chapter are examples of how important teamwork is for long-term care and rehabilitation and restoration of individuals with disabilities.

All three professions have had relatively similar development, albeit from different backgrounds. The trends in development for these three professions have been to accredit educational programs to set minimum standards for education and gradually advance these standards to graduate level, and to use entry-level clinical doctoral degrees as a continuing way for these particular professions to develop. As the responsibilities of these professions have increased, the length of time needed to educate a person to function in these professions has also increased. This growth in many ways is equivalent to existing clinical doctoral programs and, therefore, it is not surprising there has been a trend in this direction. The continued well-being of these programs will continue to depend on teamwork with other health professionals and attention to the quality of educational programs.

All three of these professions have worked together at the level of their professional associations in addressing inequities in care of patients who need their services and this alliance will continue to strengthen as the population ages and the demand for services increases.

## THE ROLE OF RESEARCH

Based on the publications and activities of professional associations, it is clear that research is emphasized in physical therapy, occupational therapy, and speech language pathology. The primary purpose for individuals entering these professions, however, is not to be researchers but to be clinical practitioners. Even so, as their education has expanded and improved, these clinical practitioners are all exposed to current research methodology and therefore, with the appropriate assistance of academic institutions and sophisticated help from their professional organizations, they are expanding their roles in research in important ways. As payers have insisted that interventions provided by health care professionals show some possibility for success, the demands by clinical practitioners to provide evidence for this success has increased. Also, the notion of evidence-based practice for health care professionals has pushed the research envelope so much that evidence must not only be provided, but must be available to clinical practitioners so they can make the best judgments about the interventions they can provide to patients and clients. The role of research will become increasingly important and the role of collaboration in research across health disciplines, as an example of teamwork, will also become an important part of future research efforts.

## BIBLIOGRAPHY

Dikengil, A.T. (1998). *Handbook of Home Health Care for the Speech-Language Pathologist.* San Diego, CA: Singular.

Ghikas, P.A. and Clopper, M. (2001). *Case Studies in Rehabilitation.* Thorofare, NJ: Slack.

Hagedorn, R. (1995). *Occupational Therapy: Perspectives and Processes.* Edinburgh: Churchill Livingstone.

Kielhofner, G. (1997). *Conceptual Foundations of Occupational Therapy,* Second Edition. Philadelphia: F.A. Davis.

Lubinski, R. and Fratalli, C. (2001). *Professional Issues in Speech-Language Pathology and Audiology,* Second Edition. San Diego, CA: Singular.

Pagliarulo, M.A. (2001). *Introduction to Physical Therapy,* Second Edition. St. Louis, MO: Mosby.

Sabonis-Chafee, B. and Hussey, S.M. (1998). *Introduction to Occupational Therapy,* Second Edition. St. Louis, MO: Mosby.

Scott, R. (2002). *Foundations of Physical Therapy.* New York: McGraw-Hill.

Silverman, F.H. (1995). *Speech Language and Hearing Disorders.* Boston: Allyn & Bacon.

Silverman, F.H. (1999). *Professional Issues in Speech-Language Pathology and Audiology.* Boston: Allyn & Bacon.

Sladyk, K. and Ryan, S. (2001). *Ryan's Occupational Therapy Assistant.* Thorofare, NJ: Slack.

Stanfield, P.S. (1995). *Introduction to the Health Professions,* Second Edition. Boston: Jones and Bartlett.

Van Riper, C. and Erickson, R.L. (1996). *Speech Connection: An Introduction to Speech Pathology and Audiology,* Ninth Edition. Boston: Allyn & Bacon.

Chapter 5

# Health Care Management

## Joan M. Kiel

Dan Arkman answers the telephone, listens for a full two and one-half minutes, and then says, "I'll get back to you." It is 4:15 p.m. and another late night is setting in. On the telephone was the hospital board chairman for Davick Hospital in Michey, California. She is concerned about the recent merger of three area hospitals and their announced plans to expand services and market share, and to aggressively recruit physicians. At the next board meeting, she wants Dan to present some response to the board to quell her fears and perhaps those of other board members. Dan immediately tells his assistant to clear his calendar for tomorrow. He needs a day or two to utilize his health care management skills in planning, organizing, controlling, and decision making.

### *HEALTH MANAGEMENT DEFINED*

The health care industry is ever changing and volatile. It is an industry that seemingly includes every person in its customer base and operates twenty-four hours a day, seven days a week. Given such daunting responsibility, it is no wonder that health care managers have a challenging, yet interesting job. Management is a process that through the delegation (decision making) and supervision (organizing) of work to others achieves organizational goals effectively, efficiently (control), and with high quality while considering internal and external factors (planning), and the organization's mission. Planning, organizing, controlling, and decision making are the four functions of management that will be elaborated in this chapter.

Managing is many times used synonymously with leading. Peter Drucker defines three tasks of managing:

- To set and act upon the purpose and mission of the organization.
- To make the work productive and the worker achieving.
- To manage the organization's social impacts and social responsibilities.[1]

Rosabeth Moss Kanter generalizes the three tasks by saying that all managers have two jobs, "handling today's issues and getting ready for the future."[2]

Although they are not health care managers, both Drucker and Kanter describe the role of the health care manager. Missions lead organizations and this has been demonstrated in religious-based health care organizations. In turbulent times of mergers, many faith-based organizations have put their mission ahead of money and remained solo or partnered with other faith-based organizations. Bottom-lines are constantly being squeezed by reimbursement; thus, workers are being cross-trained and retrained to meet the new skills of today. Health care organizations are intimately tied to society's impacts and responsibilities. The health care manager's role includes a multitude of tasks done for today and tomorrow.

## *The Importance of Health Management*

The health care industry is a trillion-dollar, double-digit gross domestic product (GDP) industry. It touches the life of every person and is a truly personal and emotional industry. The Health Care Financing Administration (HCFA) projects that national health expenditures will reach $2.2 trillion and 16.2 percent of the GDP by 2008.[3] Comprised of hospitals, outpatient facilities, mobile units, allied health workers, doctors, and researchers, the health care industry is ever growing and ever challenged. New therapies, technologies, and regulations drive the health care industry. Daily, rather than minute by minute, changes are the norm.

The need for keen health care management is paramount as changes abound in the industry. Technology is being added to improve telecommunications and real-time information retrieval. Mergers, affiliations, and buyouts are being tested in every region. Regulations from the Joint Commission on the Accreditation of Healthcare Organizations (JCAHO) to the Healthcare Insurance Portability and Accountability Act (HIPAA) are challenging managers to work in different ways. Consumers are getting more involved in their own health care, much of which is driven by the Internet. Costs, both individual and societal, must be controlled. While controlling costs, the format of the delivery network must be established. Should mergers and acquisitions continue, or should physicians return to solo practices? Should specialty hospitals be the norm, or should hospitals build continuums of care? The answer must satisfy not only the cost issue, but also the access to care issue. Resources must be allocated so that everyone can have access to care. The importance of health management is escalating in light of the various issues that managers face.

## *Who Delivers Health Management?*

Health care management can be referred to as the "three-legged stool of management." Health care institutions are managed by three prominent groups: health care executives (such as allied health practitioners who have taken management positions), physicians, and board of trustee members.

The Public Health Service Act defines an allied health professional as someone who has received a certificate, associate's degree, bachelor's degree, master's degree, doctoral level preparation, or postbaccalaureate training in a science related to health care and has responsibility for the delivery of health or health-related services.[4] Allied health care personnel have specialized training on a particular body system and thus work in conjunction with physicians and other health care providers to deliver care. Their job titles include therapist, technician or technologist, or practitioner (see Table 5.1).

Allied health workers are skilled in the clinical aspects of their discipline. With advanced training, such as a master's degree, clinicians are moving into the administrative ranks. The Commission on Accreditation of Allied Health Education Programs is the accrediting body for programs in the allied health profession. With this accreditation, graduates can sit for certifying examina-

TABLE 5.1. 1999 National Occupational Employment Statistics

| Occupation Title | Number Employed |
|---|---|
| Dieticians and Nutritionists | 41,320 |
| Audiologists | 12,950 |
| Occupational Therapists | 78,950 |
| Physical Therapists | 131,050 |
| Radiation Therapists | 12,340 |
| Respiratory Therapists | 80,230 |
| Speech Language Pathologists | 85,920 |
| Medical/Clinical Laboratory Technologists | 145,750 |
| Medical/Clinical Laboratory Technicians | 142,090 |
| Dental Hygienists | 90,050 |
| Nuclear Medicine Technologists | 17,880 |
| Medical Records and Health Information Technicians | 142,720 |
| Athletic Trainers | 16,670 |
| Physician Assistants | 56,750 |

*Source:* Bureau of Health Professions (2001). *Bureau of Health Professions Occupational Employment Statistics.* Washington, DC: Bureau of Health Professions.

tions. Specifically, the Association of University Programs in Health Administration (AUPHA) accredits eighty-one programs nationally and others exist beyond those accredited in health administration.[5] Health administration or health management curricula focus on the functions of management—planning, organizing, controlling, and decision making—with such courses as:

- Strategic Planning
- Human Resources Management
- Operations Management
- Organizational Management

In addition, many programs allow a student to specialize in an area such as finance or information technology with such courses as:

- Financial Management
- Cost Accounting
- Budgeting Techniques
- Insurance and Reimbursement
- Systems Analysis and Design
- Database Management
- Health Care Information Systems
- Networking and Telecommunications

Allied health educational programs teach both the theory and the practice of their respective professions and many times students have an opportunity to complete an internship with an organization under the guidance of both an organizational mentor and a faculty mentor. These internships provide valuable experiences to students, who can receive feedback and develop a greater understanding of health care management in a supportive setting. Students are also learning the latest concepts and technologies and can truly contribute to the organization.

Physicians are the second leg of the three-legged stool. With new opportunities in health care management, some physicians are opting for positions in managed care organizations, utilization review, or legal and regulatory affairs. Physicians can receive additional management training from the American College of Physicians Executives. In addition, many physicians enroll in masters in business administration (MBA) programs or masters in health management systems (MHMS) programs.

Boards of Trustees are the third leg of the three-legged stool. Trustees are community members with a special skill or affiliation who act on behalf of health organization's mission. They come from many backgrounds, some from outside health care, including information technology, law, finance, and business development. Board members act as a unit in shaping the future of an institution.

The three-legged stool can only remain standing if each leg is sturdy. Given this model, one must understand the outlook of each leg or group. Allied health care executives want to provide quality care while preserving the bottom line of an institution. They also want to forge ahead and enhance the institution's market share. Physicians want to provide quality patient care. Board members want to maintain close community relations and enhance the mission of the institution. Sometimes the goals of each group seem at odds with each other, although they are all aligning with the overall goal of providing quality patient care. It is in those times that the future focus emanates the strongest. The future calls for an interdisciplinary approach to health care delivery. This will mean more opportunities for allied health professionals as each discipline will be represented "at the table."

## HEALTH CARE MANAGEMENT ORGANIZATIONAL STRUCTURE

The three-legged stool represents the major players in health care management, but what guides their work activity is the structure of the organization. The health care management organizational structure is the formal arrangement of workers, work groups, departments, and divisions, as well as the tasks, roles, responsibilities, reporting relationships, lines of authority, and communication channels of the workers. The organizational structure is routinely depicted by an organizational chart. This organizational chart is based on the type of departmentalization or segmentation that the organization chooses. The four types of departmentalization are:

- Functional
- Product
- Geographical
- Process

Functional departmentalization organizes a structure according to specific department functions or duties. For example, a hospital is organized into medical, surgical, purchasing, admitting, and other departments.

Product departmentalization organizes a structure according to related services or products. For example, a hospital or health care system may offer long-term care services. Within the product line of long-term care, the structure may include assisted living, personal care, nursing home care, and hospice care. Each of these support the main product line.

Geographical departmentalization organizes a structure by location of the task or personnel. This is critical for health care as health systems merge and expand to outlying areas and physicians develop offices in all four geographic locations of the United States.

Process departmentalization organizes a structure by the complete line of tasks involved to meet a goal or produce a product. Think of it as an assembly line with several different tasks involved in producing a product. In the health care environment one can think of inpatient or outpatient processes and the specific tasks that are integrated into those processes.[6]

In the organization's structure and germane to health care is the role of the physician. The physician-hospital relationship can take on many different arrangements, each creating a new structure. Physicians can be salaried employees of the hospital and thus receive benefits and abide by the policies and procedures of their employer. Physicians may be involved in the managed care structure known as a physician hospital organization (PHO). Here physicians and hospitals have an arrangement whereby physicians utilize hospital services and in turn hospitals include physicians in managed care contract negotiations. Physicians may also be on hospital staff and thus admit patients without compensation from the institution. The loosest arrangement, but one gaining in popularity, is where physicians moonlight for hospitals as their schedule permits.

Organizations have five parts that make up their structure:

- Strategic Apex
- Middle Line
- Operating Core
- Technostructure
- Support Staff

The strategic apex is the administrative personnel who have accountability and responsibility for the entire organization. These personnel are few in number, yet they are responsible for planning, organizing, making decisions, and controlling, the four functions of management. Much of their time is spent defining and guiding the organization toward its mission goals, and assessing the strategic nature of the institution. They will network with external constituents and constantly reinvent their organization to stay in touch with changing times. The strategic apex manages the upper-middle line of personnel, those who fall directly below them. Strategic apex job titles that allied health students can aspire to include chief executive officer (CEO), hospital administrator, chief operating officer (COO), and vice president.

The middle line serves as liaison for the organization. Situated between the strategic apex and the operating core, the middle line communicates information throughout the organization and manages those in the operating core who produce and deliver products and services. The middle line confers with the strategic apex to operationalize strategic plans. The middle line also acts as head of their own department, thus performing the four functions of management on a departmental level. Middle line titles that allied health students can aspire to include director, manager, and administrative supervisor.

The operating core includes personnel who produce and deliver products and services. They are on the front line interacting with customers on a daily basis. It is their responsibility to ensure customer satisfaction is maintained. The operating core consists of physical therapists, occupational therapists, nutritionists, and all other allied health patient care deliverers.

The technostructure is responsible for standardizing the work of the organization. Technostructure personnel include trainers, analysts, and consultants. They can be internal or external to the organization and work with all of the other parts of the organization. Technostructure personnel will be found wherever there is a need to have a process examined and standardized. Health care entities are subject to numerous regulations and it is the technostructure's responsibility to help ensure compliance with JCAHO and HIPAA.

The support staff works with all levels of the organization in assisting with work necessary to carry out the mission of the organization. Support staffs act as buffers to ensure that other parts of the organization can concentrate on the core mission and values targeted by the strategic plan.[7]

Health care organizations integrate the five parts of an organization into an organizational structure. The structure of a health care organization is best defined as a professional bureaucracy. In examining this term, professional indicates the credentialed members who work in the organization. In health care, professionalism is an important concept since allied health personnel, doctors, and nurses, etc., must hold licenses and registrations from professional accrediting bodies. Bureaucracy indicates the standardized tasks that are completed to deliver a product or service. Here again bureaucracy is critical for health care. Protocols and clinical pathways are standardized frameworks for delivering care. Joint Commission on Accreditation of Health Care Organizations (JCAHO) and state departments of health regulations assess whether standards are in place to deliver quality care. Personnel hired by the institution may have trained at multiple facilities and schools, but their skills are transferable and they are guided by the standards and policies of their new institution.

Looking at an example of a hospital, one can integrate the five parts of the organization with the professional bureaucracy structure. The strategic apex is the hospital's administrators. This level usually includes the chief executive officer, chief operating officer, chief financial officer, medical director, and various vice presidents. The apex develops the mission and strategy for the hospital. The middle line is comprised of departmental managers. It is here that allied health practitioners make an entry into management ranks. For example, an occupational therapist with the most seniority becomes the departmental manager. Challenges can abound at this level as clinicians move into management. Although they may know their role as clinician extremely well, they must now acquire knowledge on planning, organizing, decision making, and controlling. Many practitioners return to school for advanced training and find fulfilling careers in the middle line. The operating core is comprised of credentialed personnel such as physicians, nurses, and allied health personnel. At this level, location of one on the structure does not equate to salary, but rather the task or responsibility one has. Operating core personnel follow their own professional standards in addition to institutional policies when delivering their care. The technostructure is a critical level of hospital organization since standards must be maintained at all times. Medical records, information technology, human resources, billing, etc., are all examples of departments that standardize work processes in hospitals. Managed care organizations and the government are calling for further standardization in terms of medical errors, privacy of medical records, and managed care negotiations, thus the work of the technostructure will likely increase. Support staff are critical in a health care organization in terms of both cost benefit and productivity. Higher paid credentialed workers are assisted by lower paid support staff so the workload can be maximized. For example, if a physical therapist has to get a wheelchair, go to the patient's room, escort the patient to the physical therapy department, and then administer treatment, excessive time is taken. Production is enhanced by having the physical therapist remain in the department and continue to work with patients while support staff wheel the next patient to the therapy session. Thus integrating the five parts of an organization into the organizational structure provides the framework for managing a health care entity.

## HEALTH CARE MANAGEMENT FUNCTIONS

In his seminal article, "The Manager's Job: Folklore and Fact," Henry Mintzberg noted that managers do a variety of tasks at a fast pace, with many tasks occurring simultaneously or disjointedly as one task interrupts the other and then is completed later on.[8] All the duties, tasks, and responsibilities that managers encounter on a daily basis can be cumulatively accounted for by the four functions of management—planning, organizing, controlling, and decision making.

## *Planning*

To Do List:

- Meet with community group to determine need for day care.
- Keep posted on union negotiations at neighboring hospital.
- Call health science school to assess number of allied health graduates available for hire.

The health care industry is the second most regulated industry after nuclear power. To contend with these numerous regulations, health care managers must be adept at planning. Planning is defined as decreasing the gap from where an entity desires to be and where the entity presently is at. Planning involves determining one's goals, objectives, mission, and strategy.[9] Managers must try to anticipate the future and then align organizational resources to respond to the future. Peter Drucker defines planning as "determining the futurity of present decisions."[10] Here, everything a manager does in the present will have an impact on the future. Managers must act with reason and rationale based on the direction their organization desires to take.

Planning is often used simultaneously with strategic planning. We will discuss strategic planning in depth, but operational planning must also be considered. Operational planning is the day-to-day decision making that guides the tasks of workers. Operational planning encompasses a short time frame, generally less than six months. Health care managers are constantly involved in operational planning. Examples include staff schedules, physical therapy treatment room schedules, budgeting for occupational therapy resources, the manager's daily meeting schedule, and patient schedules. Operational planning occurs simultaneously with strategic planning and is predominantly done by the middle line.

Strategic planning is a systematic process that addresses the overall direction of the institution. It has a two- to three-year time frame, but given the volatility of the health care industry, some organizations plan for one to one and one-half years. More stable industries can plan for longer periods of time, but five years is usually the maximum. Strategic planning is conducted by the strategic apex with input from the middle line.

*The Six Steps of the Strategic Planning Process*

Strategic planning is a process, thus managers can follow six steps to achieve their goals:

1. Complete an external analysis
2. Complete an internal analysis
3. Complete an issues analysis
4. Determine options
5. Create or recreate the mission statement
6. Write a business or operational plan

These steps are formatted into the "Y Diagram" (see Figure 5.1) and will be discussed as follows.

*External Analysis:* External analysis is an ongoing assessment of factors outside of the organization, i.e., determining the impact or future impact of these forces on the organization. External analysis consists of seven subcategories—demographics, economy, laws and regulations, personnel, competition, needs, and trends. From these seven subcategories, health care managers collect and analyze data. The key is to ask relevant, piercing questions when gathering the data.

*Demographics:* Demographics are population characteristics of the organization's market and potential market. Managers must gather information from census statistics and surveys on age, education, sex, income, marital status, and children.

*Economy:* Managers need to ask if the external environment (e.g., their geographic area) is in an inflationary or recessionary period. What are the interest rates? Is this a viable time for building or expanding?

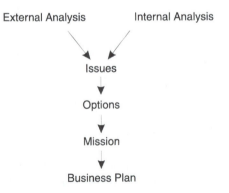

FIGURE 5.1. Y Diagram of the Strategic Planning Process

*Laws and regulations:* As previously mentioned, health care is a highly regulated industry. Health care institutions must not only be aware of regulations, but must also take measures to influence present regulations and create future regulations. Managers must be constantly aware of how laws affect their institutions. For example, if the federal government mandates health insurance coverage for all workers, how would that affect care access and delivery?

*Personnel:* Personnel will also be discussed in the internal analysis, thus there are two different approaches to personnel. In external analysis, health care managers ask broader questions such as: Can unions affect our organization? What is the unemployment rate? Are there shortages in the field or are people available for hire?

*Competition:* Competition focuses on others who offer the same or similar product. Managers want to increase market share by offering unique services within a specified service area. Using maps or zip code analysis, managers plot where other organizations are located that produce the same product. If a competitor offers a different product or service, managers should determine if their organization can replicate it, depending on market conditions. Of course, one could also produce the same product but do it with much higher quality. Managers must also try to assess the market and financial positions of their competitors to determine if they can expand or venture into new areas.

*Consumer needs:* Health care consumers are often asked to complete surveys on their needs and satisfaction with care services. Some data are required for JCAHO accreditation and other data are used to plan services. In looking at consumer needs, managers need to assess their clients' preferences, what they can afford, when they can utilize services, and what their greatest needs are.

*Trends:* Trends are a broader category of needs. Trends assess consumer lifestyle and cultural factors. For example, how does the surge of technology affect a person's life and living patterns? How can health care organizations incorporate that and other trends into their service delivery?

Using external analysis, managers can better understand the forces acting on their organization.

*Internal Analysis:* Internal analysis looks only at the manager's own organization. It is comprised of six categories—utilization (or sales), facility assets, finances, personnel, organizational structure, and tax entity.

*Utilization:* Health care managers must collect and analyze data on the utilization of services they offer. How busy is the organization? Are certain services not being used? Are they losing money or taking up valuable resources such as space? After the data are collected, trends must be analyzed. Are there hourly, daily, or seasonal trends that can help a manager plan staffing patterns? Are there any loss leaders, i.e., services that lose money, but point consumers to other services? For example, the hospital day care center may not be profitable, but when a child is sick, they are referred to a hospital pediatrician.

*Facility assets:* Health care organizations need to understand and justify all of their capital goods. What does the health care organization own in terms of buildings and key equipment? What are its capital investments and resources? These give an indication of the financial health and where growth can occur. For example, if a hospital owns ten acres of adjacent land, room is available for future expansion.

*Finances:* Finances represent the organization's budget. Managers must be knowledgeable of the revenues and expenses of the entire institution and each department. Are certain areas not profitable? Are they managed by the same person? An institution's loans and debts must also be assessed to determine the financial health of the organization.

*Organizational structure:* This is where the organizational chart is assessed. How does work flow? What are the communication patterns? Are there too many or too few layers? Managers must assess the organizational structure to ensure that work is completed effectively and efficiently.

*Personnel:* As mentioned earlier, personnel is evaluated both externally and internally. Here though, the manager takes a more finite picture. Organizations complete a personnel inventory which tracks their personnel resources. Who works in the organization by job title, tenure, and skills? Are they cross-trained or specialized? Who is promotable? How effective is the organization at recruitment and retention? By looking at personnel assets, the manager can determine organizational needs.

*Tax entity:* Organizations are affected by type as categorized by the tax code. Is the entity a for-profit, not-for-profit, or private company? The answer will have implications for finance and management.

*Issues*

The collection of information from internal and external analyses is continuous. However, at some point the health care manager must collate the data and make sense of it. What do the data indicate? What conclusions can be drawn? This takes place in the issues analysis phase. As Figure 5.1 shows, external and internal analyses lead into issues analysis. Thus, issues analysis is a series of broad statements of the major points, both positive and negative, from the two analyses. For example, if external analysis determines the hospital has two competing hospitals within a ten-mile radius, this becomes a major negative issue. However, if the hospitals are fifty miles apart and offer different services, competition would not be an issue (or one could say it is a positive issue of no competition). Not all issues are either positive or negative since some cannot be affected by the health care manager. For example, personnel would not be an issue in areas where union presence was low and managers had good rapport with workers. Managers define issues and then prioritize those that need direct attention. Managers will brainstorm with their colleagues and the organization's board to reach a consensus on issues.

## Options

Options are taken directly from the issues. Now that managers have some direction on priorities, they must determine different scenarios or options for addressing each issue. Here the organization must determine the feasible choices, i.e., a realistic plan for the organization. Managers again brainstorm and analyze data to determine the best and worst-case scenarios. For each issue, managers list three to four options. For example, if the issue is strong competition from nearby hospitals, some viable options are:

- The hospitals could merge.
- The hospital could shut down similar services.
- The hospital may look into recruiting a physician champion.

Notice that the options are written as choices, not as goals. Options are just that, choices that will be further explored in the business plan, which will be discussed later.

## Mission

Mission is the defining purpose of an organization. Many managers begin planning by writing a mission statement and then rewriting it as data are collected. Other managers collect data first and then write. This author recommends combining the two philosophies: Begin with an idea of the desired mission, then collect data, and finally compose a formal mission statement. A mission statement has an aura of fluidity and should be assessed every six months or less if major changes occur in the environment. When managers write a mission statement, they must consider the following elements:

- What does the organization do? Here the manager can view sales and utilization data.
- What does the organization have the resources to do? The manager can assess the facility assets, finances, and personnel data.

- What are the needs and preferences of the target audience? The manager can examine the consumer needs and trends data.

The mission statement should give readers clear indication of how an institution operates and what its values are.

*Business Plan*

The business plan is the last step of the strategic planning process. In retrospect, however, strategic planning is a process; thus, the cycle is always revolving. When writing a business plan, the internal and external analyses may change, or the mission may redirect the business plan. The business plan or operational plan, is a document of stated goals, objectives, and means to meet these goals based on the previous five steps of data.

The business plan has five parts—goals, objectives, actions, time frames, and personnel. The goal is the broad, overall statement of activity, e.g., deliver inpatient care. The objective is based on the goal, but is more specified and follows three rules: it must be quantifiable, include a time frame, and identify the responsible party. For example, to turn the goal of delivering inpatient care into an objective, a manager could write, "deliver inpatient care with an average monthly census of 80 percent by all of the medical and surgical units." Using the goal and objective, the manager must specify how they will achieve them by outlining the actions, time frame, and person responsible. The actions are detailed statements on how objectives will be met. The time frame specifies the deadline. The person responsible is singular and shows who is accountable. If more than one person is listed, finger pointing may occur.

Using the goal and objective example as provided earlier, a sample business plan looks as follows:

**Goal:** Deliver inpatient care
**Objective:** Deliver inpatient care with an average monthly census of 80 percent by all of the medical and surgical units.

| Actions | Time Frame | Person |
|---|---|---|
| Recruit physician champion | December 1, 2002 | Medical Director |
| Advertise hospital services | Fall, 2002 | Marketing Director |
| Benchmark services | January 1, 2003 | QA Supervisor |
| Assess patient satisfaction data | Ongoing | Marketing Analyst |

The business plan is based on the data previously collected and also contributes new data and information to the ongoing strategic planning process. This rejuvenation keeps managers and health care organizations on the cutting edge.

## *Organizing*

To Do List:

- Set up education sessions for cross-training clerical staff.
- Realign respiratory therapy department.
- Hire second director of physical therapy and divide workers into two divisions.

The second management function is organizing. Organizing is the process by which resources, mainly personnel, are positioned to achieve the goals and objectives of an organization. Health care managers must assess their personnel, their roles and responsibilities, inputs and outputs to the work, and how best the work can be accomplished.

When organizing, the manager decides the most efficient and effective way to position resources. To do this, one must consider four management principles, i.e., the principles of organizing:

- Specialization of work
- Unity of command
- Manager's span of control
- Structure: centralization or decentralization

Specialization of work or the division of labor refers to how work is divided among employees. Are workers doing one task (specialized) or multiple tasks (generalized)? Health care organizations are inherently specialized due to personnel licensure and certification. The highly regulated health care industry dictates what employees can and cannot do. For example, registered nurses can administrator intravenous medication, but licensed practical nurses cannot. Physicians are board certified in various fields and care only for patients within their particular field.

Managers not only need to look at the processes for completing a job, but also the people completing it. What are their preferences? Some employees prefer to be specialized because they can then become experts at a certain task and feel good about their contributions to the end product. Others prefer to be generalized because they believe doing a variety of jobs can help dispel boredom. In small organizations, generalists can do multiple tasks, which saves money and allows work flow to be more efficient. When specialists are out or busy with another task, no one can take their place and the work then waits. This can lead to frustrated customers. The last benefit of having generalists is that they see the entire organization and the process of their work. For example, when an emergency room nurse treats a patient and then transfers the patient to an inpatient unit, they rarely hear of the outcome. But if the institution had a rotating group of nurses, there would be opportunities to follow-up on patients.

Unity of command is where each employee reports to one manager. In the organizational structure, an employee should have only one boss to prevent any confusion when prioritizing tasks. This does not always happen in health care since physicians have various relationships with hospitals and hospital staff serve both physicians and the other hospital personnel. Support staff also work with multiple personnel and sometimes multiple departments.

Span of control refers to the number of people a manager is in charge of, i.e., a downward reporting structure. As previously explained in the section on organizational structure, managers in the strategic apex have a smaller span due to their other responsibilities. Theorists have not found an optimal number, but four factors can guide how large or how small a group should be. The first two factors depend on the manager's and worker's experience and knowledge of the job. With a more knowledgeable manager and staff, the span size can be larger as each person is attuned to his or her job. But with people just fresh from orientation or school, more nurturing is needed and thus managers need to have smaller spans to ensure individualized attention. The third factor is the type of work. Consider an intensive care unit with highly technical, changing work. Here the span size must be small as the unit's complexity demands more attention. With routine work, the span size can be larger, but not so large that the managers cannot pay close attention to their workers and prevent boredom from setting in and production from dropping. Last, and increasingly important today, is the use of technology to communicate with workers. If workers can be connected electronically, managers can have a higher span since meetings do not have to take place in person and work can be done virtually twenty-four hours a day.

Span of control is directly related to structure—whether it be centralized or decentralized. Centralization occurs when authority and control are at the top of the organization. This resembles a bureaucratic organization wherein managers are watchful of employees. The structural diagram for a centralized organization is tall with multiple layers, thus indicating a low span of control.

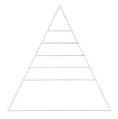

Information flows downward with little input from the middle line or operating core. In health care, centralization is used in highly structured departments such as information systems, intensive care units, and finance.

Decentralization occurs when authority and control are delegated or distributed throughout the organization. The manager is ultimately accountable, but employees are encouraged to contribute and be a part of the process. The organization is a flatter structure with few layers; thus indicating larger spans of control.

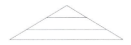

Decentralized structures are used in departments where employee participation is critical to the process and where the organization's mission encourages employee development. It is also used when managers and workers are experienced and do not need a centralized framework. Each manager has responsibility for setting the tone of the organization. The key is to work efficiently and effectively, and the four factors of organizing will become a natural part of managing.

### *Controlling*

To Do List:

- Assess medical supply vendor contract.
- Complete therapy room utilization report.
- Continue to collect outcomes benchmark data.

The third management function is controlling which is also known as measurement science, benchmarking, and quality management. Controlling is the evaluation process whereby an organization compares its actual output or performance against set goals, standards, or benchmarks. In the health care environment, control is a key function because evidence of quality outcomes must be demonstrated for reimbursement in many cases. Accreditation standards from the JCAHO and state agencies also mandate evaluation methods.

The control process has three steps:

1. Determine the goal or standard.
2. Assess performance.
3. Correct any deviation, both positive and negative.

In the first step, the health care manager utilizes the goals established during the strategic planning process to determine the priorities of the organization. The goals or standards must be written quantitatively so positive performance can be differentiated from negative performance. For example, the standard can be written as "the nutrition department will complete 80 percent of all patient dietary assessments within twenty-four hours of admission." Thus 80 percent is the standard and it is that number which determines good performance.

In the second step, the performance is measured. This is a continuous process since managers must be attuned to the performance of their workers. This is where managers assess output in terms of both quality and quantity. Managers should also assess how work is being done, i.e., the process. Quality of work can be high as well as the quantity, but are the workers satisfied? Are safety standards being met? Are processes up to date? For example, are nutrition personnel interrupting other patient care procedures in order to complete their dietary assessments?

In the third step, performance output is compared to the standard and any differences are noted. Differences or deviations can either be positive or negative. A positive deviation occurs when a standard is met, but the goal may have been set too low. A negative deviation occurs when the goal is not met, whether it be for a legitimate reason or not. For example, nutrition staff could have achieved 70 percent because of a lack of staff training or because patients were not in their rooms because of emergency procedures. In correcting the deviation, managers can return to step one and establish the next goal. In the event that staff were not trained, the next benchmark could be established as "95 percent of nutrition staff who conduct dietary assessments will be trained within three weeks of their hire date." Thus the control process continues.

In order to make the control process more effective, control must be simple, relevant, timely, and cost effective.[11] Managers and personnel must be able to understand and apply controls or standards, thus simplicity is key. In health care, this is very important because the field utilizes many abbreviations and medical terms that may not be universally defined. Controls must be relevant and based on current data. Questionable standards should not be set, but rather the best measure based on data should be established. Controls must be preventive or timely, especially in health care where quality and safety are paramount. Last, controls must also be cost effective to a point. In health care, as previously stated, safety and quality are paramount, but cost must still be considered. Additional frontal cost will negate back-end cost such as litigation or additional medical care. It is the manager's role to analyze controls and ensure they meet these criteria. In addition, the manager must educate the staff on the standards.

During the control process, an organization will utilize quantitative methodologies or continuous improvement methods. This includes breakeven analysis, economic order quantity inventory systems, Pareto charts, Gantt charts, and PERT analysis. Breakeven analysis will be expounded here since it is a common instrument used at all levels of management.

Breakeven analysis determines the size an organization or operation should be to make or lose dollars or be at breakeven. It also measures what the level of production should be to not make or lose money. Health care managers utilize breakeven analysis for building projects, staffing, and profit analysis. The formula for the breakeven point *(BEP)* is:

$$BEP = \frac{FC}{P - VC}$$

Fixed costs *(FC)* are costs inherent to the organization and do not change with the size of the operation. For example, health care facilities must heat, air-condition, and light their buildings. If the emergency room has a low census one evening, they cannot turn off the heat. The same is true for a patient unit, regardless of patient occupancy.

Price *(P)* is the unit cost for product or service. Due to reimbursement, the true cost of health care is not always apparent, but per diem costs, capitation rates, or average costs based on diagnosis can be used. For products or services not covered by reimbursement, price reflects the selling price to the consumer.

Variable costs *(VC)* are costs that change or vary with the volume of services. Variable costs cover tangible items such as supplies. For example, more sheets will be used if there is an increase in inpatients. Thus, usage is associated with volume. The higher the volume, the higher the usage, the higher the variable costs.

The following is an example of breakeven analysis: Dr. Marone is assessing a lab culture testing device. Before she purchases it, she wants to be sure it will not negatively impact her finances. The cost of the device is $2,750.

The price for each drug culture to be tested is $1.50 and the variable costs, namely a test tube, swab, and slide are .30.

$$BEP = \frac{\$2,750}{\$1.50 - .30}$$

The breakeven point is 2,292 drug culture tests. (The dollar signs cancel each other out, leaving the answer in units.)

Dr. Marone must now determine if 2,292 tests are feasible for her practice. This breakeven point now becomes the standard for the first step of the control process. Dr. Marone must analyze the number by asking the following questions: What is her current volume? In what amount of time must she reach this amount? (One must consider the fact that technology and equipment are constantly being upgraded.) If she does not do this volume of tests, can she ask other doctors if they would be willing to pay a usage fee to reach the breakeven point? Can she negotiate to pay lower fixed and variable costs? Can she raise the price for tests and still be competitive?

Any volume above 2,292 tests brings in a profit and any volume below 2,292 tests results in a loss.

Those questions are the essence of the control process using breakeven analysis. Health care managers must ask tough questions while keeping quality care in mind. One would not want to buy less expensive supplies if they would not be of high quality. One must also consider wastage or spoilage. For example, if the hospital purchases low quality swabs that are prone to breakage, technicians might use more than one swab making it more expensive to complete the job. This is why it is critical for managers to be aware of the process as well as outcome.

### Decision Making

To Do List:

- Convene board of trustees and finalize budget.
- Allocate larger space for occupational therapy department.
- Give 3.5 percent merit raises.

Decision making is the fourth management function and is utilized with the previous three functions. Decision making is defined as choosing between competing alternatives. In order to make an effective decision, health care managers need both information and a supportive environment in which to implement the decision. Managers collate information from both internal and external sources. Certainly all of the data gathered in the planning process is ripe for the decision-making process. In addition, operational data collected from others within the organizational structure and one's own observations are key. Health care managers also need to create an environment that is supportive of open decision making. This is a challenge given the three-legged stool structure previously discussed, but the decision-making process presented in this section can help guide managers to success in nurturing an open environment.

Before going through the decision-making process, health care managers need to understand the intricacies and intangibles of decision making. When analyzing how people make decisions, health care managers are encouraged to do a cultural comparison between the Americans and Japanese, the latter's unique decision-making style is now being shared with Western managers.

Japanese and American managers differ in two vital decision-making areas—first, what a decision means to the managers in each country and second, how much time is involved in decision making. In America, managers often distribute agendas for meetings with specific topics for discussion and time frames. There is a protocol for this process and although there may be open discussion and brainstorming, there is also a sense of formality or structure. The meeting begins and ends at a specific time. A question raised at the end of the meeting, especially on a Friday afternoon, is not well received. This sense of agenda does not allow open discussion and thus limits the quality and quantity of information contributed to the decision-making process. Americans define decisions as "the end." Americans are quick to make decisions, encouraging people to take sides or else be labeled indecisive. Americans make a decision and the meeting is over.

On the other hand, the Japanese believe that a decision defines a question.[12] In Japan, managers encourage participants to ask further questions and enliven the discussion. The Japanese define a decision as the beginning and the process in which further questioning is welcomed. Managers are seen as creative and effective when they use multiple viewpoints to gain a greater understanding of the questions they must answer. No one is labeled indecisive.

The second difference between American and Japanese decision-making styles is the time involved in making decisions. There are two parts to making a decision. First is the discussion period when a decision is reached and second, the implementation period for the decision. In the United States, the discussion period is often hurried. Those who can be heard in the time allotted are given an opportunity to speak, while those who can't are bypassed. Also, the environment may dissuade people from contributing their ideas for fear of retribution, embarrassment, or banishment. Thus, the time involved in making decisions in the United States can be very controlled.

In Japan, workers are encouraged to speak without a clock in the room. Many times meetings go well into the evening with stimulating conversation welcomed. Everyone's views are heard and rebutted if necessary. This period of intense discussion and openness is necessary for the second part of decision making, implementing the decision.

In the United States, when a decision is made in the aforementioned fashion, everyone may not agree with or even want to state their disagreement. This makes implementation very difficult. For example, physicians who disagree with health care administrators on hospital admission policies may simply admit their patients to another facility and not bother to discuss with management the reasons why, or they may negotiate the decision with management. This process becomes time consuming when additional time is taken to discuss decisions or even revise them after they have been made.

In Japan, the intense up-front discussions negate the need for further negotiations when implementation takes place. Everyone's questions and concerns have already been answered, and everyone knows what others think of the decision. Thus, acceptance or implementation is literally automatic (see the following diagram for illustration).[13]

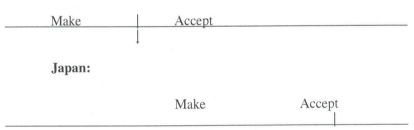

**United States:**

Make | Accept

**Japan:**

Make Accept

Not only is the total amount of time taken to make and implement decisions greater in the United States, but more important, the amount of effort expended is greater. Many times this effort falls on the shoulders of one health care manager. Certainly a great degree of effort and energy is involved in Japanese meetings, but it is spread amongst all participants. Thus, the Japanese system has been shown to take less time and energy, and have greater acceptance from all involved parties.

Health care managers must think about effective decisions and how to implement them. Effective decisions are made with the aforementioned issues in mind and follow a process that is both organized and dynamic enough to allow participation. The decision-making process follows four steps:

1. Identify the problem or issue.
2. Formulate alternatives.
3. Select and implement an alternative.
4. Evaluate the selected alternative.

When identifying the problem, health care managers must gather information to ensure their decision will be credible. In health care, the key is to benchmark or compare an institution with those that are similar. Managers can then accurately measure how their organization is performing. Managers must also look at trends and deviations to determine why something is occurring. Is it a natural phenomenon or something with a causative factor or factors? One key issue at this stage is to have everyone agree on what the problem or issue is.

Second, the manager must formulate alternatives. Here, in concert with others in the organization, brainstorming sessions and open meetings are held so everyone can share their ideas. The manager may have to set boundaries, such as budgetary restrictions, but if these are defined and rationalized at the start, they may be readily accepted. In fact, participants may even discover solutions to boundaries. Health care managers must also consider the risks to quality patient care if an alternative is implemented. Quantitatively, costs and benefits must be examined, especially in this era of tight reimbursement. As the second most heavily regulated industry, health care must consider what it can do under current laws. Given these factors to consider, an organization can develop a list of alternatives that would all be feasible solutions to the identified problem or issue.

The third step is to select and implement an alternative. Many times the selected alternative emerges during thorough analysis or others simply do not meet all of the standards. Sometimes, more than one alternative emerges, in which case managers must reanalyze the data and look to the organization's mission to assess which one fits best without doing harm. If no feasible alternative is found the manager must return to step one and collect further data.

Now that the alternative has been selected and implemented, its effects must be evaluated. Is the problem subsiding? Are participants comfortable with the decision? Managers can try another alternative if feedback is not positive. The key is to continue to collect pertinent data.

In health care, crises occur often, and managers will have to make decisions without the luxury of consultation. Effective health care managers rely on the four functions of management to help them do their job. Young managers sometimes find it inconceivable, but managers plan, organize, control, make decisions, and so much more as they lead their organizations in delivering quality health care.

## MEETING THE CHALLENGE

Dan Arkman is similar to every other health care manager. His fast-paced days include balancing a variety of tasks and the needs of both internal and external constituents. However, the responsibilities of the job are encapsulated in the institution's organizational structure and the manager's skills in planning, organizing, controlling, and decision making.

The four functions of management are pertpetually in motion. Managers use the planning process to set goals, objectives, and missions. To meet those objectives, managers must simultaneously organize and decide how to utilize resources. Once plans are underway and resources are being used, managers must evaluate their actions via the control process.

Managers who are transitioning from the clinical arena to the allied health management arena are bolstered by their clinical knowledge and the fact that they can speak the same language as those whom they will manage. Marry that with the four functions of management and they will be able to meet the challenge.

## NOTES

1. Drucker, Peter (1974). *Management Tasks, Responsibilities, Practices.* New York: Harper and Row Publishers, p. 40.

2. Kanter, Rosabeth Moss (1997). *On the Frontiers of Management.* Cambridge, MA: Harvard Business Review Book, p. 3.

3. Health Care Financing Administration (2000). *National Health Expenditures Projections: 1998-2008.* Washington, DC: HCFA, p. 1.

4. Shi, Leiyu and Singh, Douglas A. (1998). *Delivering Health Care in America: A Systems Approach.* Gaithersburg, MD: Aspen Publishers, p. 30.

5. Association of University Programs in Health Administration (n.d.). <http://www.aupha.org>.

6. Robbins, Stephen and Coulter, Mary (1999). *Management.* Upper Saddle River, NJ: Prentice-Hall Publishers, pp. 300-304.

7. Mintzberg, Henry (1979). *The Structuring of Organizations.* Englewood Cliffs, NJ: Prentice-Hall Publishers, p. 19.

8. Mintzberg, Henry (1975). "The Manager's Job: Folklore and Fact." *Harvard Business Review,* July-August, p. 51.

9. Robbins and Coulter, *Management,* p. 212.

10. Drucker, *Management Tasks,* p. 127.

11. Ibid., pp. 498-499.

12. Ibid., p. 467.

13. Ibid., pp. 467-468.

# BIBLIOGRAPHY

Association of University Programs in Health Administration (n.d.) <http://www. aupha.org>.

Bureau of Health Professions (2001). *Bureau of Health Professions Occupational Employment Statistics,* Washington, DC: Bureau of Health Professions.

Drucker, Peter (1974). *Management Tasks, Responsibilities, Practices.* New York: Harper and Row Publishers.

Health Care Financing Administration (2000). National Health Expenditures Projections: 1998-2008. Washington, DC: HCFA.

Kanter, Rosabeth Moss (1997). *On the Frontiers of Management.* Cambridge, MA: Harvard Business Review Book.

Mintzberg, Henry (1975). The Manager's Job: Folklore and Fact, *Harvard Business Review,* July-August, pp. 49-61.

Mintzberg, Henry (1979). *The Structuring of Organizations.* Englewood Cliffs, NJ: Prentice-Hall Publishers.

Robbins, Stephen and Coulter, Mary (1999). *Management.* Upper Saddle River, NJ: Prentice-Hall Publishers.

Shi, Leiyu and Singh, Douglas (1998). *Delivering Health Care in America: A System's Approach.* Gaithersburg, MD: Aspen Publishers.

## Chapter 6

# Chemical and Dietary Therapies

### Barbara F. Harland

## CASE STUDY OF TESTIMONIALS OF EFFICACY OF CERTAIN THERAPIES

Mrs. H., a thirty-eight-year-old single mother with three children, had a family history of breast cancer (her sister was currently being treated for it, and her mother, after a long struggle, died from its effects). Because Mrs. H. was now the sole support for her children, she felt a strong need to take good care of herself and would do anything to maintain her health. She breast-fed her children for a short time, believing that it was protective. She was aware of the controversy surrounding mammograms (some women had developed breast cancer even though their mammograms had been negative), so she avoided them. She had heard that selenium supplements were helpful, so she began taking two 100-microgram tablets a day. Mrs. H. also read that ginseng, garlic, and St. John's wort might be helpful, so she purchased bottles of these supplements and took one pill of each per day. Even though she was unemployed outside the home, in order not to become too stressed, she began taking afternoon naps to reduce her stress levels. As a result, she began to stay up late to watch TV, indulging in her favorite snacks beyond the eyes of her children. Mrs. H. believed there was enough mandatory physical activity around the house, so she seldom took walks or engaged in any exercise. She had discontinued service with her health management organization because she thought she was being overcharged.

Mrs. H. was close friends with the manager of a health food store who told her "everything she needed to know" about nutrition. She believed she was in good health except for her constant fatigue. However, she was sure she would feel better when her supplements kicked in.

It was time for an allied health professional to step in.

## COMPLEMENTARY AND ALTERNATIVE MEDICINE

Even though it has been more than twenty years since Doll and Peto (1981) declared that one-third of cancer deaths are related to diet, it remains unclear which dietary components are responsible. Consumers as well as scientists continue to search diligently for answers. In 1998, the federal government established the National Center for Complementary and Alternative Medicine to help in the search.

Use of complementary medicine in the United States has increased dramatically in recent years. More than 50 percent of the general public are trying alternative medicines. These two descriptive words (complementary and alternative) are used interchangeably and describe any medical practice or intervention that is not widely taught at U.S. medical schools or is not generally reimbursable by health insurance providers. However, more than seventy-five medical schools in the United States now offer courses in complementary medicine and some insurance providers support complementary medical therapy for the treatment of chronic diseases, possibly because it is usually lower in cost than traditional therapy (Lee and Georgiou, 2000). One of the most popular therapies concerns changes in diet, and the addition of nutritional supplements and herbal medicine, but such practices are considered sometimes risky by health care professionals because of possible unintended drug interactions and contamination. There may be only limited scientific evidence of the safety and efficacy for such products. Originally there were four acceptable reasons for trying alternative therapy: (1) maintenance of good health, (2) prevention of chronic illness, (3) treatment of chronic illness, and (4) treatment of acute illness.

However, the list of reasons has since mushroomed. Users are now seeking complementary medicines for cosmetic contributions to youthfulness, body building, and sexual enhancement. These desires have been part of the human psyche for thousands of years, but in our modern culture, products (both efficacious and harmful) are strongly advertised and readily available via the media, or Internet.

Currently, there are no standard, validated testing methods to analyze foods and beverages for the presence and concentration of most alternative therapeutic agents. With this new field of therapy, several new terms have emerged.

*Functional food* (Milner, 2000): a food that provides a physiological benefit in addition to its nutrient content and that may prevent disease and/or promote health (e.g., soybeans, garlic, oats, fish oil, broccoli, cranberry juice); *nutrient supplement:* a nutrient taken to supplement the diet for the purpose of enhancing health (e.g., calcium, vitamin C, vitamin E, folic acid, selenium); and *herb:* a plant with leaves, seeds, flowers, or roots used for enhancing health rather than as seasoning (e.g., echinacea, St. John's wort, ginseng, ginkgo).

Fabricated foods referred to previously contain bioactive compounds. From a manufacturer's standpoint, these are agents that are safe, easily measurable, nontoxic with no unpleasant side effects, and are preferably low cost, stable in the laboratory, and environmentally friendly to produce. They are chemical or genetic markers that are used as surrogates to identify risk factors for disease. For example, tissue and serum levels of n-3 and n-6 phospholipid fatty acids have been used as biomarkers to reflect dietary intake of fish (Greenwald, Milner, and Clifford, 2000).

In a consumer survey, the following benefits were sought by functional food users listed in descending order of desirability: energy enhancement, illness protection, heart benefits, anticancer benefits, relaxation, stomach soothing, mood enhancement, and sexual enhancement. "Functional foods, nutraceuticals, pharmafoods, and designer foods" are all marketing terms. So how should foods that go beyond basic nutrition to confer beneficial effects such as disease resistance be regulated? According to the Food and Drug Administration (FDA), the agency currently does not have the authority to regulate these new hybrid "functional" foods. The agency contends that it cannot act until Congress passes a bill charging the agency to take action. To date, Congress has not recognized that foods can have a therapeutic or restorative effect. A difficulty in assessing effectiveness of these agents is that how you feel is very subjective and is a reflection not only of what you have eaten or drunk but also your lifestyle, emotional state, and expectations. In addition, the current environment of managed health care has forced consumers to take more responsibility for their own health. They are misguidedly looking for a few creatively fabricated foods that will supply everything they need, such as an energy bar that advertises immediate relief. These instant fabricated foods supply increased energy, convenience, and portability, very important to the grazers among us who are always on the go and do not take time for an appropriate meal. For a functional food or a nutriceutical to be successful, it must meet four consumer demands: have a memorable and pleasant taste, be convenient, send a clear health message, and be reasonably priced.

Studies of the mechanisms of chemoprotection have focused on the biological activity of plant-based phenols and polyphenols: flavonoids, isoflavones, terpenes, and glucosinolates. Enhancing the phytonutrient content of plant foods through selective breeding or genetic improvement is a potent dietary option for disease prevention.

Although the primary function of food is to provide nutrients, its secondary function concerns sensory attributes such as taste and flavor. The tertiary function, said to be independent of the previous two, is to prevent disease. For the most part, plant-based phytochemicals are bitter and therefore aversive to the consumer. Sensitivity to bitter taste was an essential part of evolution and survival. These characteristics present additional challenges to fabricators of functional foods (Drewnowski and Gomez-Carneros, 2000).

## DIETARY SUPPLEMENTS

### Prebiotics and Probiotics: Are They Useful?

Prebiotics are nondigestible food ingredients that encourage the growth and activity of favorable intestinal bacteria. The two most commonly used are inulin and oligofructose. At present supporting data is scarce, and only studies involving the inulin-type fructans have generated sufficient data for a thorough evaluation regarding their possible use or grounds for tentative claims. Among the claims are: constipation relief, suppression of diarrhea, reduction of the risk of osteoporosis, atherosclerotic cardiovascular disease associated with dyslipidemia and insulin resistance, obesity, and possibly type 2 diabetes (Robertfroid, 2000). Probiotics are live microbial food entities that beneficially affect the host by improving its intestinal microbial balance. Food products containing probiotics are almost exclusively dairy products—fluid milk and yogurt—due to the historical association of lactic acid bacteria with fermented milk. The most commonly used bacteria in these products belong to the *Lactobacillus* and *Bifidobacterium* species (Kopp-Hoolihan, 2001).

Many factors affect the composition and quantity of bacteria present in the intestines: age, nutritional needs, immunological status, antibiotic use, stress, alcohol consumption and the pH, transit time, and the presence of material in the gut. The selection of probiotic strains has been in large part historical, based on years of use with no harmful side effects. Appropriate strains are selected because of their ability to: (1) exert a beneficial effect on the host, (2) survive transit time through the intestinal tract, (3) adhere to the intestinal epithelial cell lining, (4) produce antimicrobial substances toward pathogens, and (5) stabilize the intestinal microflora.

Claims that have some scientific support include: improving intestinal tract health, enhancing the immune system, synthesizing and enhancing the bioavailability of nutrients, reducing symptoms of lactose intolerance, decreasing the prevalence of allergy in susceptible individuals, and reducing risk of certain types of cancer.

Modulation of gut flora may also have an effect on urogenital health in women, as urinary and genital tract infections are often associated with colonic bacteria. Preliminary evidence indicates that probiotic bacteria or their fermented products may also play a role in blood pressure control, with animal and clinical studies documenting antihypertensive effects of probiotic ingestion. The mechanisms by which probiotics exert their effects are largely unknown, but may involve modifying gut pH, antagonizing pathogens through production of antimicrobial and antibacterial compounds, competing for pathogen binding and receptor sites as well as for available nutrients and growth factors, stimulating immunomodulatory cells, and producing lactase.

There is a critical need for long-term, well-controlled human studies to evaluate the benefits of prebiotic and probiotic consumption. Due to their long history of use in food fermentation, the FDA has designated many probiotics to be generally recognized as safe (GRAS). Even for those without GRAS status, the industry has used probiotic bacteria in food fermentations with the assumption that their history of use implies their safety. The food industry will need to carefully assess the safety and efficacy of all new species and strains of these substances before incorporating them into food products.

It would be prudent to introduce these unfamiliar adjuncts into one's diet gradually, building up to an effective daily level over a period of two or three weeks, to minimize any potential deleterious effects.

### *Flavonoids and Their Failings*

Flavonoids are a general category of chemicals occurring naturally in plants which act as antioxidants, reducing the risk of cancer. This category includes carotenoids, β-carotene, α-carotene, β-cryptoxanthin, lutein, zeanthin, and lycopene (Arab and Steck, 2000). Foods notable for their carotenoid content are deeply pigmented fruits and vegetables (carrots, sweet potatoes, tomatoes, spinach, broccoli, cantaloupe, pumpkin, and apricots).

Lycopene has some characteristics that set it apart from the usual carotenoids: it has no provitamin A activity but has significant antioxidant potential in vitro, and may play a role in preventing prostate cancer and cardiovascular disease in humans. Tomato products, including ketchup, tomato juice, and pizza sauce are the richest sources of lycopene in the U.S. diet, accounting for greater than 80 percent of the total lycopene intake of Americans. Lycopene may have a cholesterol synthesis-inhibiting effect and may enhance low-density lipoprotein (LDL) degradation. Also, intimal wall thickness and risk of myocardial infarction are reduced in persons with higher adipose tissue concentrations of lycopene. Definitive answers can only arise from a human trial specifically evaluating its effectiveness.

It has been shown that lycopene has the strongest singlet oxygen-quenching capacity of several carotenoids, with α-carotene, β-carotene, and lutein showing less antioxidant capacity. Lycopene is a fat-soluble pigment that gives tomatoes, guava, pink grapefruit, and watermelon their red color. Lycopene from tomato products appears more readily in the circulation if the tomato product is heated and a source of fat is included with the meal.

In a recent study, it appeared that lycopene was working by some other mechanism than as an antioxidant. All of this needs further human trials to pinpoint the specific therapeutic action. Men with the highest concentrations of lycopene in their adipose tissue biopsy had a 48 percent reduction in risk of myocardial infarction when they were compared with controls. Flavonoids also include isoflavones, lignans, and phytoestrogen compounds that bind to estrogen receptors and have weak estrogenic and antiestrogenic properties (Lamartineire, 2000).

Breast cancer is the most common cancer in women. Because genetics is believed to account for only 10 to 15 percent of breast cancer cases, the environment, including nutrition, is thought to play a significant role in predisposing women to this cancer. Asian women have a low incidence of breast cancer and it is thought to be attributed in part to their consumption of genistein, an isoflavone found in soy. Moreover, the greatest protection is found in women who began their consumption of genistein during early childhood.

A third type of flavonoids acting as antioxidants are the polyphenols found in teas. Teas are cultivated in more than thirty countries and are claimed to reduce the risk of a variety of illnesses, including cancer and coronary heart disease. Most research has involved green tea, however, a greater number of the world population prefers black tea. Studies using rats, mice, and hamsters showed that tea consumption protects against lung, esophagus, duodenum, pancreas, liver, breast, colon, and skin cancers in these mammals. Other animal studies showed the preventive effect of green tea consumption against atherosclerosis, coronary heart disease, high blood cholesterol concentrations, and high blood pressure. Human clinical trials will become necessary to assess the real benefits, because in addition to polyphenols, teas contain caffeine, phytate, and tannins. The latter two bind minerals, making them less available for absorption into the body (Mukhtar and Ahmad, 2000).

### *Homilies About Herbs*

The suggested benefits of herbs are based only rarely on scientific study, but more surely on years of informal observation: mint helps indigestion;

ginger helps nausea and motion sickness; lemon perks appetite; chamomile helps ease insomnia. However, if you are considering using an herb, remember this important rule of thumb: any herb that is strong enough to help you, can be strong enough to hurt you. As with any medicine, herbs can have side effects, and can be contraindicated because they may interfere with standard medicines. The following are some popular herbal supplements (Foster and Tyler, 1999):

- *Gingko biloba* to combat cerebral vascular insufficiency
- Ginseng (Asian) for energy and mood improvement
- Garlic to reduce cholesterol and blood pressure; has anticoagulant properties
- Echinacea to stimulate the immune system prior to and during the cold and flu season
- St. John's wort to treat mild to moderate depression
- Saw palmetto to promote prostate health and treat benign prostatic hyperplasia
- Cranberry to treat urinary tract irritations and infections
- Valerian as a mild sedative and to treat insomnia
- Kava as a tranquilizer and sedative
- Milk thistle to detoxify the liver
- Feverfew to relieve migraine headaches

Herbal blends marketed for specific conditions, such as healthy bone formula or female blend do not always make sense in light of current scientific knowledge (McGuffin et al., 1997). Quality control is a big issue in herbal medicines. A common problem is poorly standardized strength or potency. To guarantee quality, each step from field to market must be carefully monitored. Herbs are grown and harvested in remote areas of the world. Extraction or preparation of the herbs may take place elsewhere. Herbs may be mixed and marketed in capsules, tonics, or teas. Table 6.1 lists possible adverse effects of some herbs.

Three of the most popular herbs will now be discussed in detail: garlic, ginseng, and echinacea.

*Garlic*

Early in the eighteenth century both English and French priests tended to the fevered and ailing during a severe plague. Only the English priests caught the disease. It has been said that the massive amount of garlic eaten by the French protected them. The ancient histories of India, China, and Egypt, reveal that

TABLE 6.1. Possible Adverse Effects of Selected Herbs

| Herb | Possible Adverse Effects |
| --- | --- |
| Chamomile (tea) | Allergic reaction, digestive upset |
| Chaparral | Liver toxicity |
| Comfrey | Liver and kidney disease |
| Echinacea | Allergic reaction, stimulation of immune system. Not for use by those with systemic/autoimmune diseases |
| Ephedra | Insomnia, headaches, nervousness, seizures, increased blood pressure, stroke, death |
| *Gingko biloba* | Inhibits blood clotting. Do not take with aspirin, anticoagulants, vitamin E |
| Ginseng | Headaches, insomnia, diarrhea, heart palpitations, vaginal bleeding |
| Kava | Slowed reaction time, scaly dermatitis |
| Licorice | Headaches, fluid retention, increased blood pressure, electrolyte imbalance, heart failure |
| Pau d'Arco | Severe nausea, vomiting, anemia, bleeding tendencies |
| Pennyroyal | Liver damage, convulsions, abortions, coma, death; oil is very toxic |
| St. John's wort | Adverse interactions with antidepressant medication, possible photosensitivity |
| Senna | Laxative dependency, diarrhea, cramps, electrolyte disturbances |
| Valerian | Headache, excitability, insomnia |

*Sources:* Adapted from McGuffin et al. (1997); Sarubin (2000); and Foster and Tyler (1999).

garlic served as a culinary herb and was a valuable therapeutic. In Roman times, Pliny advised it for treatment of more than sixty illnesses. The Latin name is *Allium sativum.* The Soviet government once ordered 500 tons of garlic to fight a flu epidemic. Garlic and onion eaters have reportedly been able to lower cholesterol levels by 17 percent. Diabetics may prevent the wide fluctuations of blood glucose during garlic therapy.

Garlic research began in the United States in 1944 when the bactericidal oil from crushed garlic appeared helpful during a flu epidemic. The active compound in the oil was termed allicin, short for diallyl sulfide, one of garlic's many odiferous sulfur-containing components. In addition to lowering cholesterol in rats, investigators have since shown that garlic can reduce levels of blood fat and blood sugar, and can increase blood insulin level. Despite their findings, these investigators do not plan to continue their garlic studies. The garlic is too odoriferous, too all pervasive, and patients must consume large amounts before a therapeutic effect is demonstrated. Other agents in the marketplace are more efficacious.

## Ginseng

The edible part of the ginseng plant is the root. Russian cosmonauts took it on space flights to combat the rigors of space travel. Some American elite runners believe it gives them a boost, and the Chinese take it to give them youth, virility, and optimum health.

Ginseng's efficacy, as an energizing and revitalizing agent, however, is under question. Most ginseng research has been conducted overseas in Russia, Japan, and Britain, in studies that lacked controls and were unable to be duplicated. The FDA does not consider ginseng to be a drug, so there is no quality control over ginseng products. A recent study showed that more than half of the ginseng products analyzed were worthless and one fourth contained no ginseng at all.

## Echinacea

Echinacea is the name given to a group of wildflowers native to the United States from the daisy or aster family. It was one of the most important medicinal plants to the Native Americans of the Great Plains, used to stimulate the immune system and treat everything from coughs and digestive problems to blood infections and gonorrhea. It developed a reputation as a blood purifier and as a treatment for dizziness and rattlesnake bites. By the twentieth century, echinacea was the country's best-selling herbal remedy. But in 1909, the American Medical Association deemed it to be valueless and unworthy of future consideration. Echinacea fell into disuse just as antibiotics began to take its place.

No single ingredient or class of ingredients appear to be responsible for echinacea's purported health benefits. In addition, knowledge of the biochemistry and physiology of many of echinacea's constituents is limited, as is the ability to assess the various amounts of healing constituents. Echinacea appears to work primarily by stimulating various components of the body's immune system to mount a vigorous defense against invading viruses and bacteria. But the scientific evidence for benefits tends to be preliminary, weak, inconsistent, theoretical, or at best, suggestive. Clinical trials have been rare, and in a 1996 study it was advised that echinacea not be taken routinely, chronically, or on a preventive basis.

## Facts and Fictions of Phytosterols

Phytosterols (PS) are natural chemicals found in plants, in high concentrations in plant oils, seeds, and legumes such as peanuts. They are found in lower concentrations in fruits and vegetables, and their consumption may protect against heart disease, colon, prostate, and breast cancer. Phytosterols include plant sterols and plant stanols. The three most common forms in foods are β-sitosterol, campesterol, and stigmasterol. Only 5 to 10 percent of phytosterols are absorbed by the human body, compared with 50 percent for cholesterol.

The β-sitosterol (SIT) concentration in peanut butter is 135 mg SIT/100 gm of peanut butter. A much higher incidence of colon, prostate, and breast cancer occurs in Western societies where consumption is 80 mg PS/day than in Japanese society where consumption is 400 mg PS/day. Another compound in the phytosterol category is resveratrol. This is also found in grape skins and red wine. It may be one of the compounds that supports stories of the benefits of wine drinking. However, peanuts contain almost thirty times more resveratrol than grapes.

Phytosterols were first recognized in the 1970s for their ability to absorb dietary cholesterol thereby protecting against cardiovascular disease. They lower cholesterol in two ways: by blocking the absorption of dietary cholesterol circulating in the blood, and by reducing the reabsorption of cholesterol naturally produced by the liver (Awad et al., 2000).

# FACTS ABOUT FOOD

## The Myths of Smoked and Blackened Foods

We are swayed by image. If our grilled products have color, and the darker the better, we think they are more nutritious and delicious. Forget this. Enough research has been conducted to show that blackened foods are potentially carcinogenic. There is little food value in the blackness or in the color changes from sauces or marinades that have been chosen to enhance blackening. There is potential danger from carcinogens, which are either present in the sauces or created by the intense heat of the grilling process. Cooking until the meat is done is healthy; cooking until the meat, poultry, fish, or accompanying vegetables or fruits are pitch black is harmful (this includes blackened marshmallows). During this process free radicals are formed. The aromas and smoke created by grilling foods may be air pollutants which can damage the lungs. Surely there should be some lasting carry-over from the antismoking campaigns that have warned consumers of dangers to lung health.

### *Hidden Artificial Sweeteners and Fat Substitutes*

Fifty percent of the population in the United States is obese. Since 1991, adult obesity has increased by 60 percent (USDHHS, 2001). Even before it was at this level, there was controversy about developing sugar and fat substitutes. When it was finally decided that it might be a healthy innovation to make these products available, ostensibly to help diabetics, hyperglycemics, or hyperlipidemics gain dietary control, lo and behold the majority of the population thought it would be a splendid way to maintain weight and still consume their favorite foods. The idea also was to give those who were dieting alternative choices. It has not worked. Sugar consumption has increased, and caloric consumption has increased dramatically. Many new low-fat foods contain more sugar, and sugar-free or reduced sugar foods contain more fat. One has to be a detective and an avid label reader in order to see what is going on. The other side of the equation is energy expenditure. When we buy the same old foods in a new package, we make no change in our weight maintenance effort. It appears that instead of substituting artificial sweeteners for sugar, and artificial fats for fat, people are choosing to consume both, thus consuming far too many calories.

All of the artificial sweeteners and fat substitutes have continued to prove physically and psychologically safe for the general population. There are isolated complaints, but manufacturers hasten to address them to keep customers happy and sales up. On the strength of their successes, they are developing even more products to tempt us.

The following sweeteners have remained on the market: acesulfame-K, alitame, aspartame, cyclamate; the sugar alcohols: maltitol, mannitol, sorbitol, xylitol; saccharin, and sucralose. This list may change as some sweeteners are banned, and others take their place.

Fat substitutes are not as numerous. Olestra is a sucrose polyester, and Simplesse is a protein which contributes just four calories per gram. Other methods manufacturers use to reduce fat include adding water, or whipping air into foods; adding nonfat milk to creamy foods; using lean meats and soy protein to replace high-fat meats; and baking foods instead of frying them. To gain FDA approval for using a new fat replacer in the food supply, U.S. manufacturers must prove that their fat replacer contributes little food energy, is nontoxic, is not stored in body tissues, and does not rob the body of needed nutrients.

Oatrim, Nutrim, and Z-Trim are products developed and patented by the USDA that can easily be incorporated into commonly consumed foods, replacing fat in low-fat or fat-free products (Inglett, 1999). More direct evidence of developing obesity comes from population studies. In many countries, the incidence of obesity increases as sugar consumption rises. Wherever sugar intake increases, fat and total calorie intakes also rise. Simultaneously, physical activity declines. Concentrated sweets and fats make it easy for people to consume large amounts of calories quickly, so most diet plans recommend these artificially sweetened products be avoided. Sometimes eating small amounts of sweet-tasting foods triggers binges. In short, the effects of sugar and fat substitutes on a person's eating style and body weight depend on the user.

## Caffeine Additives in Foods and Beverages

Four out of five Americans drink, eat, or consume caffeine, knowingly or unknowingly, every day. It is the most popular drug consumed worldwide. The primary sources of natural caffeine are coffee, tea, and cocoa. Artificially caffeinated beverages and medications also contribute to daily intake (see Table 6.2). Caffeine occurs naturally in more than sixty plants. Even though more people drink tea worldwide, the major contributor of caffeine is coffee, since there is 50 to 70 percent more caffeine in coffee than in tea. Consumption patterns in the United States have changed recently: less coffee drinking, more tea drinking, or tea mixed with fruit beverages. Decaffeinated cola drinks are available, yet caffeinated waters are also available. Unless consumers read labels carefully (frequently there is no label for caffeine content), they do not know what to drink. For a comprehensive table of caffeine content in foods, beverages, and medications, see Harland, (2000). It is of interest that although the pattern of beverage consumption has changed, it is rarely based on solid knowledge of the effects of caffeine on the body.

The earliest behavioral effects of caffeine include increased mental alertness, a faster and clearer flow of thought, and restlessness (see Table 6.3). Fatigue is reduced and the need for sleep is delayed. Caffeine consumption stimulates the heart muscle, secretion of gastric acid, and urine output. Increased mental awareness may result in sustained intellectual effort for a short period without significant disruption of coordinated motor activity. However, tasks that involve delicate muscular coordination and accurate timing or arithmetic skills may be adversely affected.

Caffeine also causes bronchial restriction and constriction of cerebral blood vessels, thus compromising blood flow to the brain. Such action can afford striking relief from headaches, especially migraines. Cardiac arrhythmias after

TABLE 6.2. Caffeine Content of Medicinals

| Product | Serving Size | Caffeine (mg) |
|---------|--------------|---------------|
| No-Doz/Vivarin | 1 tablet | 100 |
| Anacin | 1 tablet | 33 |
| Excedrin | 1 tablet | 65 |
| Midol | 1 tablet | 33 |
| Vanquish | 1 tablet | 33 |
| Coryban-D | 1 tablet | 30 |
| Triaminicin | 1 tablet | 30 |
| Aqua-Ban | 1 tablet | 100 |

*Source:* Adapted from Harland, 2000, and Spiller, 1998.

TABLE 6.3. Caffeine Intakes and Physiological Consequences

| Caffeine Amt. | 6 oz. cup Coffee | Consequences |
|---------------|------------------|--------------|
| 100 or 200 mg | 1 or 2 | Increased mental alertness, faster thought flow, wakeful, restless, fatigue reduced, sleep need delayed |
| 1 g | 5-10 | Anxiety, insomnia, mood changes, cardiac arrhythmias, GI distress |
| 2-5 g | 16-40 | Spinal cord stimulated |
| 10 g | 100 | Lethal dose |

*Source:* Adapted from Harland, 2000, and Spiller, 1998.

ingesting caffeine are not uncommon, although rarely serious. Unless consumed in excess quantities, caffeine, a colorless, odorless powder at room temperature, is considered to be relatively nontoxic.

Athletes who consume two cups of coffee before an athletic event seem to improve their performance. When caffeine stimulates the release of fatty acids into the body, it conserves glycogen. Better than caffeine for this purpose, however, is a warm-up activity, which not only stimulates fat release but warms the muscles and fatty tissue deposits.

Chronic use and disuse of caffeine may produce withdrawal symptoms. Those who consume large quantities (ten cups of coffee per day) complain of headaches, drowsiness, fatigue, and a generally negative morning attitude. A potential danger exists to pregnant women who are advised to limit their caffeine intake to no more than 300 mg/day in order to avoid prolonged labor, premature offspring, or babies of less than normal weight (Hinds et al., 1996).

## *The So-Called Fruit Beverages*

Long ago fruit beverages were drinks made from squeezed, pressed, or crushed fruits. Now there are many "fruit" beverages on the market that barely contain fruits. A bottle, can, or carton labeled "grape juice" may actually be a blend of apple, grape, and pear juice containing only 20 percent juice. The rest is water plus high fructose corn syrup, with color and flavor enhancers added. In addition, to attract consumers to this product, calcium, which normally occurs in this product in marginal amounts, and vitamin C have been added to bring it to 100 percent of the daily value for these nutrients. The greater the fortification, the greater the price—when all consumers wanted or needed was fruit juice as it came from the fruit.

There is an emerging market for alternative beverages, those ubiquitous juices, teas, caffeinated waters, and sports and energy drinks packed with exotic herbs and vitamins that are overwhelming store shelves. Some juices contain the herb kava, touted as a mood elevator, or valerian root, a mild tranquilizer. Visionade claims to prevent blindness.

American consumption of carbonated soft drinks has actually declined. Beverage makers are feverishly working to invent cola alternatives that promise to be healthy, not just refreshing. Juice and tea mixtures abound. There are caffeine- and herb-laced "energy drinks." SoBe, a soy-based product, and Gatorade are currently the most popular "nutritious" drinks. However, this is a constantly fluctuating market. Consumers are becoming more promiscuous in their tastes. These beverages may turn out to be a fad—New Age snake oils for people who do not realize they are simply drinking a different kind of sugar water. The admonition for the consumer is to read the label, consider the price, and look for nutritional and monetary value.

## *Some Truths About Wines*

Moderate drinkers have lower rates of heart disease than heavy drinkers *or those who abstain completely.* Still, because of alcohol's risks, figuring out just how much (if any) to incorporate into your diet can be tricky. According to national statistics, 90 percent of drinkers drink moderately—at most two drinks per day. The U.S. government recommends that women have no more than one drink per day. Not enough scientific information supports one type of alcoholic beverage over another. Excessive consumption of alcohol is *never* recommended. Alcohol is a carcinogen. Two of the most famous wine-producing nations which include wine with their meals, Italy and France, have high rates of alcoholism and alcohol-related traffic accidents. The mechanism may be explained by the fact that moderate consumption of wine raises beneficial blood lipids (HDL), and prevents blood clot formation. These benefits are most apparent in people over the age of fifty as well as those most likely to develop heart disease from other contributing factors. Whites consume alcohol more frequently than blacks, but when black women drink, they do so more heavily. Worse yet, women are more affected by alcohol than men, making them susceptible to conditions such as alcoholic hepatitis, cirrhosis, brain damage, and possibly breast cancer.

The first hard data suggesting that moderate drinking was not inherently unhealthy appeared in 1974 when Kaiser Permanente researchers found that teetotalers suffered more heart attacks than those who drank. The 1977 Honolulu heart study showed that lifetime abstainers had more than twice as many cases of cardiovascular disease as people who had three or more drinks per day. However, countries, lifestyle, activity levels, and temperament are contributing factors in addition to alcohol consumption and dietary intake. Urinary zinc excretion was greater during alcohol consumption compared to nonalcoholic beverage consumption (McDonald, 1979). Alcohol may affect the renal conservation mechanism for zinc. Fecal zinc excretion was also significantly higher with alcohol consumption. Two-thirds of the subjects were in negative zinc balance during four eighteen-day experimental periods. The zinc-containing enzyme, alcohol dehydrogenase, is essential for the metabolism of alcohol. Aside from the contribution of alcohol, nonalcoholic constituents in fruit beverages may make healthful contributions (McDonald and Margen, 1980).

Wines are composed of ethyl alcohol, several other alcohols, sugars, other carbohydrates, polyphenols, aldehydes, ketones, enzymes, pigments, at least half a dozen vitamins, and fifteen to twenty minerals, more than twenty-two organic acids, and a number of unidentified substances. The possible variations in composition are infinite depending on the variety of grape, climate, soil, and the processes of fermentation and aging. It has been said that wine has a unique ability to relieve emotional tension because it contains tranquilizing substances other than ethanol, such as aldehydes and hydroxybutyrates (this remains unproven). Unlike pure ethanol, wine possesses a natural acidity that perhaps makes some nutritional elements more soluble and thus more readily absorbed. The average pH of table wine is 3.5, which is close to that of gastric juice. Wine may certainly stimulate appetite for psychological reasons. The association of good wine with good food, the increased sociability that wine drinking may create, and reduction of emotional tension, which in itself may depress appetite, are all important factors.


## SUMMARY

There are many approaches to the challenge of achieving optimum health, and preventing, treating, and curing disease. The existence of a National Center for Complementary and Alternative Medicine is evidence that the national government is actively engaged in screening and processing the multitude of substances purported to be effective. Allied health professionals must be aware of the constantly changing therapies that influence policy and clinical practices. The primary focus is to find what really works without interfering dramatically with optimum nutrition or lifestyle practices. The therapeutic field is rife with pseudobeliefs that have not been adequately tested for efficacy or safety. Seldom is an alternative therapy able to address a specific malady. Complementary and alternative medicine is a complicated field and must be approached with reasonableness as an adjuvant to proper nutrition and a healthy lifestyle, not a replacement for it.


## REFERENCES

Arab, L. and Steck, S. (2000). Lycopene and cardiovascular disease. *American Journal of Clinical Nutrition 71:* 1691S-1695S.

Awad, A. and Fink, C.S. (2000). Phytosterols as anticancer dietary components: Evidence and mechanism of action. *The Journal of Nutrition 130:* 2127-2130.

Doll, R. and Peto, R. (1981). The causes of cancer: Quantitative estimates of avoidable risks of cancer in the United States today. *Journal of the National Cancer Institute 66:* 1191-1308.

Drewnowski, A. and Gomez-Carneros, C. (2000). Bitter taste, phytonutrients, and the consumer: A review. *The American Journal of Clinical Nutrition 72:* 1424-1435.

Foster, S. and Tyler, V.E. (1999). *Tyler's Honest Herbal: A Sensible Guide to the Use of Herbs and Related Remedies.* Binghamton, NY: The Haworth Herbal Press.

Greenwald, P., Milner, J.A., and Clifford, C. (2000). Creating a new paradigm in nutrition research within the National Cancer Institute. *The Journal of Nutrition 130:* 3103-3105.

Harland, B.F. (2000). Caffeine and nutrition. *Science 16*(7/8): 522-526.

Hinds, T.S., West, W.W., Knight, E.M., and Harland, B.F. (1996). The effect of caffeine on pregnancy outcome variables. *Nutrition Reviews 54:* 203-207.

Inglett, G.E. (1999). Nutraceuticals: The key to healthier eating. *Chemtech 29:* 38-42.

Kopp-Hoolihan, L. (2001). Prophylactic and therapeutic uses of pro-biotics: A review. *Journal of the American Dietetic Association 101:* 229-238, 241.

Lamartineire, C.A. (2000). Protection against breast cancer with genistein: A component of soy. *American Journal of Clinical Nutrition 71:* 1705S-1707S.

Lee, Y. and Georgiou, C. (2000). The knowledge, attitudes, and practices of dietitians licensed in Oregon regarding functional foods, nutrient supplements, and herbs and complementary medicine. *Journal of the American Dietetic Association 100:* 543-548.

McDonald, J. (1979). Not by alcohol alone. *Nutrition Today,* January/February, 14-19.

McDonald, J. and Margen, S. (1980). Wine versus ethanol in human nutrition: IV. Zinc balance. *The American Journal of Clinical Nutrition 33:* 1096-1102.

McGuffin, M., Hobbs, C., Upton, R., and Goldberg, A. (1997). *American Herbal Products Association Botanical Safety Handbook.* Boca Raton, FL: CRC Press.

Milner, John A. (2000). Functional foods: the U.S. perspective. *American Journal of Clinical Nutrition 71:* 1645S-1659S.

Mukhtar, H. and Ahmad, N. (2000). Tea polyphenols: prevention of cancer and optimizing health. *American Journal of Clinical Nutrition 71:* 1698S-1702S.

Robertfroid, M.B. (2000). Prebiotics and probiotics: Are they functional foods? *American Journal of Clinical Nutrition 71:* 1682S-1687S.

Sarubin, A. (2000). *The Health Professional's Guide to Popular Dietary Supplements.* Chicago, IL: The American Dietetic Association.

Spiller, A.G. (Ed.) (1998). *Caffeine.* Boca Raton, FL: CRC Press.

United States Department of Health and Human Services (USDHHS) (2001). *Surgeon General's Call to Action to Prevent and Decrease Overweight and Obesity.* Washington, DC: U.S. Government Printing Office.

# Chapter 7

# Diagnostic Services

Veronica A. Clarke-Tasker
Marguerite E. Neita
Marvin Barnard

Diagnoses may be determined by physicians, physician assistants, and in many states, nurse practitioners. Diagnoses are methods used to identify, recognize, and/or analyze the cause or nature of a condition, situation, or problem. Clinicians utilize various techniques before making a final diagnosis. The extent of the diagnostic evaluation is dependent upon the extent and type of injury, and known or suspected pathology. Advances in technology have increased clinicians' understanding of the human body and aid in identifying underlying pathology when it occurs.

## MULTIDISCIPLINARY HEALTH CARE TEAM

A multidisciplinary health care team may include physicians, nurses, physician assistants, nutritionists, occupational and physical therapists, as well as laboratory and X-ray technologists. Specialists such as orthopedic or vascular surgeons, may also join the team. In today's health care environment, depending on the client's health care insurance, pre-approval would have to be obtained prior to scheduling a consultation. The insurance provider may deny the requested procedure if they deem it unnecessary or inappropriate. Visits to emergency rooms are often discouraged. In nonemergency situations, clients may see their primary care clinician at the clinic. If care is required after office hours, clients may have to report to a medisurgical site prior to being admitted to a hospital for treatment. Care offered at these alternative sites are usually diagnostic in nature, i.e., blood work, urinalysis, and X rays. Clients requiring more extensive treatment are either referred to their primary care clinician or transferred to a hospital.

In emergency situations, emergency medical technicians (EMT) may be the first contact clients have with the health care team. Basic skills of EMTs include oxygen administration, simple first aid, intravenous installation (IV), cardiopulmonary resuscitation (CPR), and in some cases defibrillation.

## CASE STUDY

Mr. Arnold is a sixty-five-year-old male who was involved in a single motor vehicle accident. A witness to the accident activated the Emergency Medical System by calling 911 from her cellular phone. When EMTs arrived, Mr. Arnold was unresponsive, with his seat belt securely fastened and his chest pinned against the steering wheel. Mr. Arnold's wife was located in the front passenger seat. She was startled, but had no apparent injuries. On initial assessment Mr. Arnold' s vital signs were as follows: respiration 22 and labored; pulse 135; blood pressure 115/60; and temperature 99.5. He remained unconscious with multiple bloody wounds to his upper body. An oral airway was inserted and oxygen was delivered via Venturi mask and bagging of the patient. A soft cervical collar and short spinal board were applied for immobilization of the neck and back prior to moving him to a gurney. Two intravenous lines of Ringers lactated solution were started in his left and right upper extremities. He was immediately transported to the emergency room.

### *History and Physical Examination*

On arrival at the hospital, Mr. Arnold was triaged and transferred to the emergency health care team. His temperature, pulse, respiration, blood pressure, and level of pain were reassessed and an in-depth physical evaluation followed. Mrs. Arnold was able to provide additional information regarding her husband's medical history. Mr. Arnold had diabetes and hypertension. Mrs. Arnold had the medication bottles for both of his conditions. She stated he had no prior surgical procedures and no known allergies to food or drugs. Medications, both prescribed and over-the-counter, dosage, and time they were last taken provides pertinent information about the client that aids in diagnosis.

A physician, physician assistant, nurse practitioner, or registered nurse may triage the patient in addition to obtaining a complete medical history and performing physical examination. A systematic approach is used and all findings are documented. Because the client was unconscious, the consent to treat would have to be signed by his wife or next of kin.

The following diagnostic procedures and preoperative tests were ordered by the clinician:

*Arterial blood gases*—evaluate effectiveness of ventilation and perfusion of blood

*Complete blood count (CBC)*—identify presence of infection, oxygen carrying capacity of blood

*Chemistry studies*—cardiac enzymes, renal function, liver enzymes

*Blood coagulation studies*—prothrombin time, partial thromboplastin time

*Urinalysis*—detection of bleeding, renal disease, and infection

*Type and cross-match for four units packed red blood cells*—replace blood lost

*X rays*—(chest, abdominal, spine, and lower extremities) identify injuries

*Magnetic Resonance Imaging (MRI) of the brain*—detect any underlying pathology

*Electrocardiogram (ECG)*—detection of cardiac abnormalities

## Preparation of Client for Diagnostic Testing

The phlebotomy, which is the aspiration of blood by venipuncture with a sterile catheter or needle, can be performed by doctors, nurses, physician assistants, and phlebotomists. Veins on the back of the hands, arms, or the antecubital fossa are preferred. The patient and/or next of kin would be advised of the procedure and verbal consent must be obtained. Universal precautions are followed unless the patient's condition warrants additional protection.

## FACTORS IN SELECTING LABORATORY TESTS

An appropriate request for laboratory testing initiates diagnostic procedures for every patient. Selection of the correct test provides physicians with valuable data that will guide their approach to handling patients. The procedure for returning accurate results to patient care providers in a timely manner requires that every step be controlled for quality. Factors that impact laboratory testing procedures are divided into three groups: preanalytic (before testing), analytic (during testing), and postanalytic factors (test results). Described by Barr (1999), the following outline provides a step-by-step process for the best use of the clinical laboratory, and prevents a hit-or-miss approach to laboratory testing.

## Preanalytic Factors

### Clinical Questions

Prior to ordering any laboratory and/or diagnostic tests clinicians will review clients' medical records. Completed histories, physicals, and other information included in charts will prompt clinicians to ask clinical questions appropriate to their clients' history, as well as any known or suspected underlying pathologies. In many instances, questions asked on admission may be repeated. Clinicians should explain why the questions are being repeated, as well as the reason for further examination if indicated. Clients should be told in the simplest terms how the information will be used to assist clinicians in making appropriate correlations with previous and/or similar cases. Clinical questioning is important. It enables practitioners to determine the necessity of a particular procedure. A combination of the test results and the assessment of their client's condition will enable physicians to make a more accurate diagnosis.

### Test Selected

The following factors must be considered when selecting diagnostic tests.

1. The clinicians' experience, their expectations, and the patient's condition will determine which test(s) are useful in confirming a diagnosis.
2. Practice guidelines for the particular institution also govern the types of tests ordered. In some institutions a clinical pathway and/or standing orders may be available for a variety of conditions. Such orders usually include a list of diagnostic procedures that should be requested for a particular condition. For example, if a client has a fracture, as is the case with Mr. Arnold, a preoperative checklist of tests to be ordered may be available. Space would also be provided for any additional test deemed appropriate for the client.
3. Usefulness of the test in evaluating a particular condition must also be considered. This may seem simple, but it's not. For example, an X ray or CT scan of Mr. Arnold's brain may have been appropriate in the past. However, with advances in technology and the ability of the MRI to detect pathology in greater detail, the MRI would provide a more accurate diagnosis.
4. Malpractice issues—tests are often added to cover every possibility. Clinicians are often wary of lawsuits. Therefore, every possible test

available may be ordered even though he or she knows that only one or two would provide the needed information.

5. Cost of the procedures—testing is expensive, and insurance companies will not reimburse and/or approve the performance of a test if it is believed that a less expensive test would provide similar results. Clinicians would have to present strong arguments to insurance providers in order to override decisions for less costly procedures.

## *Ordering the Test*

In some hospitals clinicians can order test(s) directly from laboratories through an integrated computer system located at the nursing units. Clinicians order test(s) on physician order forms and unit secretaries and/or nurses will enter the information into the system. Orders are usually reviewed for accuracy before nurses sign that they are completed (i.e., transcribed). In other cases clinician orders are placed in charts and transcribed to laboratory request forms. The latter procedure has a greater risk for error and often results in tests not being done (Barr, 1999).

## *Preanalytic Specimen Collection*

This is one of the most important steps in the evaluation of patient samples. Personnel collecting the samples are trained to adhere to the specific guidelines for the collection of different types of patient specimens. One mantra of clinical laboratory testing is that "a result is only as good as the specimen received." To ensure reliable results, it is essential that the following factors be controlled:

1. Preparation of the patient before collection
2. Appropriate collection techniques and containers
3. Collection of appropriate volumes for testing
4. Proper timing of collection
5. Proper identification of the patient
6. Correct and adequate labeling of the sample
7. Timely delivery to the laboratory

Some laboratory tests require patients to be NPO (nothing by mouth) before blood can be drawn. A sign may be placed outside the patient's room. The food services department is usually notified via computer. Nursing is responsible for patient teaching and the administration of some postprocedural medication. If the patient is having a test requiring contrast dye, a technologist usually comes to the floor. The clinician would have had to speak with the client prior to the procedure and consent is signed and witnessed.

## *Analytic Factors*

Prior to testing, each specimen must be properly entered into the laboratory system. The date and time of receipt are noted, specimens are given a laboratory number, and a worksheet is generated for the laboratory. Computerization of these procedures in the laboratory has reduced transcription and other errors associated with specimen processing. Once the specimen is logged into the laboratory system, testing by trained clinical laboratory scientists can begin. The responsibilities of clinical laboratory scientists and technicians under their supervision include:

1. Evaluation of the specimen for suitability (volume, storage, container selection, etc.)
2. Evaluation of testing methodology for sensitivity, specificity, accuracy, efficiency, and reliability
3. Evaluating the performance of the laboratory equipment and reagents
4. Provision of adequately trained personnel
5. Reduction of testing turnaround time

The clinical laboratory is a busy environment. Highly trained technologists are responsible for ensuring that all results leaving the laboratory meet quality assurance criteria. Technologists must work quickly and accurately, using complex instruments and procedures to analyze patient samples. They must determine the accuracy of results and be prepared to troubleshoot both instruments and procedures when problems occur.

## *Postanalytic Factors (Verification and Reporting of Results)*

Before results are reported, all laboratory test results must be verified by utilizing known quality control samples. Results are reported to the patient care area in a variety of ways. Trained clinical laboratory scientists can recognize test values that are grossly abnormal. Because these values, known as panic values, usually require immediate attention, they must be immediately reported to the physician or the client's floor by telephone. The name and title of the person receiving the test result(s) from the laboratory along with the date and time of the call may be recorded directly into the computer. Other values are logged into laboratory computers that transmit results directly to the floor.

In the case outlined at the beginning of the chapter, several laboratory test procedures were needed to immediately evaluate the patient. Preparation of the client for diagnostic blood work was necessary to determine any underlying pathology. In many instances, the clinician may not have told the patient he or she will be having blood drawn for diagnostic purposes. The nurse or clinical laboratory scientist may educate the patient about aspects of the procedure such as how it will be performed and what will be required from the patient. The reasons for conducting the test should be explained to the patient by the attending physician. The nurse can reinforce what was said, but only after the patient has been previously advised by the physician. Everyone should be aware that the patient has the right to refuse any procedure.

## LABORATORY AND OTHER DIAGNOSTIC PROCEDURES

Various laboratory and diagnostic procedures are required to make a diagnosis. The following is a list of procedures followed by questions clinicians should ask when evaluating results.

### Hematology Procedures

A complete blood count (CBC) includes hemoglobin, white cell and red cell count, platelet count, and red cell indices (see Table 7.1).

### Clinical Questions

- How effective is the oxygen-carrying capacity of the blood?
- What is the extent of blood loss due to trauma?
- How much blood needs to be replaced?
- Are there any underlying conditions?

### Specimen Collection

Specimens are collected in a purple-top tube which contains an anticoagulant chemical to prevent the blood from clotting.

TABLE 7.1 Complete Blood Count

| Component | Reference Range | Possible Abnormalities |
|---|---|---|
| White Blood Count | 3,500-11,000/µL (adults) | Increased in inflammation and infection |
| Red Blood Cells | 3.8-5.2 million /µL (females) 4.4-5.9 million/µL (males) | Increased in dehydration and decreased in fluid overload |
| Hemoglobin | 13.3-18 g/dl (males) | Decreased in hemorrhage |
| | 11.7-15.7 g/dl (females) | Decreased in hemorrhage |
| Hematocrit | 40-52 percent (males) 35-47 percent (females) | Increased in hemoconcentration (dehydration) and decreased in fluid overload |
| Platelet Count | 150,000-450,000/µL | Increased in hemorrhage |
| *White Blood Cell Differential* | | |
| Neutrophils | 54-62 percent | Increased in infection and stress |
| Lymphocyte | 20-40 percent | Increased in infection, decreased in renal failure |
| Monocyte | 4-10 percent | Increased in infection |

*Note:* Values may vary slightly between laboratories.

*Source:* Adapted from Sheehy, S.B. and Jimmerson, C.L. (1994). *Manual of Clinical Trauma Care: The First Hour.* St. Louis, MO: Mosby-Year Book, Inc., pp. 175-178; Lehmann, C.A. (1998). *Saunders Manual of Clinical Laboratory Science.* Philadelphia, PA: W.B. Saunders Company, p. 869.

## *Urinalysis*

Urinalysis is the microscopic and chemical examination of urine (see Table 7.2).

### *Clinical Questions*

- Is there any renal damage (bleeding)?
- Is there myoglobin in the urine due to extensive muscle trauma?
- Does the patient have any glucose in his urine?

### *Specimen Collection*

A clean, clear tube or container is used to collect specimens from patients.

TABLE 7.2. Urinalysis

| | Reference Ranges | Possible Abnormalities |
|---|---|---|
| Color | Pale yellow to amber | Dark or red may indicate presence of blood |
| Appearance | Clear to slightly hazy | Cloudy may indicate infection |
| Specific gravity | 1.005-1.025 | Increased in shock |
| pH | 4.5-8.0 | Acidosis/alkalosis |
| Protein | Negative | Positive may indicate renal failure |
| Glucose | Negative | Positive in diabetes |
| Ketones | Negative | Positive in diabetes or starvation |
| Blood | Negative | May indicate trauma or injury to renal system |
| Bilirubin | Negative | Positive may indicate liver disease |
| Urobilinogen | 0.1-1.0 Ehrlic units/dl (1-4 mg/24 hours) | Positive or negative may indicate liver disorder |
| Nitrite | Negative | Positive indicates urinary infection |
| Leukocyte | Negative | Positive may indicate renal infection |
| Red Blood Cells | 0-3/HPF | Positive high counts may indicate trauma |
| White Blood Cells | 0-8/HPF | Positive high counts may indicate infection |
| Epithelial cells | 0-1/LPF | Positive high counts may indicate renal damage |
| Casts | Neg. Hyaline 0-2/LPF | Type and number may indicate renal damage |
| Crystals | Occasional (uric acid, urate, phosphate, or calcium oxalate) not associated with trauma | May be found under normal conditions, abnormal crystals (cystine, tyrosine, etc.) |

*Source:* Adapted from Sheehy, S.B. and Jimmerson, C.L. (1994). *Manual of Clinical Trauma Care: The First Hour.* St. Louis, MO: Mosby-Year Book, Inc., pp. 173-174; Fischbach, F. (2002). *Common Laboratory and Diagnostic Tests* (Third Edition). Philadelphia, PA: Lippincott Williams & Wilkins, pp. 700-710.

## *Chemistry Studies*

An analysis of blood glucose, cardiac enzymes, acid-base balance, and serum electrolytes will aid the clinician in determining abnormalities in organ function (see Table 7.3).

TABLE 7.3. Serum Chemistry Studies

| | Reference Range | Possible Abnormalities |
|---|---|---|
| Glucose (fasting) | 65-115 mg/dL | ↑ in diabetes, after meals, and mild exercise; ↓ with fasting, prolonged exercise, and fever |
| Blood Urea Nitrogen | 8.0-22.0 mg/dL | ↑ in renal failure, dehydration, congestive heart failure; ↓ in malnutrition |
| Creatinine | 0.7-1.5 mg/dL | ↑ in renal failure, dehydration; ↓ in malnutrition |
| Calcium (Ca) | 8.9-10.5 mg/dL | ↑ dehydration, tumors of the bone; ↓ renal failure, malnutrition |
| Sodium (Na) | 135-143 meq/L | ↑ dehydration and diabetes insipidus; ↓ congestive heart failure, nephrotic syndrome |
| Potassium (K) | 3.5-5.0 meq/L | ↑ in renal failure and acidosis; ↓ in malnutrition, alkalosis, diarrhea, and vomiting |
| Chloride (Cl) | 100-109 meq/L | ↑ respiratory alkalosis, diarrhea; ↓ vomiting and respiratory acidosis |
| Phosphate | 2.5-4.5 mg/dL | ↑ in starvation, acute illness, ketoacidosis; ↓ with refeeding after starvation, and malignancy |
| Carbon Dioxide ($pCO_2$) | 36.0-44 mmHg | ↑ in respiratory failure, metabolic alkalosis; ↓ metabolic acidosis, lung disease, and anxiety |
| Alkaline Phosphatase | 30-130 U/L | ↑ liver obstruction, cancer of the liver, bone disease; ↓ in malnutrition |
| SGOT/AST | 8-40 U/ML | ↑ myocardial infarction, liver injury, and muscle disease; ↓ chronic renal failure |
| SGPT/ALT | 6-45 U/ML | ↑ myocardial infarction, liver injury, and muscle disease; ↓ B6 vitamin deficiency |
| LDH, Total | 100-212 U/L | ↑ myocardial infarction, hepatitis, and hemolytic anemia |
| Bilirubin, Total | 0.3-1.7 mg/dL | ↑ acute liver disease, congestive heart failure |
| Cholesterol, Total | < 200 mg/dL | ↑ hyperlipidemias, chronic renal failure, and diabetes; ↓ in malnutrition, malignancy |
| Triglyceride | < 200 mg/dL | ↑ hyperlipidemias, diabetes, renal failure, and myocardial infarction; ↓ in malnutrition |
| Protein, Total Serum | 6.2-8.0 g/dL | ↑ chronic infection and inflammation; ↓ in malnutrition and nephrotic syndrome |
| Albumin | 3.7-5.0 g/dL | ↑ hemoconcentration and exercise; ↓ chronic liver disease, malnutrition, and nephrotic syndrome |
| Uric Acid | 3.0-8.0 mg/dL | ↑ gout, renal failure, tumors, and diabetes; ↓ Hodgkins disease and renal defects |

*Source:* Adapted from Dufour, R.D. (1998). *Clinical Use of Laboratory Data: A Practical Guide.* Baltimore, MD: Lippincott Williams & Wilkins, pp. 447-563.

*Clinical Questions*

- Did the patient have a myocardial infarction (heart attack)?
- Was the accident a result of his diabetes being out of control?
- Did any other underlying condition contribute to the accident?
- What was the patient's respiratory status at the time of admission to the emergency room (ER)?
- What was the blood pH at the time of admission to the ER?

*Specimen Collection*

Serum separator, red-top tube, without anticoagulant. This allows the blood to clot so serum can be separated from the cells.

## Blood Bank

Type and cross match for four units of packed red blood cells.

*Clinical Questions*

- How urgent is the patient's need for blood?
- Should the patient receive group O blood now or is there time to wait for type-specific cross-match?
- What is the patient's blood type?
- What type of blood can the patient safely receive?
- Does the patient need any other blood components?

*Specimen Collection*

A plain red-top tube without serum separator or anticoagulant is needed since blood bank procedures require both the cells and serum in the clot. The tube should be labeled with the patient's information. If blood is needed urgently, the blood bank will provide group O cells while the cross-match procedure is done for type-specific blood.

In many states, the patient must sign an informed consent prior to a blood transfusion after the clinician explains the purpose and possible risks factors. When clients have prior knowledge of the need for transfusion, they may elect to donate their own blood or have a family member donate. Once consent is given, the blood bank is notified and blood is drawn for testing. Depending on the institution, a special band may be adhered to the patient's wrist with numbers matching the tubes of blood taken for testing.

## Coagulation Studies

Coagulation studies include platelet counts, partial thromboplastin time (PTT) and prothrombin time (see Table 7.4).

### Clinical Questions

- How well does the patient's blood clot?
- Is the patient a hemophiliac?
- Is there any danger of excessive, uncontrolled bleeding?

Components and pathways of the coagulation sequence are evaluated. These tests are performed when a coagulation profile of the client is required, and prior to surgical procedures.

## Point of Care Testing

Also available in most modern hospitals are point-of-care testing (POCT) procedures, which can be used to quickly evaluate patient status at the bedside. These test procedures utilize portable, miniaturized instruments that allow health care personnel, other than clinical laboratory scientists, to perform routine procedures such as glucose, electrolyte, acid-base balance, and even coagulation studies. However, these procedures are much more expensive than routine laboratory testing and may not provide any significant reduction in test turnaround time (Burr, 1999). Nonlaboratory health care personnel, such as nurses, physician assistants, and physicians, routinely perform POCT procedures; however training, coordination, and management of POCT are within the purview of clinical laboratories.

TABLE 7.4. Coagulation Values

|  | Reference Range | Possible Abnormalities |
| --- | --- | --- |
| Prothrombin time (PT) | 10-13 seconds (adults) | 2.5 x normal indicates abnormal bleeding tendency |
| Partial thromboplastin time (PTT) | 22-32 seconds (adults) | Determines the tendency of trauma patients to bleed if abnormal values are >36 seconds |

*Source:* Adapted from Sheehy, S.B. and Jimmerson, C.L. (1994). *Manual of Clinical Trauma Care: The First Hour.* St. Louis, MO: Mosby-Year Book Inc., p. 179; Fischbach, F. (2002). *Common Laboratory and Diagnostic Tests* (Third Edition). Philadelphia, PA: Lippincott Williams & Wilkins, pp. 700-710.

## Diagnostic X Rays

When X rays are ordered, the physician indicates both the type of X ray he or she desires, but also the purpose. For example, an X ray of the abdomen may be ordered to rule out small bowel obstruction. Once tests are ordered it is the responsibility of nursing to ensure that the orders are transcribed and submitted to the X-ray department. Once received and logged, a trained patient transporter will arrive at the nursing unit. This individual will usually report to the nursing station to advise the staff that he or she will be taking the patient to the X-ray department. The nurse and/or nursing assistant responsible for the patient will report to the patient's room and assist with the patient's transfer from bed to chair/stretcher. All precautions are followed to ensure that the right patient (name check on armband as well as verbal) is leaving the unit. For patients with spinal injuries, two or more individuals may be required to ensure that the patient is transferred from the bed to the stretcher without harm. Upon arrival to the X-ray department an X-ray technician will explain the procedure(s) to be performed. Once tests are completed, a primary reading may be obtained prior to the patient leaving the unit. Abnormal results are called to the appropriate nursing unit, who in turn will notify the ordering physician of any abnormalities.

Referring to Mr. Arnold's case study, X rays of the chest, abdomen, spine, and lower extremities, including an MRI of the brain, were ordered due to traumatic injury. Clients sixty years of age and older and those with a history of respiratory disorders should also be evaluated. When determining the type of X rays needed, the physician may again refer to admissions notes and presenting symptoms. The following questions/clinical data will aid the physician in reaching a decision.

### Clinical Questions

1. Is the client sixty years of age or older?
2. Does the client have a history of chest trauma, asthma, congestive heart failure, lung cancer, or any other respiratory disorders?
3. Does the client have a history of smoking, or is currently a smoker?

Types of injuries that may occur when chest trauma is suspected:

- Fracture of the ribs
- Frail chest
- Simple, tension, and open fractures
- Pneumothorax
- Hemothorax

- Pulmonary contusion
- Pericardial tamponade
- Fracture of clavicle
- Fracture of sternum

If any of the aforementioned conditions are confirmed, the unit where the client is housed would be notified. The doctor who read the X ray may document his or her recommendations for additional diagnostic X rays, and the nurse at the unit would notify the primary physician. A copy of the X-ray report may be faxed to the primary physician's office.

### Magnetic Resonance Imaging of the Brain

If the client requires a Magnetic Resonance Image (MRI) of the brain, several questions must be asked of the client prior to treatment.

#### Clinical Questions

- Does he or she have any metal parts, i.e., metal plate in head, rod in leg, or pins?
- Has he or she ever had the procedure before?
- Is the patient claustrophobic?
- Is the patient allergic to contrast dye?

The information provided will assist the physician when preparing the client for treatment. If the client is claustrophobic, he or she may receive oral sedation prior to reporting for treatment. An MRI of the brain is usually not ordered during the acute phase of treatment.

### Electrocardiogram (ECG)

Men over age forty and women over age forty-five may require an ECG if they have a known or suspected cardiac condition. Mrs. Arnold reported that her husband had a history of hypertension. A cardiologist would read the test results and provide a written report.

### Postoperative Period

Additional diagnostic testing would be required throughout the postoperative period. Similar to the preoperative phase of therapy, the following laboratory data may be monitored until the client's condition stabilizes:

- Arterial blood gases (see Table 7.5)
- Complete blood count (CBC)
- Chemistry studies
- Coagulation studies
- Urinalysis
- Postoperative infection

Despite all precautions taken to avoid their occurrence, *nosocomial* or hospital-borne infections are a frequent, and sometimes fatal, complication for hospitalized patients. The microorganisms implicated in hospital-borne infections are usually resistant to multiple antibiotics and special care is taken to minimize the occurrence of these types of infection. Many simple, but effective procedures, such as proper hand washing and use of gloves by all personnel who come in contact with the patient, can reduce the incidence of this type of infection. Although the incidence of nosocomial infections vary with the health care institution, the majority (40 percent) are urinary tract infections, especially in the catheterized patient. Surgical wound infections comprise 20 percent of hospital-borne infections, respiratory tract infections comprise 15 percent, and systemic blood infections (bacteremia) comprise 5 percent (Delost, 1997). Patients who are already infected at the time of admission have a *community-based* infection.

TABLE 7.5. Arterial Blood Gases

|  | Reference Range | Possible Abnormalities |
|---|---|---|
| $PaO_2$ | 83-108 mm Hg | < 50 mm Hg hypoxia |
| $PaCO_2$ | 35-45 mm Hg | > 45 mm Hg hypoventilation |
| pH | 7.35-7.45 | < 7.35 acidosis, > 7.45 alkalosis |
| $HCO^-_3$ | 22-28 meq/L | ↓ in metabolic acidosi (diabetic ketoacidosis)<br>↑ metabolic alkalosis |
| $O_2$ saturation | 94-100% | ↓ hypoxemia, anemia, and abnormal hemoglobins |

*Source:* Adapted from Sheehy, S.B. and Jimmerson, C.L. (1994). *Manual of Clinical Trauma Care: The First Hour.* St. Louis, MO: Mosby-Year Book, Inc., p. 171.

*Microbiology Procedures: Microbiological Culture and Antibiotic Sensitivity of Isolated Microorganisms*

*Clinical Questions*

- What microorganism is causing the infection?
- Where is the focus of infection?
- Is the infection nosocomial (hospital borne) or community based?
- What antibiotics are best suited to fight this type of infection?
- Is the infection systemic or localized?

*Specimen Collection*

Specimens include wound swabs, samples of sputum, tissues, or exudates, blood and urine cultures. The type of specimen submitted to the laboratory is based on the clinical evaluation of the patient to determine a probable site of infection. Treatment is begun once the organism has been identified. Infections increase the length of time the patient remains in the hospital and increase the cost of the hospital stay. To reduce the incidence of these infections, home treatment may be arranged depending on the clinical feasibility and the client's health insurance.

**Discharge Planning**

Discharge planning begins on the day of admission to the hospital. Rehabilitation of the client is essential in order for him to return to the community. Occupational and physical therapy consultations may be required. Social workers usually visit the client prior to surgery in anticipation of the client requiring additional care.

Referring to our case study, Mr. Arnold would require crutches in order to ambulate. Crutch walking would be taught prior to his discharge home. Additional physical therapy treatments would be provided on an outpatient basis.

## REFERENCES

Barr, J.T. (1999). Clinical Laboratory Utilization: Rationale. In Davis, B.G., Mass, D., and Bishop, M.L. (Eds.), *Principles of Clinical Laboratory Utilization and Consultation.* Philadelphia, PA: W.B. Saunders Company.

Delost, M.D. (1997). *Introduction to Diagnostic Microbiology: A Text and Workbook.* St. Louis, MO: Mosby-Year Book, Inc.

Dufour, R.D. (1998). *Clinical Use of Laboratory Data: A Practical Guide.* Baltimore, MD: Lippincott Williams & Wilkins, pp. 447-563.

Fischbach, F. (2002). *Common Laboratory and Diagnostic Tests* (Third Edition). Philadelphia, PA: Lippincott Williams & Wilkins, pp. 700-710.

Kidd, P.S. and Wagner, K.D. (2001). *High Acuity Nursing* (Third Edition). New Jersey: Prentice-Hall.

Lehmann, C.A. (1998). *Saunders Manual of Clinical Laboratory Science.* Philadelphia, PA: W.B. Saunders Company, p. 869.

Sheehy, S.B. and Jimmerson, C.L. (1994). *Manual of Clinical Trauma Care: The First Hour.* St. Louis, MO: Mosby-Year Book, Inc.

Chapter 8

# Psychosocial Interaction and Its Therapeutic Impact on Patients' Physical and Mental Health: Implications for Health Care Providers

K. Habib Khan

## *INTRODUCTION*

The main purpose of this chapter is to provide some critical information about psychosocial phenomenon that could accelerate or hinder the healing process among patients. This chapter will briefly define the concept of health and discuss the impact of group and individual interaction on patients health. Moreover, it will identify certain personality traits of health care providers that may directly impact how quickly patients recover from their illnesses, identify important skills and personality traits that can increase the effectiveness of the health care provider's role in dealing with sick people, and provide practical suggestions for those health care providers who will assume leadership roles in health administration. This chapter will also discuss strategies and skills health care administrators must master in order to be effective and inspiring leaders, and will provide some suggestions for dealing with job-specific and everyday stresses.

In addition, the work of one of the most distinguished psychologists of the twentieth century, Abraham H. Maslow, will be discussed briefly and used to describe some of the psychological concepts related to theories of management and their impact on people's lives. Maslow believed it was human nature to be good, helpful, collaborative, and driven toward success. His teachings have emotionalized the field of management in the United States and around the world.

In his famous book *Toward a Psychology of Being,* Maslow (1962) opened a new chapter in psychology about learning through experience when he suggested:

> Here is now emerging over the horizon, a new conception of human sickness and of human health, a psychology that I find so thrilling and full of wonderful possibilities that I yield to the temptation to present it publicly even before it is checked or confirmed, and before it can be called reliable scientific knowledge.

Warren Bennis (1998) commented on this quote and stated, "It is all there in that one sentence—a sentence that sentences psychology to a new life; that has turned it inside out or more precisely outside in: to gain truth through personal experience, to be a courageous knower" (p. ix). I wholeheartedly agree with Bennis because Maslow's prediction has become a reality for most psychologists.

## TECHNICAL COMPETENCE VERSUS PEOPLE SKILLS

Health care providers have long debated the importance of people skills in the healing process of patients. Until recently, health care providers placed more emphasis on technical knowledge and competence than bedside manners, empathy, and sympathy toward individual patient concerns. This change is the direct outcome of intense competition in the health care industry and popularity of movements such as the Patients' Bill of Rights and Patients Are People Too. In addition, an abundance of information is available on the Internet related to consumers' rights and many educated and well-informed patients now consider themselves consumers of health services. They want more and better services for the money they spend on health care.

This situation has forced the health care industry to perceive their services as real business endeavors based on an open market economy. The bottom line has become an important element in expanding and sustaining medical practices in this country. In addition, with the newer concept of managed care and health maintenance organizations (HMOs), the health industry has become more vigorous, rigorous, and intense in terms of business competition in order to improve the bottom line. The ability to generate enough cash has become necessary to market, expand, and improve the quality of comprehensive health care services in the twenty-first century.

There have been many negative stories published by the press, especially during the congressional hearings held during President Clinton's first term in 1993, in which many well-known and professionally competent health care providers and well-known HMOs were portrayed as callous, uncaring, and insensitive. These stories added fuel to the fire and now the public is asking for more transparency about decision making, accountability, and civility on the part of health care providers and all agencies associated with HMOs.

In addition to these well-documented cases, we each have personal knowledge of situations in which technical competence alone did not serve the welfare of patients according to their expectations, level of satisfaction, and perception, especially when very competent health care providers lacked sensitivity, basic social competence, responsiveness, and listening skills. In these instances patients felt betrayed because their unique personal and medical needs were not addressed or met despite the fact that they had spent a fortune on their health care needs.

For example, a patient who is a friend of mine went to a renowned hospital for hip replacement surgery. A wealthy man, the patient asked for a spacious and well-furnished private room. The attending physician and surgeons knew the patient very well from his two previous major operations, hence the best and the brightest of the hospital staff were assigned to care for him. A few hours after the operation, a very experienced and technically competent nurse entered the patient's room. She did not utter a word of greeting, ask the patient how he was doing, or ask if he was in pain. Instead, she hurriedly moved his leg up higher, so it would heal properly. She was not gentle and hurt the patient more because she was abrupt and very unfriendly. This made the patient very unhappy and agitated since the nurse had increased his pain and suffering without demonstrating any sensitivity.

The next day the patient was still very upset and told his attending physician he did not wish to have that particular nurse return to his recovery room. Although the attending physician told him the nurse was the best and most experienced nurse in the entire hospital, the patient insisted on changing her. The second nurse was less experienced, but she had better people skills and demonstrated a great deal of care, empathy, and sense of service. Her presence made the patient feel welcome and comfortable. This helped the patient cope with his severe pain and discomfort. The patient told me this nurse's friendly greetings and her inquiries as to how he was feeling and recovering made him feel better. Consequently, he recovered fully and the second nurse was assigned to work with him at his home for one month during the recovery process.

## DEFINITION OF HEALTH

According to the World Health Organization (WHO, 1999), health is defined as "a state of complete physical, mental, and social well-being and not merely the absence of disease or infirmity." According to Buckingham and Smith (2001) this WHO definition of health has become somewhat illusive and controversial to define. The biggest controversy is centered on defining the "social well-being" component of WHO's definition. What does social well-being actually mean? It has a different meaning for different people. For example, it could simply mean being content, but also having a feeling of balance in social interaction during a normal day.

The rise of health promotion has led to an elaboration of the original WHO definition of health, which can be simplified as being the extent to which an individual or group is able to realize aspirations and satisfy needs, and to change or cope with the environment. According to J. M. Last (1998), health is an essential part of everyday life; however, it is not the object of living but rather a concept that stresses social and personal resources as well as physical capabilities.

The majority of psychologists and some sociologists argue that social well-being is a state of social adjustment in which a healthy balance between social expectations, economic success, and availability of social and psychological support exists. Others argue that approval from one's peers and other significant people in one's life is required in addition to economic and environmental balance. Therefore, socially adjusted individuals are capable of maintaining healthy relationships with the existing social order, thus avoiding serious negative social consequences. This situation makes them healthy and productive members of society.

## PSYCHOSOCIAL THERAPIES

It is an accepted fact that health is defined in a psychosocial context. Therefore, treating illnesses, diagnosing the causes of diseases, and even conducting epidemiological studies are part and parcel of social phenomenon. Instituting a healing process and prescribing a cure has an indisputable relationship with psychological therapies. For example, a sick person needs more than medicine to recover fully and remain a productive, well-adjusted, and contributory member of society. It is also indisputable that health care providers play a pivotal role in diagnosing disease, prescribing appropriate medical prescriptions, and developing patient recovery plans, normally starting with a list of do's and don'ts.

After dispensing medication, attending health care providers provide instructions regarding what to do and what not to do, what to eat and what to avoid, and other practical recommendations such as get enough rest, drink liquids, and include exercise, etc. However, if certain psychological concepts and principles were understood and applied appropriately by health care professionals, their effectiveness would take a quantum leap. Consequently, these health workers would be more likely to have happy patients who would recover faster and would come back to the same health care providers. In addition, patients would likely recommend that health care provider to their family and friends. This is the best prescription for a successful medical practice. Marketing research data clearly support the notion that referrals from satisfied customers is the best form of advertisement for health care providers.

Other concepts, such as the client-centered philosophy of service, support the fundamental code of ethics for health care workers, which is that the welfare of the patient comes first under all conditions. During the formative years of medical history, doctors, nurses, and other health workers were taught that all patients should be treated just like close family members. This philosophy was designed to build close emotional ties between care providers and patients so that the sense of service and sacrifice is heightened.

I assume that most twenty-first century health care providers believe in these basic premises, otherwise they would not have chosen this noble profession. However, just verbalizing this commitment on the part of health care providers is not enough. Health care providers need to prove this notion to their patients. Patients need to experience it firsthand. It is just like when someone says "trust me"—most people would not trust that person until the person is proven to be trustworthy. Feelings of trust are developed over time and are the outcome of a positive interpersonal relationship.

Most health care providers need to convey the message that patients are their number one priority, and nothing is more important than taking care of patients. If adopted, practiced appropriately, and applied skillfully, the following set of skills would contribute toward conveying this message to patients. The world-renowned psychotherapist Carl Rogers (1951) has utilized these skills very successfully in practicing client-centered psychotherapy for nearly fifty years. The basic ingredients and major salient features of this therapeutic approach include:

### Active Listening Skills

Many patients complain that their health care providers do not care about them as persons because the health care providers are too busy and do not have the time to listen carefully and attentively to patients' concerns. There-fore, I believe listening skills are fundamental for all health care providers for the following reasons:

1. If you do not listen carefully you may miss something very critical that your patient is trying to convey to you, something that may be key to the process of final and proper diagnosis.
2. It is always gratifying for the patient to experience attentive, caring concern from the health care provider.
3. Listening attentively builds trust and confidence in the relationship.
4. Listening helps patients to relieve pressures and worries.
5. Finally, it strengthens a patient's belief that this health care provider has his or her best interest at heart. If a patient experiences this intense, sincere, and uninterrupted attention from the provider, it confirms the belief that he or she is being taken care of professionally. It also boosts morale and builds loyalty.

### *Empathy (Respect)*

According to *Dorland's Illustrated Medical Dictionary* (Anderson 1988), empathy refers to intellectual and emotional awareness and understanding of another person's thoughts, feelings, and behaviors, even those that are distress-ing and disturbing. Empathy emphasizes understanding. Many health care providers think patients need sympathy, which emphasizes sharing of an-other person's feelings and experiences. But Carl Rogers (1951) believes patients need empathy from the therapist not sympathy. Rogers considers sympathy demeaning—the patient may start believing that you, the care-giver, are feeling sorry for him or her.

However, common sense dictates that patients need sympathy but from close friends and relatives, not from therapists and other health care provid-ers. Sick people need assurance and emotional support more than those who are well. This support may be provided verbally or nonverbally, but must be given sincerely because most patients are very perceptive despite their ill-nesses. Therefore, it is important for health care providers to use nonverbal cues or body language to convey their genuine empathy, sensitivity, and un-derstanding. I firmly believe most patients do not need sympathy, but would appreciate empathy. They need reassurance that everything is fine and their caregiver fully understands their illness.

Nonverbal cues may include a broad smile, eye contact, leaning toward the patient, and listening attentively while conducting routine check ups. In addi-tion, verbal reassurances may include remarks such as, "I am glad you came in time," "You are fine" or "You will be fine and everything is under control," "The disease (medical condition) is treatable with the medicine you are taking," etc. It is important to be gentle, caring, truthful, and understanding. The health care providers must avoid giving the impression that they are in a hurry by not looking at their watch and by not taking phone calls during important one-on-one sessions. Most health care providers ignore the fact that in the eyes of the patients they are the most significant person in that environment and whatever they say and do, patients take very seriously.

## *Total Acceptance (Unconditional Positive Regard)*

According to Carl Rogers (1951), unconditional acceptance of the patient by psychotherapists or by health care providers is the first step toward healing. Unconditional acceptance provides patients the comfort they are seeking. This is the first step toward establishing trust, faith, and credibility as care providers. This unconditional acceptance goes beyond racial boundaries, gender, religion, socioeconomic status, and other differentiations and stratifications. It is the responsibility of all heath care providers to ensure this feeling of acceptance is conveyed beyond reasonable doubt through verbal and nonverbal behavior (body language), and fair and friendly treatment, regardless of the environment. Carl Rogers (1951) sums up his philosophy of total acceptance as follows:

> One of the most satisfying experiences I know—is to just fully appreciate an individual in the same way that I appreciate a sunset. . . . I don't find myself saying, "soften the orange a little on the right hand corner and put a bit more purple along the base, and use a little bit more pink in the cloud color. . . ." I don't try to control a sunset. I watch it with awe as it unfolds. (p. 189)

## *Reflection, Projection, Clarification, and Summarization*

Reflection, projection, clarification, and summarization are essential concepts and techniques for learning to be an effective therapist or health care provider. These skills can only be mastered if one listens to the patient carefully, reflects, projects, clarifies, and summarizes what the patient is saying. One has to train and practice with these skills to become an efficient user. The goal is to understand the patient's feelings and pain. One must let the client talk, which helps the person cope with the situation and solve the problems. This famous quote from Jesus Christ eloquently presents the case in the following manner: "If you bring forth what is inside you, what is inside you will save you. If you do not bring forth what is inside you, what you do not bring forth will destroy you."

As a therapist or health care provider, one must be able to convey to patients that he or she understands their pain, discomfort, and worries. For example, when a patient says that he or she was awake until 4 a.m. watching television, one may project the patient's feelings by asking whether he or she is having trouble sleeping. Similarly, when a patient complains that his or her pain persists despite taking a prescribed medication, one may ask if the patient feels frustrated. If the patient says yes, it means the therapist or health care provider has accurately reflected how the patient feels. However, if the patient says no, then the therapist or health care provider has misunderstood the patient. The point is to not dismiss the patient's feelings and pain. Instead, one should always support, accept, reflect, project, respond to, and understand the patient's problems and concerns. This conveys to the patient that his or her welfare comes first and, in turn, builds loyalty.

## *Intuition*

*Webster's Collegiate Dictionary* defines intuition as an act of contemplation, quick and ready insight, immediate apprehension and cognition, knowledge or conviction gained by intuition, and finally, in summation, intuition is "the power or faculty of attaining to direct knowledge or cognition without evident rational thought and inference" (p. 615).

If we accept this definition, it can be translated as a "gut level feeling or a hunch." This innate ability appears to be a gift from God. It also means there will be individual differences among therapists in applying this skill. If we translate this phenomenon into a psychological construct, it is a decision-making power based upon one's perceptions and internal data analysis and cannot be explained in logical terms. What makes this phenomenon interesting and unique is when intuitive decisions turn out to be right ones for the patients, considering all the known and unknown facts. Above all, these decisions positively impact the welfare of the patient.

For the reasons discussed in the preceding paragraph, it is difficult to teach this skill in a classroom or in practicum seminars. It is my belief that people develop strong intuitive feelings concerning future events or results based upon their experiences, introspection, and interaction with others in different and/or similar settings, exposure to diverse groups of patients and exotic diseases. Developing this unique ability is an essential requirement for most of the health care providers because the right kind of intuition at the spur of the moment can save lives. Finally, intuition is an inner strength and insight into the possible cause of a problem or disease. It occurs when a person is perceptive enough to link a cause to an effect when there are no obvious links or clues.

It is interesting to note that during the diagnostic process when all laboratory results turn up negative and a patient is still sick and suffering, an experienced (and sometimes inexperienced) health care professional comes up with uncustomary and uncommon solutions to the problem at hand and solves the mystery. This is a valuable and unique ability to have, one that would improve the health care provider's effectiveness at all levels of the health care delivery system in this country.

## *Sensitivity*

Sensitivity is a personality trait defined as being aware of the needs and emotions of others. The sensitive person is one who is cautious, careful, tactful, diplomatic, and receptive to others' feelings, needs, aspirations, and unique personal issues such as race, gender, religion, politics, sexual preference, and abortion, etc.

All health care workers must be sensitive in order to be effective in the healing process. In a practical sense sensitivity refers to a state in which health care providers do not stereotype situations, group behavior, and persons belonging to different ethnicities, and reach conclusions based on personal beliefs and biases. In our society sensitivities to cultural differences, gender issues, racial differentiations, age-related factors, socioeconomic status, country of origin, religion, and ethnicity are very important. If health care providers do not demonstrate sensitivity when dealing with patients, their effectiveness will be compromised. Sensitivity can easily be developed through appropriate short-term and long-term training activities and exposure to diversity.

## *Superior Judgment*

It is enormously important that most health care providers demonstrate superior judgment skills. The main reason for this requirement is the fact that health care providers often have to make decisions under tremendous pressures of time and emergency conditions. The right decision would save lives, but the wrong decision would jeopardize the welfare of the patients under the provider's care. The main question is, is it possible to teach superior judgment skills? The answer is no because superior judgment skills come intuitively. It is also believed that real life experiences teach people lessons. These "lessons learned" serve as guides in similar situations. However, health care providers can be trained to be critical thinkers. This kind of training can prevent them from making hasty, impulsive, and wrong decisions.

According to Ruggiero (1999), critical thinking is an acquired ability to observe, collect, analyze, and evaluate data, to ask questions about the issue at hand, and finally, to draw conclusions based upon evidence. The highest order in critical thinking is evaluated by an individual's ability to make right and reasonable decisions in difficult and challenging situations where personal biases, distorted perceptions, and manipulations by various factions are discarded. *The decision is based on evidence and evidence alone.* Critical thinkers normally act as follows:

- They base their judgment on evidence.
- They ask questions.
- They overcome confusion by reflecting, sorting, and analyzing.
- They look for connections and relationships between concepts, arguments, and divergent views.
- They are intellectually independent and honest.
- They acknowledge complexity and avoid simple solutions to complex problems.
- They seek competing views and additional evidence.
- They test arguments and opinions for reasonableness.
- They recognize errors in thinking and selective perceptions.
- They apply critical thinking in real-life situations.
- They are honest with themselves.
- They resist temptations in the decision-making processes.
- They are more reflective as opposed to being reactive and impulsive.

In conclusion, critical thinkers are common people with an uncommon ability to make decisions and solve problems with presence of mind, logic, and common sense in real life as well as in life-threatening situations. Health care professionals must master this process in order to save lives.

## EXPECTATIONS FROM A SUCCESSFUL HEALTH CARE PROVIDER

The public in general and patients in particular expect a lot from health care workers. They perceive health care workers as educators, facilitators, coaches, mentors, cheerleaders, counselors, teachers, motivators, and leaders. It is very difficult to be all these things to all people they come in contact with. That is why is it very essential for health care workers to know themselves. They need to understand their strengths and weaknesses. They need to realize that they are not super humans. At times they might need help, they might need therapy, and/or they might need to consult with colleagues and friends. They also need to know why they have selected this challenging profession. Health care workers need to assess if they have the commitment, abilities, and stamina to cope with the challenges and earn the rewards this profession can bring to them.

Health care providers who are optimistic and caring impact their patient's recovery. It is a known fact that positive interaction with health care providers strengthens patients' immune systems because they feel good about themselves and proud of their association with their healers. When people feel good, their bodies produce chemicals that promote healing and resilience. The personality of the health care provider has a significant impact on the speedy recovery of the patient. The most desirable traits for health care providers include people-oriented personalities and love for the jobs.

As stated earlier, it is absolutely important for health care providers to use self-analysis to discover whether or not they have the strength to control their emotions in stressful and difficult situations. It is equally important that health care providers demonstrate emotions when needed, but manage such emotions appropriately.

How one thinks affects the body and soul. Positive interactions with loved ones and caregivers uplifts the spirit. This is especially true for sick people.

## HEALTH WORKERS AND STRESS

Health care providers experience tremendous stress in their working environment. The health care profession is the most challenging of all service-oriented endeavors for the following reasons:

1. Health care providers are in constant contact with sick people and individuals who are seeking both comfort and treatment at the same time.
2. They work long and irregular hours, which affects their family and personal lives.
3. Many health workers work in emergency wards and hospices. They also work with terminally ill, disabled, and/or geriatric patients with limited cognitive and psychomotor abilities.
4. Due to their extended and unpredictable schedules, health care workers do not have time to take care of themselves. They do not sleep long

enough, they do not eat right, and likely do not have time to exercise and entertain themselves.

5. Health care workers often do not know where to go when they have problems, and do not really know when to ask for help because they carry the burden of being strong for their patients and families. They perceive themselves as professionals and they wrongly assume they are not supposed to ask for help even when they are in dire need of it.

## *HOW TO HANDLE STRESS*

When a patient comes to a clinic, the first thing a nurse does is check the patient's blood pressure, temperature, pulse rate, and other vital signs. On the other hand, when a client goes to see a pyschologist, the psychologist asks questions to check the client's mental health and emotional stability. Once in a while, health care workers need to ask the following simple questions:

1. Am I happy?
2. Am I productive?
3. Do I sleep at least six to seven hours every day? Is my sleep sound or often interrupted?
4. How do I feel all day?
5. Do I accomplish a lot every day?
6. Am I frustrated a lot?
7. Do I feel dejected or discouraged a lot?
8. Do I feel depressed often?
9. Is my relationship with my loved ones deteriorating or getting better?
10. Am I having financial problems?
11. Do I find my work boring and tedious?
12. Do I find my colleagues at work unfriendly?
13. Do I have friends I can trust and talk to without worrying about their opinion of me?
14. Am I reasonably compensated for my talent and the contributions I make?
15. Do I feel unappreciated most of the time?

The honest analysis of the answers to these questions would provide a clue whether you need some professional help.

## Stress and the Immune System

According to the Reader's Digest publication *Live Longer, Live Better* (Weiss, 1995), it is commonly believed and confirmed by medical professionals that stress is linked to headaches, backaches, and gastrointestinal problems. More recently a connection has been made between stress and the immune system. Scientists are now seriously studying the interaction between mind and body in hopes of better understanding human healing.

The same publication suggests the body's natural response to stress is physical as well as emotional. In stressful situations, the brain releases chemicals that trigger the immune system to start producing defensive antibodies. When stress is too great or lasts too long, however, the immune system can stall, leaving the body more vulnerable to illnesses.

*Live Longer, Live Better* recommends trying one or more of the proven stress relievers listed below when faced with a painful emotional experience:

- Talk to a trusted friend, family member, or religious counselor about what is troubling you. Express your anger. Neither holding anger in nor blowing up is constructive.
- Cry if you like; it may relieve some tension.
- Focus on action you take alone or with others to resolve the situation or to make matters better.
- Exercise on a regular basis and maintain a healthy diet.
- Get all the sleep you need, but don't use sleep as an excuse or escape.
- Avoid nonprescribed mood-altering drugs (including alcohol which is a depressant).

The following suggestions are based upon my personal experiences and all the reading I have done on handling stress. However, keep in mind these recommendations are preventive in nature and should be considered part and parcel of the primary health care paradigm (preventive rather than curative):

1. *Pamper yourself:* After a hard day of work or after a challenging week, go and pamper yourself. This may include doing things you enjoy most, e.g., listening to music, going to the movies, playing golf, getting a massage, manicure, and/or pedicure, going to the gym, etc. It is an individual choice. Do what pleases you and makes you feel good and fortunate.
2. *Eat a healthy breakfast:* Breakfast is the most important meal of the day. Studies have shown that people who eat a healthy, balanced

breakfast every day are capable of handling stress better than those who do not.

3. *Avoid caffeine:* Caffeine does not help in coping with stressful situations. It is a fallacy that caffeine calms the nerves. Caffeine increases blood pressure and hyperactivity. It is recommended you drink no more than two cups per day.

4. *Limit alcohol:* Your liquor intake must not go beyond two drinks per day. The use of alcohol aggravates depression, anxiety, and stress.

5. *Sleep at least six hours every night:* The most recent longitudinal study results reported in *The Washington Post* indicated that people who sleep at least six hours per night live longer, while those who sleep between six to seven hours live even longer. Excessive sleep, i.e., more than eight hours, is not healthy and does not promote longer life. Adequate sleep is an important part of staying healthy and handling stress.

6. *Eat right:* Once again, this is a personal choice. However, a balanced diet that includes lots of fresh fruits and vegetables is highly recommended. In addition, avoid red meat, processed meat, TV dinners, soft drinks, and too much salt. Drink at least six to eight glasses of water per day.

7. *Exercise:* Physical activity is essential for managing stress. It is recommended that you exercise at least twenty minutes four times per week at a minimum. Maximum benefits are derived from spending about 100 minutes per week in a gym or exercising at home. If practiced regularly, exercise will likely improve your quality of life in addition to helping you handle daily stress effectively.

Some reasonable stress in your daily life serves as a work motivator. The basic human instinct is that people do things to avoid pain and/or to seek pleasure. Therefore, a moderate level of stress provides an impetus to get going and do what needs to be done.

In conclusion, stress is part of everyday living. Dr. Hans Selye (1907-1982), a Canadian endocrinologist and pioneer in the study of the effects of stress on the human body, wisely noted that humans should not try to avoid stress any more than they would avoid food or exercise.

I would like to conclude this section on stress by saying that stress is unavoidable in life. For example, the following situations often may cause stress: getting a flat tire on the highway, losing your address book, splattering tomato sauce on your shirt or tie, getting caught in a traffic jam due to an accident or rush hour traffic, fighting with your boss or significant other, waiting at the dentist or the hair dresser, standing in a slow checkout line, spilling milk on a newly waxed floor, and waiting your turn at a favorite restaurant. When confronted with a stressful situation, it is up to you how you react. You have two choices: you can try not to react negatively and accept the situation as is because you have no control over it, or react with anger, aggravation, or impatience, thus creating unnecessary stress.

## HEALTH WORKERS AS CARE PROVIDERS, LEADERS, AND MANAGERS

> Proper management of the professional life of human beings, of the way in which they earn their living, can improve them and improve the world and in this sense be a utopian or revolutionary technique. (Abraham H. Maslow, 1962)

Many health care workers who are good at their jobs and possess good people skills eventually become managers and leaders in their organizations as well as in their field. On the other hand, some health care professionals are trained to be managers, such as health management sciences program graduates.

This section will briefly discuss distinguished psychologist Abraham H. Maslow's research on management, as well as theories derived from his work. Maslow's theories of management have had a significant impact on American business practices. His research on management was originally published in *Eupsychian Management* (Maslow, 1962), which was later revised and reprinted as *Maslow on Management* (Maslow, Stephens, and Heil, 1998). However, Maslow became famous for his work on human potential and motivation. He created a hierarchy of needs and the concept of self-actualization. Maslow's basic premise is that every human being has an innate motivation to achieve self-actualization. In Maslow's own words, "Each of us is born with certain innate need to experience higher values, just as we are born physiologically with need for zinc or magnesium in our diet."

This statement argues that our needs and motivations are biologically rooted. Every human being has an instinctive need for higher values, truth, justice, and so on. However, fulfilling these higher needs is only possible when all lower-level needs are fulfilled. Maslow's hierarchy of needs includes the following (starting from the lowest level to the highest):

1. Physiological needs
2. Safety needs
3. Social needs

4. Need for self-esteem
5. Need for self-actualization

It is assumed those who have achieved the most inspired level of self-actualization are the most suitable to be effective leaders, psychotherapists, and health care providers since they are content and do not struggle to fulfill their lower level needs. These individuals have the energy, motivation, and desire to lead, care, and inspire.

Douglas McGregor, one of Maslow's contemporaries, authored the classic text *The Human Side of Enterprise* in 1960. McGregor became known as the father of Theory X and Theory Y. These theories of management referred to managerial leadership styles that portrayed the manager as authoritarian (Theory X) or as collaborative and trustful (Theory Y). McGregor used much of Maslow's research on the hierarchy of motivation to develop his assumption of Theory Y managers. The key to success for leaders depends on how they perceive their colleagues. Answers to the following questions may provide some indication as to what kind of philosophy a leader believes in:

1. Do you believe people are trustworthy?
2. Do you believe people seek responsibility and accountability?
3. Do you believe people seek meaning in their work?
4. Do you believe people naturally want to learn?
5. Do you believe people do not resist change but resist being changed?
6. Do you believe people prefer work to being idle?

Maslow believed in the good nature of humans. These questions may work for health care workers who assume leadership roles. The outcome of these discussions should provide insight into the thought processes and beliefs that ultimately affect leadership style and job performance.

In conclusion, this chapter has taken a position that substantial psychosocial-based therapeutic benefits are derived from positive one-on-one and group interactions, especially when participants include health care providers and other significant people in their lives. Health care providers must demonstrate unconditional acceptance of the people in their care on an "as is" basis. Health care workers who enjoy their jobs and feel good about themselves are more likely to be effective. In addition, personality traits such as sensitivity, reflectiveness, intuitiveness, ability to think critically, and collaboration are most desirable. Moreover, skills such as listening, caring, sharing, and being open and honest contribute to healing and health promotion. The best way to handle stress is to recognize the stressful situations and develop an effective and personal strategy to combat it. This includes pampering yourself, getting enough rest, eating a balanced diet, moderating use of alcohol and caffeine, and engaging in some kind of physical exercise for about 100 minutes per week. While serving as a team leader/ manager, one must develop a team based on trust, mutual respect, and a belief in people's integrity, motives, strengths, dignity, capabilities, and above all their motivation and desire to succeed and excel (as advocated by Maslow). The collaborative team approach is most relevant in the health care field. Authoritarian dictators have no place in the health care setting, since the trend is team-building and treating patients through interdisciplinary approaches.

## BIBLIOGRAPHY

Anderson, D.M. (Ed.) (1988). *Dorland's Illustrated Medical Dictionary,* Twenty-Eighth Edition. Philadelphia: W.B. Saunders Company.

Bennis, W. (1998). Foreword to the New Edition. In Maslow, A.H., Stephens, D., and Geil, G. (Eds.), *Maslow on Management.* New York: John Wiley & Sons.

Buckingham, R.W. and Smith, T. (2001). In Buckingham, R.W. (Ed.), *A Primer on International Health.* Boston: Allyn & Bacon.

Last, J.M. (1998). *Public Health and Human Ecology,* Second Edition. Stamford, CT: Appleton and Long.

Maslow, A.H. (1962). *Toward a Psychology of Being.* Princeton, NJ: Van Nostrand.

Maslow, A.H., Stephens, D., and Heil, G. (Eds.) (1998). *Maslow on Management.* New York: John Wiley & Sons.

McGregor, D. (1960). *The Human Side of Enterprise.* New York: McGraw-Hill.

Rogers, C.R. (1951). *Client-Centered Therapy: Its Current Practice, Implications, and Theory.* Boston: Houghton Mifflin.

Ruggiero, V.R. (1999). *Becoming a Critical Thinker,* Third Edition. Boston: Houghton Mifflin.

Weiss, S.W. (Ed.) (1995). *Live Longer, Live Better.* Pleasantville, NY: Reader's Digest.

World Health Organization (WHO) (1999). *World Health Organization Report.* Geneva, Switzerland: WHO.

Chapter 9

# Interdisciplinary
# and Community-Based Health Care

Ivan Quervalu

Historically, community-based health care has been mostly conducted by community health nurses. Organized public health efforts are associated with the sanitary revolution of the eighteenth and nineteenth centuries. Through the written work of Florence Nightingale, students have learned of her accomplishments and concerns about the impact of environmental contaminants on health, community assessments, and her use of statistical information regarding sanitation disposal behaviors and community census data (Nies and McEwen, 2001). In addition, public health nursing, through the concept of district nursing in England, developed by providing nursing care to the poor and by community organizing, which allowed the poor to improve their own health status. Societal health was ultimately improved through the slow introduction of health nursing and eventual establishment of nursing education.

Presently, community-based health care is focused on primary rather than institutional or acute care, with much use of epidemiological methods of data gathering in primary, secondary, and tertiary prevention. Much of this care is provided by nurses and physician assistants, with assistance from allied health services as needed. Community-based nursing models are designed to promote access to and utilization of quality health services in rural populations and underserved populations in urban areas. Community-based nursing is identified as a first priority of the National Nursing Research Agenda (NNRA) (NIH, 2001). Community-based health care can then be defined as providing a community and its vulnerable populations (the homeless, low-income individuals and families, HIV-infected individuals, the elderly, etc.) access to health care in the community as well as referrals to primary care services in hospitals. With community-needs assessment, diagnosis, and planning skills firmly embedded in community nursing training, nurses and other medical professionals are leading the charge to provide direction for needed health care services.

## INTERDISCIPLINARY BEHAVIORAL APPROACHES

From the 1960s to the present, psychologists, social workers, and community organizers became concerned about community health and collaborated with nurses to improve health conditions in "ghetto" neighborhoods (minority communities). Social workers are an integral part of this interdisciplinary approach. Social workers are trained in a wide range of services such as individual counseling, group and family counseling, community organizing, research and planning, and administration. Many social workers are stationed at hospitals alongside nursing personnel. They provide discharge planning for community reintegration, administer grant funded programs, deliver social services for HIV patients and the elderly, and write social research projects for other special populations. Another group of social service providers, psychologists provide an extensive array of services ranging from individual counseling to psychological tests for children and adults and administration of social services programs. Consequently, social workers, psychologists, psychiatrists, and nurses work side by side in team efforts in hospitals as well as in community-based health care services. They work in a variety of settings such as hospital satellite clinics, community mental health centers, foster care agencies, public and private schools, community housing advocacy agencies, nursing homes, etc.

## BEHAVIORAL SERVICES IN HOSPITALS

In most major hospitals in the United States, there is usually a *department of psychiatry* or at most a *psychiatric emergency room*. Some hospitals have both, as well as a mobile crisis-intervention team that answers 911 (police) distress calls in any part of the county or city in order to handle emergency psychiatric cases. Many patients with mental illnesses or psychiatric episodes enter the hospital through the emergency room. Often, patients with medical trauma (stabbings, spousal abuse, or car accidents) present with symptoms that require the intervention of a psychiatrist or psychiatric nurse, and perhaps some medication. Patients with severe psychiatric illnesses or psychiatric episodes may also be admitted to the psychiatric emergency room. Follow-up visits with a counselor may be required.

Some hospitals have *psychiatric inpatient units.* Most have adult psychiatric inpatient units, while others are specialized (e.g., they have an adolescent psychiatric inpatient unit). Some hospitals have inpatient detoxification units for alcohol and substance abuse (opiates). Detoxification units are designed for overnight stays, usually from seven to fourteen inpatient days. Inpatient units are sometimes limited by the number of beds available.

Within many hospitals' departments of medicine or primary care there are *consultation and liaison units.* These units provide psychiatric assessment and diagnosis for patients who have medical problems but also exhibit some behavioral problems. Consultation and liaison psychiatric services are called upon by physicians to provide assessments and follow-up services. Although physicians can prescribe psychotropic medications, usually for depression and anxiety, psychiatrists are more familiar with complicated psychiatric diagnoses as well as the interaction of psychotropic medications and medical prescriptions. Consultation and liaison services are specifically intended for the hospital's medical unit. However, they can be called for consultation by any department to determine a patient's ability to function or state of jeopardy if so indicated.

As a result, interdisciplinary team approaches with established protocol procedures are used within hospitals. These approaches are also used to provide assistance to community grassroots agencies, or public and private organizations as needed. Physicians, psychiatrists, nurses, social workers, and psychologists often hold interdisciplinary team conferences during which they formulate agreed-upon assessments and/or treatment plans for patients. Sometimes, other hospital personnel may be included in the conferences. An example is illustrated in the case of Jason.

## THE CASE OF JASON

Jason is a twelve-year-old male who was referred to a hospital's adolescent psychiatric inpatient unit following an attempted suicide in a public housing building. While in the hospital Jason would not talk to anyone and would not take any medications. He ate fairly well but had trouble sleeping through the night. Attempts by the psychiatrist to speak to him were fruitless.

One day, while undergoing a routine physical examination in the medical side of the building, Jason made friends with a CAT scan technician. It seemed Jason was interested in the computer attached to the CAT scan and began talking to the technician. After a while the technician realized Jason had a number of problems. When the nurse came to get Jason, she asked the technician how everything went. The technician said everything went fine. The nurse told him that Jason never speaks. The technician then told her how Jason had told him a number of things about his suicide attempt. Hearing this, the nurse said she would be in touch with the technician later. The nurse then informed the chief psychiatrist, who suggested that perhaps the technician could help Jason speak to him. An arrangement was made for the technician to come over during the recreational part of Jason's schedule. They met and played checkers, and eventually Jason agreed to speak to the "doctor" (the psychiatrist). A session was immediately scheduled. After a few visits, an interdisciplinary team conference was held and the technician was included to summarize his visits. The team consisted of the psychiatrist, the nurse, the psychologist, and the technician. It seemed Jason was a victim of child sexual abuse at an earlier age, and prior to his hospitalization, he was rejected by a girl he liked very much.

In a short time Jason recovered. However, his recovery could have taken longer if the nurse had not asked the CAT scan technician how Jason's procedure went. Since Jason started talking with the technician, the psychiatrist realized the technician was crucial in getting the boy to open up, to trust him, and to engage the boy to also trust the doctors. As a result the psychiatrist made the decision to include the technician as part of the interdisciplinary conference team.

Often, patients open up to particular individuals. Play therapists are often a viable source of communication with nonverbal children. Hispanic patients open up to Spanish-speaking personnel, such as a bilingual maintenance employee rather than an authoritative physician with no bedside manners. Moslem women often shy away from male physicians and prefer female physicians. These cultural competency or clinical issues are discussed in other parts of this book. The importance of the case vignette is that the team approach to include the technician was effective in the treatment process of the patient.

Another component of the department of psychiatry is the *outpatient unit*. A wide range of different outpatient units are located within the hospital setting, depending on the population needs within a community.

*Psychiatric adult outpatient clinics* are intended primarily for walk-in patients who feel they need someone to talk to about their problems or a mental health issue. Issues can range from anxiety, depression, child management and housing problems to marital and family relational problems. Staff are usually social workers, psychiatrists, psychologists, and even former patients or paraprofessionals who help with group counseling or group activities. Outpatient services are also provided for patients who need follow-up after they have been discharged from a psychiatric inpatient unit. Some outpatient clinics have housing or employment counselors as well.

*Child and adolescent outpatient psychiatric clinics* are similar in treatment modalities as the adult outpatient program. Sometimes they include after-school programs that provide both recreational and therapeutic activities alongside therapeutic counseling.

*Day treatment programs* are intended for patients who have been discharged from a psychiatric inpatient unit but have more serious mental illness and are deemed severely and persistently mentally ill (SPMI) This type of program provides a structured environment with a schedule for individual counseling, group counseling, treatment planning, lunch, day trips, and vocational and recreational activities. Some patients improve significantly, are discharged, and are referred to an outpatient unit for continued follow-up.

*Partial hospitalization programs (PHP)* are for patients with severe mental illness who would be in a hospital inpatient unit were it not for this type of day treatment program. These programs provide intensive psychiatric day treatment for children and adolescents as well. Patients move on to the day treatment program as they get better. PHPs are cost effective when compared to hospitalization or institutionalization.

*Methadone maintenance clinics* not only provide methadone on a daily basis, but also individual and group counseling, and concrete services, e.g., employment, housing, etc. If they are linked with a hospital, patients are provided with medical care as needed. Ryan White programs are linked with methadone programs because of the high incidence of HIV/AIDS among drug users.

*MICA day treatment programs* are intended for those individuals who have both mental illness and chemical abuse problems (MICA). Psychosocial educational treatment programs, which include family and individual counseling, drive some of these programs.

*Day programs* for the elderly include a wide range of services from medical problems to behavioral health services which have recreational, daily activities, and medication monitoring.

Finally, there are *hospital satellite (community) behavioral health clinics* that provide services similar to hospital outpatient psychiatric clinics but in a nonstigmatized environment within the general community. They may be situated within a health care satellite clinic or as a stand alone behavioral health clinic with a friendly user name such as the John F. Kennedy Family Care Clinic. Satellite behavioral health clinics obtain many of their referrals from their community network which includes churches, community centers, housing developments, and walk-ins.

Sometimes hospitals address particular health concerns such as:

*Therapeutic nursery services* are usually located in communities that have higher rates of infant mortality. These services are geared for young mothers and their children in order to address mothers' psychological needs as well as prenatal and young children's nutrition and medical conditions.

*Prison health services* are usually provided by a designated hospital that has a contract to provide medical and behavioral services within a prison community. Persons with serious and persistent mental illnesses are usually monitored by intensive case management (ICM) workers. Prison health services provide assistance to adults as well as to children and to adolescents with serious emotional disturbances, and their families. This service provides access to needed medical, social, educational, and other resources. Activities are geared toward enabling patients to develop their strengths and improve the quality of their lives in their community (Clark and Mazza, 1999). Sometimes behavioral health clinics need the services of a certified alcohol and substance abuse services counselor (CASAC) or an addiction specialist to deal specifically with alcohol and substance abuse services along with behavioral health service providers.

## DEPRESSION IN PRIMARY CARE

A recent innovative and effective approach which more and more hospitals have implemented is the screening of depression among patients while on a visit with their primary care physician. Many evidence-based studies have established that a significant percentage (from 12 to 20 percent) of patients in primary care are diagnosed with anxiety, depression, suicidality, or alcohol or substance abuse when screened within a primary care setting. There is a need to conduct additional research as well as provide mental health and substance abuse services, particularly for older Americans. The data indicate a significant number of the elderly are suffering from depression, alcohol abuse, and other mental illnesses (Rabins et al., 1996). Depression is the leading mental health problem among the elderly. Multiple stressors associated with aging such as physical illness, role depletion, social isolation, bereavement, and multiple losses, as well as cumulative lifelong stressors such as those related to poverty, contribute to the risk of depressive symptoms. Depression is the most common nonorganic mental disorder among persons over the age of sixty-five (Wills, 1993). Recent epidemiological studies have indicated the prevalence of mental illness among the elderly is between 20 and 25 percent compared with 15 and 20 percent for the general population (Pollock and Reynolds, 2000). According to *Mental Health and Mental Disorders* (National Institute of Health, 2000), depression rates are much higher among older people who experience a physical health problem, and 12 percent for persons who are hospitalized.

Recently, screening for depression anxiety and chemical abuse (which includes alcohol) within primary care settings has taken a firmer foothold in many hospitals as a result of federally funded studies. These studies have documented the cost effectiveness of providing behavioral services with otherwise undiagnosed populations, thus preventing further mental illness with patients who have medical ailments. The major obstacles to screening are that there are not enough personnel to screen patients and not enough time for physicians to actually screen patients for psychiatric problems, unless patients inform them of any problems or concerns (Harvard's Aging Coordinating Center, 2001). However, national studies have shown that with minimal effort, a social work assistant or other trained personnel can identify patients with possible depression or anxiety symptoms. Once symptoms are detected and treated appropriately, the efforts of the screening process contribute not only to the well-being of the patient but also become cost effective in terms of preventing mental illness and physical deterioration, and resultant medical care and medication (National Library of Medicine, 1993).

Standardized instruments used in the screening probe for disturbances in sleep, diet, work habits, relationships, and general feelings of worth, as well as alcoholism. Such instruments include the General Health Questionnaire (twelve short questions), CAGE (four questions for alcoholism), CES-D (twenty-two questions for depression), and Beck's Anxiety Scale (eighteen questions). There are usually some questions on suicide tendency, for example, "Have you thought life is not worth living anymore?" Some patients may say yes and are prompted for more information such as "Have you thought of how you would do it?" Some patients will say no, and you may stop questioning them about suicide, but others will say yes and may need to be prompted further. If the patient has previously attempted suicide and is thinking about it seriously as you question her or him, you will need to call for a psychiatric assessment or take the patient to the nearest psychiatric emergency room.

In many hospitals there are special screening days such as National Depression Screening Day held each year during Mental Illness Awareness Week. Hospital personnel, public health educators, nurses, or social workers usually set up a table where individuals volunteer to take the screening test. Patients must sign a consent form and are screened for depression using the questionnaires previously cited.

## COMMUNITY HEALTH SERVICES

The most efficient approach for hospitals to improve access to health care services, particularly to poor and vulnerable communities, is to establish satellite clinics. Satellite health clinic programs are usually geared toward an identified population that needs both health and behavioral health services. Before satellite clinics were established, patients would have no resort but to go to the nearest hospital emergency room, usually in the last stages of an illness. With the advent of satellite health and behavioral health clinics, patents can be seen and treated at a preventative level. By conducting outreach activities, patents can be identified early in their stage of illness. Ongoing outreach activities include educational promotional activities such as free screenings at street fairs, shopping malls, presentations at shelters, and distribution of flyers, etc.

Satellite clinics and the various outreach programs are necessary marketing approaches in order for hospital systems to keep up with the many different types of vulnerable populations in their community.

### Vulnerable Populations

*Minority populations,* many of which are located in poor communities, are defined as the four government-protected groups, including African Americans, Hispanic Americans, Native Americans, and Asian and Pacific Islanders. Statistics have consistently shown these groups have higher rates of health and mental health illness than white Americans (Lecca et al., 1998). As mentioned, satellite clinics are located in minority communities in order to improve access to health and behavioral health services. It is easier to go to a neighborhood clinic than to travel to a hospital's psychiatric outpatient clinic. These neighborhood clinics may also be located in communities where new immigrants have settled such as the Russian community in Brighton Beach, New York City. There are many Chinatowns, Little Italies, Korean Towns, and Spanish "barrios" in different cities throughout the United States, from San Francisco to New York. Consequently, hospital systems reaching out to new market populations must ensure that access and availability are established as new and older immigrant populations settle in their communities.

*Homeless* populations are everywhere, and many go unseen. The homeless population has been growing since the 1980s. There are several types of homeless populations: those who are poor and without shelter, those who live in a supervised public or privately operated shelter, and those who live in a temporary institution or a place not designed to be a living habitat. Projections indicate that in the future, single mothers with children will be the majority of the homeless in the United States (Bassuk et al., 1996).

*Adolescents* and young adults up to twenty-four years of age are also a growing population with health problems such as pregnancy, alcoholism, and substance abuse, sexually transmitted diseases including HIV and AIDS, depression, suicide, and serious psychiatric illness. Adolescents are often involved with the juvenile justice system in terms of criminal behavior usually associated with substance abuse and gang-related activities.

*Foster care* parents and children who are in the foster care system receive a wide range of services provided by the foster care agency that has the responsibility for caring for the child. Health and behavioral health services are provided by the foster care agency through its community referral linkages. Although some agencies have medical services on site, most clients are referred either to an outside-agency-approved physician or to a hospital clinic near the foster parent's home. Foster care social workers work with biological parents to focus on a number of agreed-upon goals. These goals are primarily geared toward helping the natural parent establish a permanent and safe home in order for the child to be discharged to them. Typically, parents must accomplish the following: parental skills training, substance abuse counseling, steady employment or welfare income stability, improved parent-child relationship, supervised home visits, and postdischarge "prevention" counseling at a local social service agency. The problem is that once they are discharged and technically out of contract service with the foster care agency, a significant percentage of parents return to their old habits and their children are reintroduced to the foster care system. Many children are placed in kinship foster homes and have a higher likelihood of thriving and remaining out of the foster care system once discharged. Kinship foster homes are linked with community social service agencies for medical and behavioral health services.

*The elderly*—One of the goals of Healthy People 2010 is not simply to increase life expectancy but to increase the number of years older adults can live healthy and independently and increase ability to participate in rewarding activities (USDHHS, 2000). The primary health problems of older adults include: arthritis (62 percent for women), hypertension (33 percent), diabetes (11 percent), visual impairment (18 percent), and hearing loss (33 percent) (Nies and McEwen, 2001). In addition, problems include proper nutrition, disability and accidents, incontinence, elder abuse, and mental disorders.

Many elderly are poor and forced to live on fixed incomes or on welfare. Fortunately many are entitled to Medicare but may fail to go to their doctor or hospital clinic when needed. Reasons for this failure may include: (1) disengagement or isolation, such as when the elderly alienate themselves by locking themselves in their apartment or house. Such behavior may also indicate psychiatric illness or high anxiety after a traumatic event such as the World Trade Center disaster, (2) Alzheimer's disease which prevents the elderly from remembering appointments, (3) physical limitations which prevent them from traveling or walking to the clinic or doctor's office, or (4) lack of funds for transportation.

Many of these obstacles can be overcome to a certain extent. Many clinics, as well as hospitals, offer transportation, wheelchair services, and/or escort services. Some offer home care services which can help the isolated once home care personnel are welcomed into the home. Methods to improve access to health care can range from home health care services to home visits by auxiliary health care workers. Visits by a senior citizen center social worker or a rehabilitation therapist from a hospital or other social service agency can be used to assess a frail, elderly patient's physical and mental condition. By taking this holistic or psychosocial approach when making a home visit, a visitor can be more aware of the patient's major problems and refer them for follow up services. If the therapist notices the patient's home is very disorderly or the patient is severely disoriented and incoherent, referrals should be made to the nearest senior citizen center or another visit with a psychiatric social worker or nurse should be scheduled. This extra step may help the patient along the road to recovery.

*Home-based health care services* are coordinated by hospitals or independent home health care agencies, and provide multidisciplinary high quality care in the home. Personnel can include nurses, certified health unit coordinators (CHUCs), health unit coordinators (HUCs), physical therapists, and home health aides. More professionals may be included as needed. In order to receive these services, a physician must write an order for home care in the patient's chart. After a needs assessment is conducted, the patient's insurance carrier determines whether the patient is eligible for services (Clark and Mazza, 1999).

At the other end of the human development spectrum are *early intervention programs (EIP)* which provide services to children from infancy to three years of age who are suspected of having severe or multiple disabilities. Early intervention programs provide equal access to a free and appropriate education. An EIP team may consist of a registered occupational therapists, a registered physical therapist, a speech and language pathologist, a special educator, a child development specialist, a social worker, and a program coordinator. EIPs provide early identification, screening, and evaluations for at-risk children and also provide services in home or community-based settings. Sometimes services are provided in nursery schools, child care centers, Head Start programs, and private schools (Clark and Mazza, 1999). Services include educational programs, psychological services for children with behavioral problems, developmental evaluations, speech and language therapy, physical therapy, nutrition services, and social services for the family.

### *Referral Process*

Most minority people will only go to the hospital for physical and/or mental problems when the problem is unmanageable and they have no other choice but to go to the emergency room (Biegel, McCardle, and Mendelson, 1985). However, after many years of prevention and health promotion activities, churches, faith-based groups, and other community agencies have formed networks with hospitals and mental health centers in their communities and have begun to refer individuals to the services they need. Many churches have pastoral counselors on staff, who in addition to their religious duties, provide basic crisis counseling and if necessary refer individuals to the appropriate social services or health agencies.

Sometimes reports of child abuse are presented to pastoral counselors or schoolteachers who are obligated to report the abuse, including elder abuse, to the appropriate child services agency or local child welfare office. This same mandate or responsibility for child or elder abuse reporting is also applicable to allied health services personnel who are presented with or have evidence of abuse. Child abuse is much easier to report (particularly if it is self-evident) than elder abuse, since the elderly are less inclined to report the abuse for fear of retaliation from the abusing person. Nevertheless, it is worth reporting these cases for corrective action.

### COMPLEMENTARY AND ALTERNATIVE MEDICINE TREATMENTS

Beyond the traditional cadre of health care professionals which includes physicians, nurses, and allied health services personnel, there has been an emergence of alternative therapy professionals and modalities which have now become part of mainstream medicine in the United States. In 1997 more than 40 percent of Americans used complementary and alternative medical treatments and therapies for a wide range of health problems (NIH, 1994). Many people began using alternative medicines because they were cheaper, effective, and generally safe. Popular complementary and alternative treatment therapies include iridology, traditional oriental medicines (including acupuncture), touch therapies, biotechnomagnetic applications, foot reflexology, and homeopathic medicines.

*Chiropractic services* are some of the first complementary therapies to merge with the mainstream medical profession. Chiropractic services, which are now very popular, are based on the chiropractic physician's ability to diagnose and treat existing pathologies and dysfunctions by specific manual and physiological procedures. They are now covered by many insurance carriers.

*Iridology* is the study of the coloration and fiber structure of the eye for indicators of an individual's inherited and acquired tendencies toward health and disease, his or her current condition in general, and the state of every organ in particular. Iridology cannot detect a specific disease, but can tell individuals if they have overactivity or underactivity in specific areas of the body. For example, an underactive pancreas might indicate a diabetic condition. Iridology is a system that leads to a provisional diagnosis on its own, and typically a very accurate one. It should be combined with clinical and differential diagnosis as well as other reliable diagnostic methods. Iridology can detect health factors related to a given syndrome that may be very difficult to determine by other, more orthodox, diagnostic procedures. In this way iridology is an excellent tool for detecting underlying health factors. Iridology can also show the course a disease or disorder is following, what factors are preventing a quick and full recovery, and indicate the most suitable therapy (International Iridology Practitioners Association, 2002).

Iridology accurately shows the inherent ability of the individual's tissues to cleanse and heal themselves, also known as constitution. It also shows where these constitutional weaknesses exist and which are the weakest links in the individual's "chain of health." Consequently, these constitutional weaknesses can be guarded to prevent potential problems, especially those that are chronically degenerative. Although iridology cannot specifically name the type of infection, it will indicate the infection's intensity and effects on both local areas and the person as a whole. More important, it can detect factors involving the immune system that may need attention to overcome the infection or illness. Howard University is currently studying iridology, it's efficiency, how it works, and its role in preventive medicine. Iridology is well on its way to becoming the medicine of the future.

*Traditional Oriental medicine* is widely known in the United States. Besides acupuncture and acupressure, it includes herbal medicines and oils, Qigong, and oriental massage techniques including cupping and moxibustion.

*Acupuncture* is another widely-used alternative therapy that is gaining popularity throughout the United States, including in schools of medicine. Acupuncture involves the stimulation of specific anatomic points in the body for therapeutic healing purposes. It is performed by puncturing the skin with special, thin, wire-like needles. However, acupuncture practitioners also use heat, pressure, friction, suction, and/or electromagnetic energy impulses to stimulate the points. It has been successfully used to help drug abusers prevent relapse. It promotes relaxation and temporary, as well as permanent, relief for a number of chronic ailments such as back pain and arthritis. Several insurance carriers provide coverage for this service and more are expected to include this treatment modality in their plans.

*Acupressure* is very similar to acupuncture. Acupressure stimulates various points and muscles through applied pressure from the fingertips or hands of the therapist.

*Qigong* is the art and science of using breath, movement, and medication to cleanse, strengthen, and circulate vital life energy (Ying and Yang) and blood. The art of Qigong is used in Tai Chi, as well as other practices of oriental physical movements that emphasize maintaining internal and external balance within one's environment. Qigong is a slow and purposeful exercise practiced by many elder Chinese Americans in Chinese-American neighborhood parks. Other types of manual therapy for the entire body system include Shiatsu and Jin Shin Jyutus (NIH, 1994), which involve applying milder pressure along eight extra energy meridians.

*Cupping* is the technique of applying suction over an ailing part of the body. A vacuum is created by warming the air in a jar, cup, or small glass of bamboo then overturning it and placing it on the body in order to disperse areas of local congestion. Cupping is used to treat arthritis, bronchitis, sprains, and other ailments.

*Moxibustion* is a common practice among Asians, and can often be seen at clinics where recent immigrants or refugees are treated. Based on the therapeutic value of heat, moxibustion is performed by heating pulverized wormwood and applying it to the skin over specific meridians. It can be very helpful for women during labor and delivery periods (Lecca et al., 1998).

*Community-based folk care practices* are varied and practiced throughout the United States. They range from Native American folk practice to immigrant and minority health care practices.

*Shamanic healing,* performed by a shaman healer, is found worldwide. Traditional shamans are usually skilled in manipulative or herbal practices that help cure spiritual and physical ailments.

*Native American health care* practices include *sweating and purging,* two spiritual cleansing and healing techniques that are usually held in a steam-filled teepee (water is poured over hot rocks to produce a saunalike atmosphere). Other Native American practices include herbal remedies, shamanic healing, healing ceremonies performed by medicine men or medicine women, and singing and chanting.

*Latin American folk practices* are used by Hispanic Americans in South and Central America, particularly in rural areas where there is a shortage of medical doctors, and in the United States. Commonly used by Mexican

Americans, South Americans, and Caribbeans, as well as individuals living in the southwestern United States, *Curanderismo* is based on healing with indigenous plants and herbs in the form of curative potions and the laying on of hands. Another indigenous healing practice is *Espiritismo* (spiritism or spiritualism). It is practiced among Puerto Ricans, Dominicans, and other Hispanic cultural groups. It is based on a belief of the existence of an invisible world of disembodied spirits that interact and communicate with the living. Espiritismo is based on the writings of Allan Kardec ([1869] 1951) who argued that people can develop their mental faculties to the point where their spirit guides can lead them through life's difficulties. *Santeria* is both an alternative religion and a folk-healing system with a *santero* and *santera* as priest or priestess. It is a religious cult practiced by Hispanics in general and Cubans in particular. Santeria is a blend of African religion and Christianity that involves witchcraft, magic, and ritualistic use of herbal potions or baths to alter the influence of spirits. Another religion similar to Santeria is *voodoo,* which is practiced in Haiti. Voodoo is conducted by an *ungar* (priest or priestess).

Among the *African-American community* prayer is one of the most common practices for treating illnesses. Many African Americans believe some people possess a power to heal and help others. There are also many healers in African-American communities, which is reflected in Maya Angelou's *I Know Why the Caged Bird Sings* (Spector, 1991). Also, many African Americans use African-American folk health practices (many of which originated in Africa), as well as some of the practices used by other racial or ethnic groups mentioned earlier. This is particularly true for low-income African Americans who live in or adjacent to other ethnic or racial communities. African-American practices can range from home remedies to putting a "fix" or "mojo" on someone. Some home remedies include the use of sugar and turpentine to rid worms or cure a backache, sassafras to treat colds, salt and pork to treat wounds, two pieces of silverware to treat a "crick" in the neck, clay placed in a dark leaf and wrapped around a sprained ankle, or garlic to remove evil spirits (Lecca et al., 1998).

### Government Promotion

In addition to the practice of alternative treatment approaches mentioned previously, many schools of medicine include courses on complementary and alternative medicines within their curriculum. Some universities, including the University of California and the University of Illinois at Chicago, have been awarded five-year federal grants of $1.5 million per year to conduct research on botanicals, including issues of safety, effectiveness, and biological action. The University of Utah's school of medicine received $6.6 million to study 1,200 patients with osteoarthritis and the use of glucosamine and chondroitin sulfate to reduce joint pain and improve mobility.

The National Institute of Health's National Center for Complementary and Alternative Medicine (NCCAM) received $68.7 million to conduct research, support research training, and disseminate information on validated therapies. Among its initiatives is a study of the demographics, prevalence, and patterns of use of complementary and alternative medicines within minority and underserved populations which have used traditional and folk medicines for centuries (NCCAM, 2002). Another major proposal includes a study on the use of *Ginkgo biloba* to prevent dementia and other intellectual dysfunctions in older adults. In conjunction with NCCAM, NIMH will conduct the first rigorous clinical trial of St. John's wort and its long-term effect on depression. Three hundred thirty-six patients at twelve clinical sites will be studied.

The nursing profession, which is credited with the community-based health practice movement, has now moved on to holistic nursing. Holistic nursing involves studying and understanding the interrelationships of the biological, psychological, social, and spiritual dimensions of the person (Dossey et al., 1995). In other words, it means treating the whole individual in an integrated manner that includes community and immediate surroundings.

Along with these promotional and research activities, there have been numerous national studies such as Boston University's Black Women's Health Study (BWHS). The BWHS is a longitudinal study of a large group of black women that will examine the causes and prevention of illness (Rosenberg et al., 1995).

Teleconferencing is a growing technology that has taken root throughout the United States, particularly at medical institutions, and has begun to spread to a number of different institutions, including forensic and prison health services. Teleconferencing is ideal for large rural areas, such as in Africa or Australia, which do not have the luxury of having health care specialists on hand. With the advent of computers, modem hardware, and video cameras, teleconferencing makes it convenient and cheaper to have a specialist or psychiatrist make an assessment (in conjunction with the primary physician) and recommend a treatment plan.

## REFERENCES

Biegel, D., McCardle, E., and Mendelson, S. (1985). *Social Networks and Mental Health: An Annotated Bibliography.* Beverly Hills, CA: Sage Publications, Inc.

Dossey, B., Keegan, L., Guzzetta, C., and Kolkmeier, L. (1995). *Holistic Nursing: A Handbook for Practice*. Gaithersburg, MD: Aspen Publishers, Inc.

International Iridology Practitioners Association (2002). *Overview of Iridology*. Retrieved from the World Wide Web: <http://www.iridologyassn.org>.

Kardec, A. ([1869] 1951). *El Libro de los Espiritos*. Mexico City: Orion.

Lecca, P., Quervalu, I., Nunes, J., and Gonzales, H. (1998). *Cultural Competency in Health, Social, and Human Services*. New York: Garland Publishing, Inc.

National Institute of Health (1994). *Alternative Medicine, Expanding Medical Horizons: A Report to the National Institutes of Health on Alternative Medical Systems and Practices in the United States*. Washington, DC: NIH publication no. 94-066.

National Institute of Health (2000). *Mental Health and Mental Disorders* (Chapter 18). Retrieved from the World Wide Web: <http://www.healthypeople.gov>.

National Institute of Health (2001). *Community-Based Models*. Retrieved from the World Wide Web: <http://www.nlm.nih.gov/pubs/cbm/cbmodels.html>.

National Institute of Health, National Center for Complementary and Alternative Medicine (2002). *Expanding Horizons of Health Care*. Retrieved from the World Wide Web: <http://nccam.nih.gov/an/research_progress/part4.html>.

National Library of Medicine (1993). *Depression in Primary Care: Detection and Diagnosis*. Vol. 1, *Detection and Diagnosis, Clinical Guideline Number 5*. Washington, DC: AHCPR publication, National Library of Medicine.

Nies, M. and McEwen, M. (2001). *Community Health Nursing: Promoting the Health of Populations,* Third Edition. Philadelphia, PA: W.B. Saunders Company.

Primary Care Research in Substance Abuse and Mental Health for the Elderly (2001). Retrieved from the World Wide Web: <http://www.hms.harvard.edu/aging/mhsa/index.html>.

Rabins, C. III, Frank, E., Perl, J., Imber, S., et al. (1996). The prevalence of psychiatric disorders in elderly residents of public housing. *Journal of Gerontology: Medical Sciences,* 51A, no. 6, M319-M324.

Rosenberg, L., Adams-Campbell, L., Palmer, J. (1995). The black women's health study: A follow-up study for causes and prevention of illness studies. *Journal of the American Women's Association,* vol. 50, no. 2.

Spector, R. (1991). *Cultural Diversity in Health and Illness*. Norwalk, CT: Appleton and Lange.

United States Department of Health and Human Services (2000). Healthy People 2010. Retrieved from the World Wide Web: <http://www.health.gov/healthy people>.

Chapter 10

# Demographic and Health Trends in the Twenty-First Century

Richard E. Oliver
Stephen L. Wilson

Roy, a seventy-one-year-old retired merchant, lives in a small rural community with his wife. His children are grown and live many miles away in other states. Roy has diabetes. His wife works at a local department store to maintain the health insurance that helps pay for Roy's medical supplies and prescription drugs which can cost more than $1,000 per month. Roy's diabetes has resulted in a below-the-knee amputation on one leg. He also has numerous other chronic conditions, but is still able to live independently with his wife in their two-story country home.

Roy is becoming increasingly concerned about maintaining his independence and the pressure he has placed on his wife to keep her job. He requires regular care from a wide range of health professionals whom he believes are not communicating with one another or with him in the most effective manner. Roy is becoming increasingly depressed and does not know how he can continue to live this way.

Roy reflects a demographic reality that is of increasing concern in this country. As an elderly person with multiple chronic conditions, he is fortunate to have a spouse who is able to help support him. Living in a rural area, he is dependent on the provision of sophisticated, coordinated health care services, which are not always available in sparsely settled areas. As the population ages and health costs increase, the challenge of providing high quality health care to all Americans, regardless of age, residence, and health status, will be a daunting task.

The health care delivery system is directly impacted by a number of demographic trends that are occurring across the United States. Several of the

We are indebted to Tracy Dranginis for providing the graphics used in this chapter and to Deborah Kennedy for providing helpful comments and suggestions.

more important trends will be covered in this chapter, along with a discussion of the implications for health care and the allied health professions.

Over several decades, many demographic trends related to population shifts have occurred. The 2000 census revealed that 281.4 million people were counted in the United States, a 13.2 percent increase from the 1990s. According to the census, every state grew in population, although the trend was toward significant increases in western and southern states with less growth in the midwestern and northeastern states. Colorado, Utah, and Idaho had the largest increases in terms of percentage of population, while California, Texas, Georgia, and Arizona had the largest increases in terms of numbers of people. Over the next two decades, the increased growth pattern in western and southern states is expected to continue (see Figure 10.1).

The population increase was most reflected in urban areas, which experienced strong growth in the 1990s. In 2000, 80.3 percent of Americans lived in metropolitan areas, up slightly from 79.8 percent in 1990. While the largest metropolitan areas continued to include such cities as New York, Los Angeles, and the Washington-Baltimore area, the fastest growing metropolitan areas included Las Vegas, Nevada; Naples, Florida; Fayetteville, Arkansas; and Phoenix, Arizona.[1] Growth in these latter cities is partly related to their attractiveness as retirement communities.

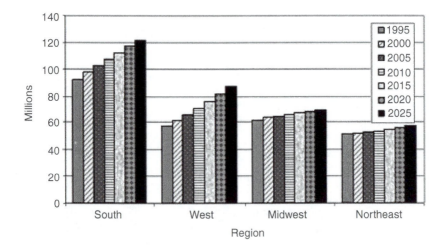

FIGURE 10.1. U.S. Population Distribution by Geographic Region 1995 to 2025 (*Source:* U.S. Census Bureau, Population Division, PPL-47).

## AGING POPULATION

Over the next thirty to fifty years, the most critical demographic in the United States will be the aging population. The baby boomer cohort (born between 1946 and 1962) will be reaching retirement age during the next twenty years. This cohort represents a segment of Americans that are getting older and living longer, a fact that will have a major impact on everything economic, social, and political in the United States.

Currently, every state and region of the country is affected by the aging population. Among the elderly (age sixty-five and older), more than 50 percent live in nine states: California, Florida, New York, Texas, Pennsylvania, Ohio, Illinois, Michigan, and New Jersey. Between 1990 and 1999, twelve states, mostly southern and western, had increases of 17 percent or more in their elderly populations: Nevada, Alaska, Arizona, Hawaii, Colorado, Utah, New Mexico, Delaware, South Carolina, North Carolina, Wyoming, and Texas. Many of the elderly represent significant levels of poverty in several states, including Mississippi, Louisiana, the District of Columbia, Arkansas, West Virginia, New Mexico, Texas, Alabama, New York, and North Carolina.[2]

All states have significant portions of the elderly who live in rural areas. In general, people age sixty-five and older are slightly less likely to live in metropolitan areas than younger people. Currently, nearly 15 percent (61 million people) of the United States' rural population is age sixty-five and older.[3]

In 2000, the population age sixty-five and older numbered 34.5 million and represented 12.7 percent of the United States population. This meant that one of every eight Americans was over age sixty-five. Of this number, 20.2 million were older women and 14.3 million were older men.[4] Future projections are even more significant. The older population will continue to grow, particularly between the years 2010 and 2030, when the baby-boom generation reaches age sixty-five. While the population age eighteen to sixty-four will decline by more than 6 percent from 2000 to 2050, the population age sixty-five and older will increase to nearly 25 percent of the total population by 2050 (see Figure 10.2).

Over the next fifty years, the population landscape will be transformed to the point that one person in every four will be age sixty-five and older. Furthermore, significant numbers of this population are expected to represent minorities; 25.4 percent of the elderly population in 2030 will represent an ethnic group compared to 16.1 percent in 1999.

As the aging population increases, the differences within this cohort will become more striking. From 2000 to 2050, the cohort age sixty-five to seventy-four will more than double in number, while the cohort age seventy-

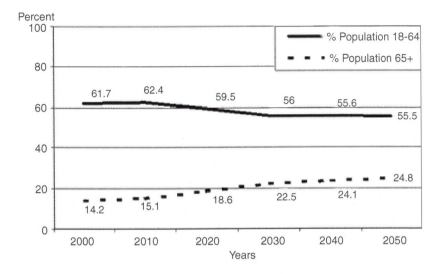

FIGURE 10.2. Percent of Population by Age Group, 2000 to 2050 (*Source:* U.S. Census Bureau, Current Population Reports, P25–1130, *Population Projections of the United States by Age, Sex, Race, and Hispanic Origin 1995 to 2050*).

five to eighty-four will increase more than 150 percent. However, the major change will be reflected in the cohort age eighty-five and older (old-old) which will nearly quadruple in size and comprise about 5 percent of the population in 2050 (see Figure 10.3).

The impact can be best understood by examining the numbers in this cohort, which will increase from about 35 million people in 2000 to nearly 82 million in 2050. Such an increase emphasizes the size and longevity of this cohort. With regard to health care, both acute care and chronic care expenses will increase, but extended longevity, particularly within the cohort age eighty-five and older, could result in much greater spending for long-term care. The financial impact will be profound.[5] There is considerable concern the United States will not be able to respond and provide the services needed for this population through traditional programs currently in place, such as Medicare.

An aging population presents significant challenges for the health care system. A greater incidence of health problems and greater need for assistance are an inherent part of the aging process (see Figure 10.4). Particularly, aging inevitably results in an increase in chronic health problems such as diabetes, congestive heart failure, stroke, Alzheimer's disease, and arthritis. The impact of these conditions on the health care system will intensify

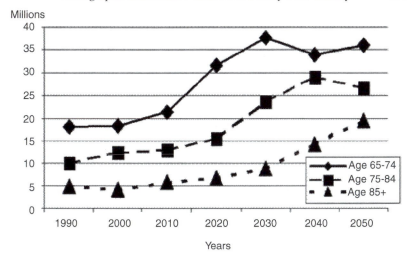

FIGURE 10.3. Population of Persons Age Sixty-Five and Over: 1990 to 2050 (*Source:* U.S. Census Bureau [NP-T4], *Projections of the Total Resident Population by 5-Year Age Groups, Race, and Hispanic Origin with Special Age Categories Middle Series 1999 to 2100*).

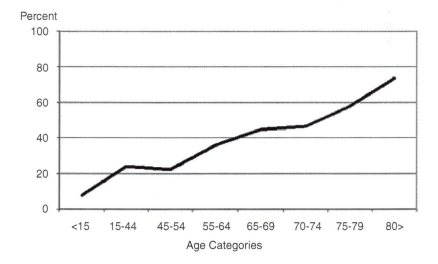

FIGURE 10.4. Percent of Population Needing Assistance by Age, 1997 (*Source:* U.S. Census Bureau Survey of Income and Program Participation, August–November 1997).

as both the longevity and number of persons over the age of eighty-five put additional stress on earmarked resources and other budgetary reserves.[6]

As the elderly increasingly challenge the resources of the health care system, health practitioners will, more than ever, have to be prepared to practice in an environment of geriatric care. This means developing sensitivity to the needs of the elderly, as well as recognizing that as chronic conditions increase, there may be less support that can be reasonably provided through the traditional health care system. Attending to end-of-life issues will be imperative. It is said that a person in the final weeks of life can often consume health care resources equal to those consumed during his or her entire life span. As the population ages, the health care system will be stretched to its limits. The art of making symptoms manageable and helping patients to live fully within the constraints imposed by disease will be key to successful health care.[7]

Maintaining independence will be an important goal since the older population will desire to have maximum freedom in the least restrictive environment. For the most part, the older population will continue to reside in their own homes for as long as possible, which will sometimes make it difficult to provide coordinated services. Community-based support systems will be needed since this population will, in many cases, require partial care that does not have to be provided through the traditional health care system. Home modification programs and alternative housing such as assisted living residences and continuing care retirement communities will become important options for elders. Alternative and complementary modes of care, such as adult day care and day hospitals, will also become more popular. Providing accommodations to support elderly populations living in rural communities will be particularly difficult, where in addition to the usual challenges of chronic disease and functional decline, this population often faces significant geographic isolation.

Another important demographic trend is that as the population ages, women will steadily increase their influence within the health care system. Women tend to live longer than men and, as the baby boom cohort ages, the senior age groups will be increasingly represented by females.[8] Recently, there has been acknowledgment that women have specific health needs that have not been well addressed within the health care system.[9] Over the next three decades, the significant size of the female baby-boomer cohort will clearly impact on the direction of health care.

Except for the unsuccessful efforts of the Clinton administration, the United States government did little to address policy issues related to improving the health care system during the last decade of the twentieth century. During the next two decades of the twenty-first century, the true impact of the increasing aging population will confront the health care system. Clear policies that ensure proper health care for the elderly will be required.

Policy issues must ensure the Medicare program is adequately funded to provide benefits for an increasing population that will require health services longer than any other previous generation. Complex questions related to providing a drug insurance benefit and addressing the high costs of long-term care are only a few of the issues that need to be resolved. Finally, as the elderly population increases, the number of people within the younger cohorts will decrease. The health care industry will recruit workers from an increasingly smaller work force at a time when significant numbers will be needed with the education, skills, sensitivity, and commitment to care for the elderly.

As the United States prepares for an aging population that will consume more health resources, every state will experience an increase in numbers of aging in cities, towns, and rural communities. The burden will be greater in southern and western states where more of the elderly population will be located. This will place a significant strain on the health care systems and educational systems that must prepare the health workforce in these parts of the country. It will be the responsibility of both state and federal governments to address these challenges early in the twenty-first century.

## *RACIAL AND ETHNIC DIVERSITY*

Traditionally, the United States has attracted myriad cultures from around the world. This racial and ethnic diversity has provided a rich heritage for the country with an impact that will be even more profound in the twenty-first century. From 1990 to 1999, the United States became more ethnically diverse than ever before, with significant growth among racial and ethnic groups. However, not all segments of the population grew at the same rate. Rapid growth occurred in the Asian and Pacific Islander and Hispanic populations, fueled by immigration. Although the Asian and Pacific Islander population accounted for only 4 percent of the total population, it was the fastest growing racial or ethnic group over the ten-year period, with a growth rate of 45 percent and a total of eleven million people. During the same period, Hispanics were the second fastest growing racial or ethnic group with a population increase of 40 percent. This raised the Hispanic cohort from 9 percent to 11.5 percent of the United States' population, with a total of 31 million people. The black population in the United States increased by a rate of 14 percent to a total of 35 million people. The growth rate of whites was only 4 percent with a total of 196 million people.[10] The Latin American, Indian, and Alaskan Native populations also experienced population growth, but at a lesser rate.

From 2000 to 2050, the minority and ethnic demographics will continue to change. While the white population will gradually decrease from 75 percent of the population in 2000 to a little over 50 percent of the population in 2050, minority and ethnic populations will increase. From 2000 to 2050, the black population will continue to increase slightly, while the Asian and Pacific Islander population will increase by about 6 percent. Perhaps most dramatic will be the continuing increase in the Hispanic population. Over the next fifty years, the Hispanic population will increase to almost 30 percent of the population in the United States. By 2050, the Asian, black, and Hispanic populations will nearly equal the white population in the United States (see Figure 10.5). As noted in the discussion on aging demographics, many people within these racial and ethic groups will comprise part of the cohort age sixty-five and older.

As society becomes more multicultural, the health care system will have to face the challenge of caring for people of diverse cultures who speak different languages and have different levels of acculturation, socioeconomic statuses, and unique ways of understanding illness and health. Most health systems, as well as the health care workforce, are inadequately prepared for providing care to these populations. Health care organizations must offer a culturally sensitive environment in which potential clients and families feel comfortable that their unique values and beliefs are understood and respected.[11] The health care workforce must be prepared to work within a care

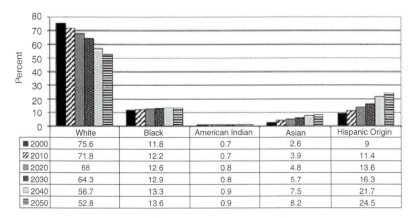

| | White | Black | American Indian | Asian | Hispanic Origin |
|---|---|---|---|---|---|
| ■ 2000 | 75.6 | 11.8 | 0.7 | 2.6 | 9 |
| ▨ 2010 | 71.8 | 12.2 | 0.7 | 3.9 | 11.4 |
| ▥ 2020 | 68 | 12.6 | 0.8 | 4.8 | 13.6 |
| ■ 2030 | 64.3 | 12.9 | 0.8 | 5.7 | 16.3 |
| ▢ 2040 | 56.7 | 13.3 | 0.9 | 7.5 | 21.7 |
| ▤ 2050 | 52.8 | 13.6 | 0.9 | 8.2 | 24.5 |

FIGURE 10.5. Percent Distribution of Population by Race and Hispanic Origin, 1990-2050 (*Source:* U.S. Census Bureau, Current Population Reports, P25–1130, *Population Projections of the United States by Age, Sex, Race, and Hispanic Origin 1995 to 2050*). Persons of Hispanic origin may be of any race, but do not include citizens of Puerto Rico. American Indian represents American Indians, Eskimos, and Aleuts. Asian represents Asians and Pacific Islanders.

environment in which cross-cultural competency conveys a sensitivity to different racial and ethnic backgrounds.[12] Equally important is the fact that the United States health care workforce does not reflect the racial and ethnic makeup of those being served. It is imperative that greater attention be given to creating a multicultural work force capable of meeting the demands of the twenty-first century.

## POVERTY AND UNDERSERVED POPULATIONS

Another demographic that has an impact on many dimensions of health care is the large segment of the United States population that is living in poverty. Individuals in this category include significant numbers of the elderly, urban poor and homeless, and rural populations that live below poverty levels. The underserved and poor populations are also disproportionately represented by minority and ethnic populations.

Although the number of persons living in poverty has declined recently, the reasons that cause these conditions remain (see Figure 10.6). It can be expected that addressing problems related to those living below poverty levels will be a national priority for decades to come. Many of those living at poverty levels are dependent upon state and federally subsidized programs, such as the Medicaid program, for access to health care. Others, many of whom work at low wage jobs, have limited or no health insurance.

Many are women and children, who have existed on the periphery of the traditional health care system. About 44 million Americans are currently

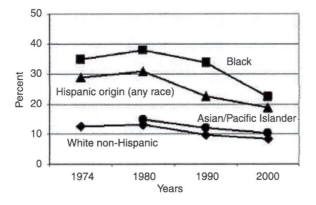

FIGURE 10.6. Persons older than 65 Living in Poverty by Race and Hispanic Origin, 1974-2000 (*Source:* U.S. Census Bureau, *Poverty in the United States, 2000*, P60–214).

uninsured. Of these, approximately 60 percent live in families with incomes below the federal poverty level. Assuming current trends related to employee-based health insurance, immigration, and income support programs continue, it is expected that the number of uninsured will increase over the next decade. This group is particularly prone to poor health, financial hardship, and family dysfunction.[13]

Although the poor access traditional health care sources, they receive much of their medical care from hospitals, clinics, and physicians that are separate and distinct from the facilities used by those who are insured. Currently, much of the medical care for the poor is delivered through emergency rooms and neighborhood clinics supported by voluntary agencies, hospitals, and government programs. Despite the availability of such care, there is a disparity since the uninsured are less likely than those who are insured to have a usual source of direct care. Although the health care system has traditionally allowed the uninsured to receive uncompensated care through hospitals and physicians, financial pressures have eroded these sources of care.[14]

Efforts have been made to provide organized and cost-effective care to the poor. Medicaid HMOs have tried to deliver care to the underserved but with mixed results. Inner-city hospitals and university-based medical centers have, for many years, provided medical care to the poor. More recently, these institutions have run into financial difficulty as federal reimbursements have decreased and health care costs have increased. Many of these institutions have relocated to suburbs while others have simply closed.[15] Academic health centers, many of which are located close to poverty populations, have helped provide care to the uninsured but this has not been enough. Furthermore, the health care system has not been successful in locating health care providers, particularly physicians, in communities in which the poor live.[16]

The reality of poverty will not be solved in the twenty-first century but it is imperative that these populations, including those with low income and the uninsured, have access to the same level of health care as others in the United States, something that has not always been the case in the past. There are major policy issues that will need to be addressed regarding how states and the federal government will provide health care to those unable to pay for it.

## CHANGES IN THE FAMILY STRUCTURE

Over the past three decades, changes in the American nuclear family structure have been significant with a shift toward nontraditional families, including dual workforce and single head of household families. One major dimension has been the movement of women into the workforce while still maintaining traditional responsibilities within the family unit. The participation of women in the workforce tripled from 1950 to 1985.[17] In 1988, 64 percent of families were characterized as dual workforce families, a trend that is continuing into the twenty-first century.[18]

Other changes have occurred for women. A significant shift has occurred in women's roles to increasingly include that of head of the family. In 1991, 19 percent of white families were headed by single mothers, while 58 percent of African-American families and 29 percent of Hispanic families were headed by single mothers. These households share fewer economic resources than those of dual workforce families. Over 50 percent of families headed by single mothers live below the poverty level.[19]

In both dual workforce families and families headed by females, women usually assume the role of caregiver for both children and increasingly, for aging parents.[20] All of these changes have resulted in a combination of factors, e.g., stress, lack of money, more responsibility, and less time, that contribute to unique health issues experienced by women. In addition, the expense and challenge of raising children is enormous and many times there are insufficient health care systems for these families. There is sufficient evidence to show single mothers, as well as their children, are at risk for health problems that are not always well addressed by the health care systems.[21]

Following the trends in the latter part of the twentieth century, it can be expected that the United States will experience continuing changes in family structures. Through 2010, traditional families will continue to decline, while households headed by single persons will increase in frequency (see Figure 10.7). Changing family structures will force the health care delivery system to adapt to more nontraditional populations where such issues as access and continuity of care will be critically important.

The nontraditional populations of both dual workforce families and single head of household families will require convenient primary care that is available outside of traditional work hours, ideally on a 24/7 basis. Many working households, particularly among poorer populations, may have difficulty even accessing care sites. Although it is unlikely, the possibility of home visits by physicians or other primary care professionals would certainly improve access to care. It can be expected that large numbers of working families will be required to provide support for aging parents and other relatives as well, further necessitating a flexible health care system. Families will require job flexibility to be able to provide support for family members during periods of sickness or disability. Transportation systems may have to be in place so families can easily travel to and from appointments.

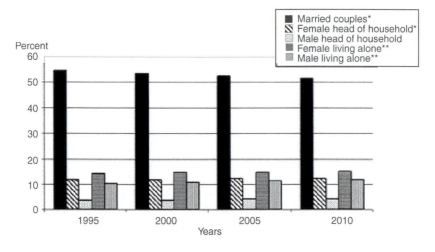

*Family Households
**Nonfamily Households (individuals living alone or nonrelated individuals)

FIGURE 10.7. Projections of Household Type, 1995–2010 (*Source:* U.S. Census Bureau Current Population Reports, P25–1129 *Projection of Number of Households and Families in U.S. 1995-2010*).

The health care system will have to respond to changing family structures in the United States. Federal support programs such as the Children's Health Insurance Program (CHIP) and Special Supplemental Nutrition Program for Women, Infants, and Children (WIC) will need to be more fully advertised. Policy opportunities for the twenty-first century might include increasing Medicaid support to more children and providing better compensation for health professionals who work with Medicaid recipients. Finally, access to quality health care will be a continuing challenge for populations in underserved urban and rural areas.[22]

## DEMOGRAPHIC CHANGES
## AND THE ALLIED HEALTH PROFESSIONS

This chapter identifies several demographic shifts occurring in the United States that will have major impacts through the next century. These changes will affect the total social, political, and economic fabric of the country. For the health care delivery system, these impacts will be tremendous as systems will have to adjust and new systems will have to be devised to address the changing needs of the population. For the allied health professions, it will be a time of challenge and change as these shifting demographics result in different patients/clients entering the health care system.

Perhaps the most dramatic shift will be the impact of the aging population over the next twenty years. In terms of sheer numbers, allied health professionals can expect their patient/client population will be comprised mostly of the elderly. An aging population that is living longer with increasing acute and chronic health problems offers both challenges and opportunities every allied health profession must be well prepared to respond to. Professionals such as rehabilitation specialists, dietitians, and physician assistants will have to ensure the aging population remains functional and productive, even as more of the aging enter the old-old (age eighty-five and older) cohort. Other professionals such as clinical laboratory scientists, respiratory care providers, and radiography technicians, will have to ensure they provide the highest quality care as the elderly utilize the health care system. Allied health professionals will have to be more than technically prepared to serve an older population. They will have to be particularly sensitive to the physical and psychological aging process, demonstrate a positive professional attitude toward this population, and understand that aging is a normal life process and the elderly can be happy, fully functioning individuals who continue to add value to society.

It is important to note that a significant part of the health care workforce, and certainly the allied health workforce, belongs to the baby-boomer cohort. The possibility of a shrinking workforce and particularly of a smaller allied health workforce within the next two decades is very real. Between 2000 and 2030 the ratio of potential workers (age eighteen to twenty-four) to older adults (age sixty-five and older) will dramatically decrease from 4.8 to 1 to 2.8 to 1.[23] The decrease in the workforce will have an impact on virtually every economic sector of the country, including the health care workforce. Unless incentives are put in place, many allied health professionals will leave the health care workforce when they reach the age of retirement. The volatility of the health care system during the late 1990s helped create low levels of satisfaction among health practitioners. If this situation continues in the twenty-first century, there may be few incentives to remain in the workforce. As these practitioners retire, they will likely leave major staffing shortages within the health care system. Besides providing incentives to stay in the workforce, the challenge for the educational sector must be to insure that a sufficient supply of competent, well-educated professionals will be available for the health care workforce. Opportunities must be provided for educational institutions to prepare enough practitioners to meet the health care needs of an increasing older population, and replace retiring practitioners.

An equally important demographic trend will be the increased ethnic and minority populations in the United States. As the white and ethnic/minority populations change in size, health care systems will be responsible for providing accessible, sensitive care. Allied health professional programs will need to include curricula based on cultural sensitivity, and allow students to practice providing care to those with individual and cultural differences. This also virtually mandates that all allied health professions give serious attention to diversifying the workforce and prepare multilingual practitioners who can communicate and care for expanding patient populations. For instance, in allied health educational programs, minorities represent about 20 percent of enrollment,[24] yet the populations allied health professionals serve will increasingly represent ethnic and minority groups with different values and beliefs that can directly affect the quality of the care given. The need for all health professions to ensure a multicultural workforce is put in place to care for an increasingly diverse population is absolutely essential.

Allied health professionals will need to be particularly sensitive to the needs of the underserved and those living in poverty. Professional programs will need to educate future allied health professionals on the importance of working in underserved communities, and provide clinical opportunities to practice in these settings. Curricula should also include material and experiences that teach students cultural sensitivity. Educational programs will need to prepare graduates for work in nontraditional environments such as community-based clinics and other ambulatory care sites. Many colleges and universities are already encouraging or requiring students to complete service learning opportunities as part of their curriculum. Opportunities for allied health students to work in underserved areas and with poor populations can provide exciting experiences that sensitize as well as excite students about working in underserved environments. Since many of the underserved and poor live in less populated and poorly served areas of the country, clinical experiences should be extended to rural areas.

In summary, allied health professionals will have to be educated differently to provide health care to an older and increasingly diverse population. With workforce shortages potentially impacting all sectors of the United States' economy, every effort must be made to ensure that allied health professions are seen as stimulating, enjoyable careers and that the health care industry is a satisfying, prestigious place to work. While allied health professionals' technical skills will certainly change over time, particularly with advances in technology or research, the real challenge will be to provide professionals with the interpersonal skills they need to care for an increasingly diverse population. These demographic changes are occurring now and will become more pronounced over the next two decades. How the allied health professions address these realities will determine the extent to which the care they give is caring, sensitive, and humane in the twenty-first century.

## REFERENCE NOTES

1. U.S. Census Bureau, *Census 2000 Brief: Population Change and Distribution, 1990 to 2000*, pp. 3-6. Retrieved from the World Wide Web: <http://www. census.gov/prod/2001pubs/ c2kbr01-2.pdf>.

2. U.S. Administration on Aging. *Profile of Older Americans: 2000.* Retrieved from the World Wide Web: <http://www.aoa.gov/aoa/stats/profile>.

3. Thomas C. Rosenthal and Chester Fox. Access to Health Care for the Rural Elderly. *The Journal of the American Medical Association 284*(16):2034-2036.

4. U.S. Administration on Aging. *Profile of Older Americans: 2000, p. 1.*

5. Brenda C. Spillman and James Lubitz. The Effect of Longevity on Spending for Acute and Long-Term Care. *The New England Journal of Medicine 342*(19): 1409-1415.

6. U.S. Administration on Aging (2000). *Older Population by Age: 1990 to 2050.* Based on data from the U.S. Census Bureau. Retrieved from the World Wide Web: <http://www.aoa.gov>.

7. Joanne Lynn. Learning to Care for People with Chronic Illness Facing the End of Life. *The Journal of the American Medical Association 284*(19):2508-2511.

8. MHS Staff. Women's Health: Marketing Challenges for the 21st Century. *Marketing Health Services 20*(3):4-11.

9. Bernadine Healy (1995). *A New Prescription for Women's Health.* New York: Penguin Books, pp. 24-25.

10. The U.S. Census Bureau. *Population Profile of the United States: 1999.* Retrieved from the World Wide Web: <http://www.census.gov/population/www/pop-profile/profile1999.html>.

11. Bettie Jackson. Subtle and Not So Subtle Insensitivity to Ethnic Diversity. *Journal of Nursing Administration 28*(12):11-14.

12. J. Emilio Corrilio, Alexander Green, and Joseph Betancourt. Cross-Cultural Primary Care: A Patient Based Approach. *Annals of Internal Medicine 130*(10): 829-834.

13. Institute of Medicine (2000). *Informing the Future: Critical Issues in Health.* Washington, DC: National Academy Press.

14. Steven A. Schroeder. Prospects for Expanding Health Care Insurance Coverage. *The New England Journal of Medicine 344*(11):847-852.

15. Eli Ginzberg. Improving Health Care for the Poor: Lessons from the 1980s. *The Journal of the American Medical Association 271*(6):464-467.

16. Eli Ginzburg, Miriam Ostow, and Anna B. Dutka (1993). *The Economics of Medical Education.* New York: Josiah Macy Jr., Foundation.

17. Howard Hayghe (1986). Rise in Mother's Labor Force Activity Includes Those with Infants. *Monthly Labor Review 109*(2):43-45.

18. Jane Riblett Wilkie (1991). The Decline in Men's Labor Force Participation and Income and the Changing Structure of Family Economic Support. *Journal of Marriage and the Family 53*(1):111-112; Bernadine Healy (1995). *A New Prescription for Women's Health: Getting the Best Medical Care in a Man's World.* New York: Penguin Books, pp. 15-16.

19. Frank F. Furstenberg. Divorce and the American Family. *Annual Review of Sociology 16:*379-403.

20. Cynthia M. Logsdon and Karen Robinson. Helping Women Caregivers Obtain Support: Barriers and Recommendations. *Archives of Psychiatric Nursing 15* (5):44-248.

21. Healy, *A New Prescription for Women's Health;* Rosemarie Tong. Just Caring About Women's and Children's Health: Some Feminist Perspectives. *Journal of Medicine and Philosophy, 26*(2):147-162; J. Popay. Being a Woman Is Hard Work: The Policy Implications of Poor Health Among Lone Mothers. *Journal of Epidemiology and Community Health 53*(12):749.

22. Tong, Ibid.

23. Lynn Martin. *Who Will Care for Each of Us? America's Coming Health Care Labor Crisis: A Report from the Panel on the Future of the Health Care Labor Force in a Graying Society.* Chicago: University of Illinois, School of Nursing, p.17.

24. U.S. Department of Health and Human Services (1994). *Minorities and Women in the Health Fields.* Washington, DC: U.S. Department of Health and Human Services.

Chapter 11

# New Directions for Accreditation of Allied Health Education Programs

John E. Trufant

Accreditation, widely endorsed and supported by faculty and administrators in the nation's colleges and schools of allied health, is typically also among their major concerns. Unlike sister professional schools, e.g., business, engineering, law, medicine, and others, that are accredited by a single agency, schools of allied health must prepare for as many accreditations as they have programs within their schools. With the majority of schools having multiple programs, the frequency, costs, and preparations for accreditation represent significant investments, both direct and indirect. It is not uncommon for an allied health dean to lament in exaggeration, "An accrediting team just left last week; one is here this week; and another is due next week."

Despite both positive and negative opinions that schools may harbor about accreditation, a discriminating public that is investing growing proportions of both personal finances and public taxes in higher education is demanding evidence of value for its investment. Without question, accreditation has become an essential threshold criterion that students, parents, legislators, government agencies, and the community use to measure school and program quality. Yet few who rely on this measure understand what it means and, as a matter of fact, most of the process and the outcomes that surround the rather complex system of accreditation are shrouded in secrecy and confidence.

Of the thousands of schools and programs that seek accreditation, nearly all are successful. Consequently, one might ask, "If the process does not discriminate among best and worst schools and programs and eliminate the worst, is it not failing in its major purpose?" Proponents would respond that because most succeed in the accreditation process, it is working as it should because it raises all, or nearly all, to an acceptable level of quality and provides mechanisms for the worst to correct their problems and also cross the bar.

Higher education in America over the past two decades has expanded dramatically; as a proportion, the allied health sector has grown at a higher rate. Emulating its sister health professions in medicine, nursing, and others, allied health has embraced accreditation and adopted similar processes, most of which are firmly entrenched across health professions accreditation.

Simultaneously during these past two decades of expansion, higher education was also being subjected to great public pressures for reform as well as increasing competition from innovative institutions, especially through the use of technology. The old concepts about what constituted a college education and how it would be achieved were changing rather dramatically. Distance learning, the virtual campus, online courses, credit for life experience, and a host of nontraditional innovations were changing everyone's attitudes about postsecondary education. Overlaid on the system was accreditation. Was it adapting to keep pace?

The need for developing new directions for accreditation of allied health education programs is auspicious and the time is opportune.

## PART I: OVERVIEW OF ACCREDITATION

### Purposes of Accreditation

A cursory examination of various accrediting agencies' statements of accreditation purposes shows both commonality and divergence. Formal statements have wide general acceptance and agreement. Through the years, however, accreditation has been forced to accept other purposes and, in some instances, has been misused to achieve other ends. The following, although not exhaustive, demonstrates the evolving and expanding list of these purposes.

*Assure Quality.* Nearly all accrediting agencies include *quality assurance* as the major purpose of accreditation. To be accredited assures various levels of government, other educational institutions, internal and external constituencies, and others that the institution/program meets minimal standards of quality by which similar programs are evaluated.

*Provide Public Accountability.* The United States maintains the most diverse system of higher education in the world, one that is largely autonomous of governmental controls, especially in the determination of curricula. The American system of accreditation, rather unique in the world, has countered the need—indeed, opposed the idea—to establish a method of governmental assessment and ranking by which the public can judge whether an institution or program is one of recognized quality. In the eyes of the public, *accreditation* is the imprimatur of a responsible and respectable school or program.

*Encourage Improvement.* Across all health professions, the knowledge base to enter practice continuously expands. Also, new research demonstrates more effective methods that faculty may employ to educate their students. Accrediting agencies reflect these alterations in their accreditation standards, which are the criteria by which programs are judged. Accreditation standards undergo revision periodically to reflect current professional practice. Because accreditation is cyclical, i.e., it is time-limited, programs must continuously improve to meet new standards.

*Promote Shared Governance.* American colleges and universities are distinguished by a long history of shared governance in which administrators and faculty, and to a certain extent students, participate in the institution's decision-making processes. Accrediting teams, especially for institutional but also increasingly for programmatic accreditation, often address the question of the role of faculty in decision making and by doing so reinforce and promote the principle of shared governance.

*Provide Consultation.* Accreditation focuses primarily on whether and how well a school/program meets each of the accreditation standards, and some agencies allow, or even encourage, accreditation site visitors to provide consultation on means of meeting standards judged to be deficient and/or to advise on improving other aspects of program operations that may not be included in the standards. On the other hand, some agencies strictly forbid site visitors from commenting on any aspect of program operation that is not specifically in the standards.

*Leverage Resources.* Included among the accreditation standards for nearly all health professions programs are those that address the adequacy of resources, including numbers of faculty, space to house the program, instructional equipment, financial resources to support the program, and other resource components. Accreditation can be used to leverage institutional and college administrators to provide more resources to a program.

*Gain Eligibility for Financial Aid.* Students who need federal student financial aid must ensure they enroll in a school/program that can provide access to such aid. If the school/program is accredited by an agency recognized by the federal government's Department of Education, the school/program will be able to provide such access. With the increasing dependence of students on federally guaranteed loans, the link of their availability to accreditation questions the time-honored principle of the "voluntary" nature of accreditation.

*Strengthen the Profession.* During the last several decades, significant maturation has occurred in most of the allied health fields. Positions that once depended on informal preparation or on-the-job training now require associate degree training and many former associate degree programs have advanced to the baccalaureate level. More recently, some professions now require master's education for entry into practice, and it is not uncommon in a number of fields to find doctoral level programs preparing clinical practitioners. Professional organizations in these fields have strengthened the profession as a whole through the influence they have exerted on accreditation standards and revised educational requirements. However, the close relationships between governing boards of professional organizations and their respective accrediting agencies have raised serious questions about the independence of accrediting agency decision making.

*Improve Salaries and Working Conditions.* Although attribution to accreditation of any relationship to employment conditions for faculty is overtly anathema, the connection is more direct than most will recognize. Standards that deal with provisions such as student class size, class loads, and program director qualifications at the least indirectly affect working conditions and more likely play a direct part on them.

*Limit Programs and Graduates.* Any accusation that accreditation has been used to limit the number of programs or graduates in any field is instantly disavowed by the accreditation community. Of course, most would agree that such an objective is a malevolent divergence from the ethical foundation of accreditation. Although limiting the field is not a recognized purpose of accreditation, it nonetheless appears to have had that effect from time to time across some of the allied health areas.

### Institutional and Programmatic/Specialized Accreditation

Accreditation of higher education in the United States falls into two categories: *institutional* and *programmatic/specialized*. In its 1994 *Handbook of Accreditation*, the North Central Association of Colleges and Schools defines and contrasts these as follows:

> Institutional accreditation evaluates an entire institution and accredits it as a whole. An institutional accrediting body evaluates more than the formal educational activities of an institution; it assesses as well such characteristics as governance and administration, financial stability, admissions and student personnel services, institutional resources, student academic achievement, institutional effectiveness, and relationships with constituencies outside the institution.

Specific programs within an educational institution can also seek accreditation. This specialized (or program) accreditation evaluates particular units, schools, or programs within an institution and is often associated with national professional associations, such as those for engineering, medicine or law, or with specific disciplines, such as business, education, psychology, or social work. (p. 1)

Most allied health educational programs at the associate degree level and above reside in institutions of higher education and are included under the institutional accreditation umbrella. This is a major advantage, for it enables students to access federal financial aid resources. However, either all or most of the programs in the allied health school must also seek programmatic accreditation since access to licensure, certification, or registration is linked to completion of a program accredited by a specific profession-based agency. In those fields that do not link accreditation to practice credentials, directors of educational programs must also seek accreditation, in order to recruit students and faculty, improve their programs' reputation within institutions and communities, identify with the larger profession, use accreditation as an assessment tool, and gain access to programs and resources of the accrediting agency and others.

One of the questions allied health educational program administrators raise is why institutional and programmatic/specialized accreditations are not more coordinated and integrated. Many specialized accreditation documents require either identical or similar information, and/or data required for institutional accreditation, e.g., campus resources, student support services, administrative policies, etc. Could the means be identified to standardize and incorporate the data requirements of institutional accreditation to avoid duplication for programmatic accreditation? Of course, the accreditation cycles of institutional and specialized accreditations rarely converge and so the data compiled for institutional accreditation may be dated for specialized accreditation. Then too the same question is raised for a school of allied health that has multiple specialized accreditations, each of which requests different data in variable formats. The burden on allied health schools of managing multiple data requirements is not insignificant, and the value added to the accreditation process of responding to these differences has to be questioned.

### Historical Overview of Accreditation in the United States

Early written accounts on education in the United States provide evidence of oversight of schools' educational staff and curricula. As education became more widespread and publicly supported, local officials assessed their schools, teachers, and administrators. However, while such processes were related to quality assurance, their relationship to what is today defined as accreditation was distant.

It is generally acknowledged that accreditation began at the turn of the twentieth century. Fauser (1989) reported that "the North Central Association of Colleges and Secondary Schools began accrediting high schools in 1905. By 1909 standards were drawn up for colleges, and by 1913 the first list of accredited institutions appeared." These early efforts were so successful that accreditation expanded to all regions of the country and many established and developing disciplines over the next several decades.

The American Medical Association (AMA) played an instrumental role in allied health accreditation for much of the twentieth century through its Committee on Allied Health Education and Accreditation (CAHEA). Many of the largest allied health professions and numerous other allied health fields organized their accreditation activity through CAHEA. In the early 1990s, the AMA determined it would no longer sponsor the accreditation of allied health programs. During the transition to a new, freestanding accrediting agency, several allied health programs made the decision to develop independent accrediting agencies. The others formed a new accrediting agency, the Commission on Accreditation of Allied Health Education Programs (CAAHEP). Of course, many allied health professions were never sponsored by CAHEA and thus have been independent agencies from the outset of their accreditation activity. In the twenty-first century, CAAHEP has become the accrediting agency for seventeen allied health professions, while another twenty have remained independent agencies.

### Current Organization of the U.S. Accreditation Systems

The organization of accreditation in America has two dimensions: institutional and specialized (i.e., professional). Institutional accreditation applies to the entire university/college, which serves as the umbrella for all of the institution's programs. The six regional accrediting agencies, e.g., Middle States Association of Colleges and Schools and Southern Association of Colleges and Schools, are the best known of the institutional type. Accreditation by one of these agencies makes the university eligible to participate in certain federal student financial aid programs. Its importance in this respect makes accreditation almost mandatory for most institutions of higher education. Other agencies also accredit entire institutions.

Professional/specialized accreditation exists in parallel with institutional accreditation. By and large, the two systems operate independently of one another. A number of allied health accrediting agencies, however, require that the programs they accredit must be in institutions that have regional accreditation. Although the standards each type of accreditation uses have little overlap, the basic processes of self-study and site visits are similar. Programmatic/specialized accreditation assesses individual programs to determine compliance with a unique set of standards. Nearly all allied health fields have specialized/programmatic accrediting agencies. Again, although accreditation by these agencies is considered voluntary, many states adopt legislation that links licensure/registration to practice to graduation from a program accredited by a specialized/programmatic accrediting agency. When this is required, it essentially removes the voluntary nature of the activity.

Accrediting agencies have a form of their own accreditation, which is called *recognition.* They may be recognized by the United States Department of Education (USDE) or the Council for Higher Education Accreditation (CHEA), or by both. To be recognized by either organization, an agency must apply for and meet the criteria that both have established. USDE recognition enables institutions/programs accredited by a USDE-recognized accrediting agency to have access to certain federal student financial aid funds. All of the institutional/regional accrediting agencies have USDE recognition. An accrediting agency cannot seek USDE recognition if all of the programs it accredits are in institutional/regional accredited institutions. However, if some of its programs are in hospitals, laboratories, or other institutions that are ineligible to apply for institutional/regional accreditation, the agency may seek USDE recognition as well as CHEA recognition.

## PART II: ACCREDITATION IN ALLIED HEALTH

### Accrediting Agencies

The term *allied health* refers to a broad grouping of health professions and is not itself a profession, such as medicine, nursing, or optometry. The number of professions and health occupations included in allied health is controversial with some sources citing nearly 200 fields. Many of these, however, are not considered professions. They do not have specialized/programmatic accreditation and, therefore, do not have accrediting agencies. Nonetheless, the number of independent accrediting agencies in allied health is substantial, which has many implications for the schools that house such programs.

With the emergence of many new health professions over the past half-century, nearly all of which fall under the rubric of allied health, agencies to accredit them have also proliferated.

After the AMA removed its control over accreditation of allied health programs, several professions that fell under the CAHEA umbrella used that organization's dissolution to establish independent accrediting agencies, e.g., Clinical Laboratory Sciences Occupational Therapy, and Nuclear Medical Technology. Others collaborated to form a new agency, CAAHEP, which was founded on July 1, 1994. CAAHEP then became one of the largest specialized accrediting agencies in the United States with more than 1,800 programs in more than 1,300 institutions. Today, the eighteen professions that belong to CAAHEP for accreditation purposes include:

- Anesthesiologist assistant
- Athletic trainer
- Blood bank technology specialist
- Cardiovascular technology
- Cytotechnology
- Diagnostic medial sonography
- Electroneurodiagnostic technology
- Emergency medical technician—paramedic
- Health information administration/technician
- Kinesiotherapy
- Medical assistant
- Medical illustrator
- Ophthalmic medical technologist/technician
- Orthotic and prosthetic practitioner
- Perfusion
- Respiratory therapy
- Surgical technology

Many other allied health fields have their own accrediting agencies, such as the following:

- Occupational therapy
- Physical therapy
- Physician assistant
- Art therapy
- Genetic counseling
- Orthoptist
- Dietetics

- Audiology and speech-language pathology
- Therapeutic recreation
- Rehabilitation counseling
- Radiation therapy
- Nuclear medical technology
- Clinical laboratory sciences
- Music therapy

### Accreditation Processes

Although myriad variations in the processes used to accredit allied health programs exist across the multiple accrediting agencies, one will also find many similarities. In general, the accreditation process includes the following steps: the program conducts an assessment of how well it meets the accreditation standards; the program produces a self-study document based on the evaluation data used in its assessment; through the accrediting body, the program invites a group of peers to review the self-study and conduct a site visit to the campus; the site visit team conducts an assessment and writes a report of its findings on whether and/or how well the program meets accreditation standards; the program reviews the site-visit report and comments on inaccuracies, if any; the accrediting body considers all of the evidence and reaches a decision on the program's accreditation status; finally, the program and other administrators are notified of their status. In the event the program disagrees with the decision, it has opportunities to appeal.

Increasingly, accrediting agencies are exploring and implementing approaches to streamline various aspects of the process, especially administrative features. Information technology provides multiple opportunities to increase efficiency, improve communications, reduce costs, and decrease time intervals. For example, some programs are now producing self-studies on floppy discs or compact discs rather than hard copies; others are posting their studies on institutional Web sites. Self-study appendixes, which have been notoriously voluminous, are simply referenced as materials available through the institution's library, archives, or in a program's electronic files. Site visitors can contact the institution online to obtain assessment information about the program.

Of course, the advent of distance learning has forced new thinking about accreditation processes, including a reexamination of many of the standards that are used to assess the quality of an academic program. Traditionally, a critical element of the process has been the campus site visit. Many distance learners are never on the campus; in fact, a distance learning program may not have a physical campus location. Consequently, the site visit may need to become a "virtual" visit over the Internet or through other electronic means.

One can anticipate that the use of information science in accreditation processes will accelerate in the years ahead, will significantly challenge traditional approaches, and will alter many of the timeworn conceptions about how those processes must be managed.

## Accreditation Standards

What factors are used by accrediting agencies to judge a program's quality and to determine whether to award or withhold accreditation? Through the years, agencies have used various terms to refer to these factors, including, for example, *criteria* and *essentials*. It appears the current trend is to use the term *standards*, although other terms continue to be used.

Standards can vary from explicit statements that identify the presence or absence of an educational resource, for example, to broad statements that encourage considerable interpretation in individual cases. CAAHEP has adopted a template for its accreditation standards and guidelines, to which all of its eighteen programs will conform as required revision cycles occur every five years. However, a review of non-CAAHEP programs' standards identifies multiple similarities across many different disciplines/programs.

Typically, the first section of a set of standards contains some boilerplate information the program must address, such as the accreditation status of the institution within which the program operates, resources (personnel, financial, clinical, and physical) that support the program, demographic and descriptive information about the students, and operational policies (such as fair practice, and maintenance of student records). The second section most often addresses the curriculum and its assessment. In some cases, curricular content standards are very detailed; in others, they are more general. The final section frequently deals with the maintenance and administration of accreditation, and specifies responsibilities of the program and the accrediting agency and how program changes are to be handled.

## Costs of Accreditation

For an allied health academic unit (e.g., a college or a division), the costs of programmatic accreditation can be significant. Direct costs include fees, usually levied on an annual basis, charged by each agency that accredits a program and the fees charged by each agency for undergoing an accreditation cycle. Throughout the period during which a program prepares for an accreditation visit, other costs will be incurred. Such costs could include released time for someone to lead the accreditation effort; preparation, administration, and analysis of surveys and interviews for the self-study; duplication expenses, and more.

The larger cost—and the one most difficult to measure—is the time faculty, administrators, and others devote to the entire accreditation effort. Although one could argue that the assessment activities one undertakes should be part of every program's continuous improvement efforts, even where that is true accreditation adds another level of activity. Most agree the benefits far outweigh the costs. However, as educational institutions are being required to increase efficiencies and decrease costs, minimizing the costs of accreditation while maximizing accreditation's value looms as an imperative task for all involved in accreditation.

## PART III: ISSUES IN ALLIED HEALTH EDUCATION

The near-universal acclamation of the positive attributes of accreditation by multiple stakeholders in allied health education should not be interpreted to mean that discontent does not exist. In fact, deans and directors of allied health schools and programs register many complaints about various aspects of the process. The nine sections that follow highlight some of the more common and contentious issues in allied health accreditation.

### Lack of Agreement on the Purpose of Accreditation

Part I of this chapter reviewed a number of purposes of accreditation, some of which would undeniably be considered disdainful—at least in public affirmation—such as leveraging resources and improving salaries and working conditions. Yet disagreements exist on some purposes that would seem to be unarguably appropriate (providing consultation would be one example). In fact, some accrediting agencies explicitly state that site visitors are discouraged from consulting; others prohibit it. With so many accrediting agencies in allied health, each of which may differ not only in its stated purposes but even more in its unstated purposes, one can understand why program administrators and faculty may be both confused and disgruntled.

### Lack of Coordination Across and Within Agencies

Most schools of allied health are accredited by multiple agencies; a few may have as many as fifteen to twenty allied health programs that are accredited by separate agencies. Requirements, as well as expectations, vary greatly across these agencies. Data developed for one agency may be in a format unacceptable to another agency, or different data may be requested. Requirements for self-studies vary greatly across agencies. Some agencies limit the number of report pages, others detail the outline of the report, and still others provide no guidance at all. Some agencies assume that a college or university with regional accreditation satisfies institutional-level requirements, such as student records management, student service functions, and faculty involvement in governance. Other agencies demand that programmatic accreditation assess and report on the same factors. The upshot is that each allied health program accreditation is independent of all others.

### *Focus on Inputs, Process, and Structure Rather Than Outcomes*

Since the 1990s, evaluation of student achievement has become a more central concern of accrediting agencies. As alternatives to traditional on-campus education exploded, such as distance learning, the focus was forced to shift to outcomes of the educational process as the primary measurement of quality. Equating educational quality with library resources, number of classrooms, and amount of full-time versus part-time faculty no longer sufficed. Nonetheless, the number of standards for most allied health accrediting agencies that continue to address inputs (e.g., degree level of faculty), process (e.g., student time in the classroom), and structure (e.g., the program's administrative hierarchy vis à vis that of other programs in the academic unit) continues to dominate the accreditation process. Many of the standards are highly prescriptive regarding the content of the curriculum, even to the point of specifying how many hours of instruction a student must have.

### *Variability in Site Visitor Competence*

Although the site visit remains a core strength of the accreditation process, most school/program administrators and faculty agree that its greatest weakness is the variability of site-visitor competence, despite the provision of site-visitor training in many accrediting agencies. Of all the elements in the accreditation process, nearly all program officials would agree that the most critical is having site visitors who are prepared (i.e., they have read and are familiar with the self-study report and other materials); objective (i.e., they assess the program on the accreditation standards, not on their own independent judgment); fair (i.e., they recognize that the same goal can be accomplished in multiple ways); inclusive (i.e., they make a strong effort to speak with as many stakeholders as they can to gather multiple points of view); and collegial (i.e., they interact as professional colleagues in a friendly manner). The traditional role of the site visitor as inspector, i.e., one who is on campus to discover every weakness and identify every problem, has changed. Campus leaders want site visitors to appraise the conclusions regarding the achievement of standards reported in the self-study against visitors' observations and to identify the discrepancies along with the rationale for those decisions.

### Program Autonomy versus Accreditation Intrusiveness

The line between a program maintaining its autonomy and an accreditation agency meddling in affairs that are unrelated to its purpose is wide and blurry. Many of the appeals from campus administrators on accrediting agency decisions have resulted from their conclusion that the agency has overstepped its legitimate boundaries in ways that negatively affected some aspect of the accreditation decision. These disagreements often arise over the resources available to the program. Although outcomes assessments may demonstrate that students are strongly achieving program goals, site visitors may criticize the adequacy of resources. Or site visitors may comment that the number of students is too few or too many without relating such a conclusion to an accreditation standard or to the lack of achievement of outcomes.

### Time-Based Accreditation Intervals versus Continuous Assessment and Reporting

Most allied health accrediting agencies establish maximum time intervals between comprehensive accreditation assessments. These intervals vary across different agencies, with the maximum at ten years and the minimum at five. Of course, shorter intervals can be determined by the accrediting agency when programs have deficiencies that need to be corrected sooner. Time intervals for accreditation, especially longer ones, ignore the fact that many changes occur that can negatively affect program quality in very brief periods. Changes in leadership, turnover of faculty, shifts in the job market, limitations on resources, breakthroughs in knowledge developments, etc., can quickly affect program outcomes. With no reporting on accountability for quality between accreditations, how can an accrediting agency assure the public that the conditions on which accreditation was granted are still extant?

## Discouragement of Innovation

The question of whether accreditation discourages innovation in allied health educational programs has long been debated, and the answer may indeed be changing as the focus of accreditation shifts to outcomes. That aside, standards certainly set limits—even if perceived—on how much innovation can be implemented. Faculty, often uncomfortable with innovation, may use standards as rationale for maintaining the status quo, especially if the innovation modifies faculty roles, responsibilities, or numbers. Program administrators may also be wary of the potential reactions of site visitors to innovations, especially if the effects of the changes have not yielded results.

## Exploration of Virtual Educational Models

Accrediting agencies have recently been confronted with entirely new educational delivery models, many of which use technology in creative and dynamic ways. The traditional concept of accrediting an institution or program that has a geographic location has collided with the realities of contemporary education. Standards are being rewritten and in some cases interpreted in unprecedented ways, to accommodate these innovations in education. Accrediting agencies have recognized the need to alter methods and procedures, and it is likely that many inventive ideas will continue to reshape accreditation in the future.

## Relationship Between Professional Associations and Their Accrediting Agencies

How much influence do professional associations have on their respective accrediting agencies? Although independence is a requirement for recognition of an accrediting agency by the Department of Education and the policies of most accrediting agencies include statements about the accreditation body's independence, the close association of accrediting agencies and their respective professional societies remains a realm of suspicious collusion. Among areas that have attracted skepticism are accreditations that are used as tools to influence the economics of the profession in such areas as faculty salaries, degree levels, and limitations on the number of programs and/or students. A serious concern involves linking professional certification to graduation from a program with accreditation from the related agency.

## PART IV: NEW DIRECTIONS

One of the great strengths and attractions of America's system of higher education is its vast diversity. Today, it seems literally true that everyone who seeks postsecondary education can identify a program that fills his or her requirements. During the past decade, this diversity has expanded rather dramatically through the use of technology. Unthinkable until recently, students may graduate from an institution that has only a virtual campus. The flexibility that has allowed students to create their individual curricula has mushroomed. As students of all ages and from all walks of life seek to continue learning and recharge their careers and their lives, lifelong learning is becoming a reality. Colleges and universities have made dropping in and stopping out an acceptable pathway for students seeking enrichment, specific new skills, and simple enjoyment.

Has the accreditation system maintained pace with the dramatic changes occurring in postsecondary education? As one might expect, the answer to this question is best framed as a continuum with little/none at one end stretching to much at the other end. The profusion of accrediting agencies in allied health reflects this continuum. Some agencies have demonstrated a remarkable eagerness for innovations; others have been content to maintain traditional approaches.

The purpose of this section is to present new directions that accrediting agencies might consider as they undertake self-assessments aimed at improving their efficiency while assuring and/or enhancing their effectiveness. This section does not offer a new system but rather elaborates on alternatives that each agency may find useful. Furthermore, it seeks to encourage the generation, public discussion, and dissemination of more alternatives.

### Priority on Outcomes Standards

While higher education has devoted much attention—and many resources—to the overarching importance of identifying and measuring outcomes, i.e., student academic achievement, most accreditors continue to focus their attention on many other criteria. An analysis of any set of accrediting standards shows they can be sorted into four broad categories:

1. *Inputs*—these standards address the resources that are available for the instructional program, including personnel, equipment, facilities, etc.
2. *Structure*—these standards address how the inputs are organized to manage and govern the instructional program

3. *Process*—these standards address instructional processes, such as the use of lecture, laboratory, and clinical teaching
4. *Outcomes*—these standards address student and alumni academic achievement

Among allied health accrediting agency standards, it is common to find the overwhelming number of standards are input, structure, and process standards. Frequently, these standards are addressed independently, i.e., they are not related to outcomes of the academic program. For example, an accrediting team may find the number of computers available is inadequate for enrollment yet a review of student satisfaction questionnaires shows students have voiced no complaints about computer availability and their performance on examinations that require the use of computers is excellent. Numerous other examples could be cited that raise questions about the purposes of specialized accreditation and whether it is being used as a tool to leverage changes and bring pressures to campus administrators unrelated to student academic achievement. Many untested assumptions about the relationship of inputs, structure, and process to outcomes enter the accreditation equation. In this age of the virtual campus, many of these assumptions are not only being questioned but also discarded.

### Models of Continuous Assessment and Reporting

Most allied health accrediting agencies establish a period of time between the years of comprehensive accreditations, i.e., when the entire accreditation process must be undertaken. These time periods vary across agencies and often vary for new versus established programs. Some agencies may grant as many as ten years between comprehensive reviews. This leaves open the possibility that many changes could occur during a decade, or even during a shorter time span, that could affect the quality of the academic program. Yet in most cases such changes and the declines they may cause would go unnoticed until the next accreditation. The program would continue to be recognized during the interim as accredited, which is a strong public affirmation about quality that may have changed.

Although a number of accrediting agencies require annual or biannual reports from accredited programs, most do not request assessment data on student and alumni achievement. Rather, they focus on faculty, budgets, leadership, and other nonoutcomes standards. Should programs have to demonstrate continuously during their period of accreditation that they are maintaining, if not improving, their outcomes? Should a program whose graduates show significant declines in passing the licensure examination have no responsibility to the accrediting agency for reporting such performance? Does the accrediting agency have no responsibility to address this quality issue?

Building a system of regular reporting and verification of student outcomes data that motivates programs to preserve minimal levels of quality and results in safeguarding the public's trust in accreditation seems an essential component of a modern accreditation system.

## Site Visit Innovations

Of the three major elements of accreditation, the site visit is likely considered the most important; at the least, it seems to generate an elevated share of attention. Having a group of peers on campus to examine all aspects of one's program generally raises administrator, faculty, and student tensions, even for programs that have excellent outcomes. Typically, the two- or three-day site visit is planned many months in advance, which provides adequate opportunities for the campus to make careful preparations, such as assuring everyone's familiarity with the self-study, cleaning facilities, organizing files, etc. Although it is considered a time to show off, few would dispute the general feeling of relief when the site team departs.

Although one could argue the logic that periodic preparations to get the house in order are worthwhile, would not most agree that the house should always be in order? Is it time to consider instituting site visits that occur by surprise or with a very short period of notice, such as one or two weeks? If the results of a site visit are so beneficial, should they not occur much more frequently that at the time of the next comprehensive visit?

In a world where the virtual campus can be visited from anywhere at any time, one might question whether the physical presence of a site visitor on a program's campus is essential to verify the quality of the program. If evidence of achievement of outcomes is indisputable, what value is added to the process by having a group of peers visit one's program? With the growing interest of some allied health agencies to accredit programs in other nations, alternatives to the traditional on-campus visit are likely to gain increasing prominence in the years ahead. Certainly, it seems the time has come to test other options.

## Ensuring Competent Site Visitors

No single factor in the accrediting process can raise more ire among program administrators and faculty than site visitor incompetence. The critical importance of accreditation in allied health programs, many of which are tied to graduates' ability to be licensed, heightens the seriousness with which they approach the task of accreditation. The contrast between an excellent self-study process and ineffectual or poorly prepared site visitors discredits the entire accreditation process.

Most accrediting agencies sponsor site visitor training programs. However, the scope and depth of such training varies widely and the fact that someone is trained is no assurance of effectiveness. Furthermore, after-the-fact assessment of poor performance during a site visit does little to offset the negative impact on that program, even if it prevents future failures for other programs. Most programs are reluctant to invoke the appeals procedure on the basis of site visitor incompetence. It is difficult to prove, and few programs are willing to challenge their accrediting agencies on this issue.

Can we identify ways not only to improve but to ensure the competence of site visitors? Improvement is probable; ensurance is not. Site visitors are required to make many judgments about whether and how well a program meets accreditation standards. An aspect of their judgment is their experience in the field and their familiarity with programs they are using as benchmarks. Through training, their knowledge can be expanded, as can their ability to make fair judgments. Working on a team with a chairperson who has proven himself or herself competent can be a major positive factor. Site visitor feedback from program officials and other members of the site team can also lead to improvement. Among the criteria programs officials would rank high on the list for site visitors is predictability about what to expect.

The more difficult issue in ensuring competence is the site visitor's personal philosophy about accreditation. Many engage in the task as inspectors and define their function as identifying every possible deficiency. Their approach is negative. Their criterion is perfection; anything less is deficient. Often, they are unfriendly, demanding, and aloof. These site visitors will be universally considered incompetent.

For a task as far-reaching and essential as accreditation is to allied health, the various agencies could collaborate to establish a site visitor training program that would draw together the best practices from the various accrediting agencies to create a successful program from which all could benefit. They could introduce the concept of a certified allied health site visitor. Elements of such a program could include didactic instruction, independent study, online courses, role-playing, knowledge-based assessments, and an internship/residency. Graduates of the program would receive certificates that would demonstrate their credentials to be a site visitor.

### *Reduction of Accreditation Documentation*

The tales told among accrediting teams of the voluminous documentation submitted by programs undergoing accreditation are legendary. Self-studies that number hundreds of pages with appendixes that fill boxes have been reported. For many years, it seemed one of the assumptions in accreditation is that more is better, i.e., overwhelming the site team with information leads to a better outcome.

Fortunately, this assumption appears to be changing. A number of accrediting agencies now limit the self-study narrative to a certain number of pages. Requests for quantitative data are in tables that establish the data elements to be reported. Other agencies use a self-study form that dramatically abbreviates what needs to be reported, all of which address agencies' standards directly and concisely. Huge binders of accreditation materials are also being replaced with computer disks. Also, self-studies are being placed on program Web sites for ease of access, both for internal as well as external parties.

The periodic nature of accreditation leads to tidal program attention to self-study and documentation of performance. As an accreditation visit becomes imminent, preparations intensify; and as they do, the volume of material grows. In a preferred world of continuous planning for improvement, an accreditation team would examine the plans and assessment data programs are already using to review progress and modify curricula and other program elements. It seems feasible that all documents required for a comprehensive reaccreditation would be available at any given time with no special effort required to gather and analyze them solely for accreditation. Having such documents and data on hand would help streamline accreditation and encourage attention to continuous improvement.

### Competition in Accreditation

Allied health programs cannot choose the agencies from which they seek accreditation. In fact, many professions have secured this monopoly by influencing state legislatures to enact laws that tie licensure to graduation from programs that are accredited by a profession's accrediting agency. The results of lack of competition, well known in the corporate world, include higher prices, absence of innovation, inattention to customer satisfaction, lack of flexibility, and more. Would accreditation in allied health and perhaps all professional/specialized fields benefit from a competitive system of accreditation?

Accrediting agencies might argue that competition would be impractical because the system for establishing standards depends on the collaboration of the profession, the educators, and the public. They might also contend the close relationship between the professional society and the accrediting agency is an essential part of ensuring that programs prepare graduates who are capable of entry into the practice.

Nonetheless, it is intriguing to consider how the accreditation system might change if programs had a selection of agencies from which to seek accreditation. Would the benefits that characterize a competitive environment accrue to the accreditation system? Would accreditation become less expensive, more innovative, highly customer responsive, and very flexible, while at the same time continuously improve the outcomes of educational programs? It may well be past time for an experiment in allied health that tests the viability of a competitive accreditation system.

## *Availability of Information to the Public*

Allied health accrediting agencies make available to everyone much information about their policies, practices, and personnel. The Internet has facilitated access to this information. One can learn about who constitutes decision-making bodies and how they are selected, when and where the next review and revision of an agency's standards will be, the procedure to apply for accreditation, the costs, the meaning of various categories of accreditation (e.g., provisional, initial, continuing), the specific process the agency uses for accreditation, and much more. Every agency publishes the standards (i.e., criteria, guidelines, and essentials) by which programs will be evaluated and accredited.

However, for an individual program one can find only minimal information. All agencies provide a list of programs they have accredited. Some include the degree level (e.g., certificate, associate, bachelor's) of their programs. Others may indicate the year of a program's initial accreditation and additional dates, such as the date of the last accreditation action or when the next accreditation is scheduled to occur. Still others will indicate the accreditation status of the program, as, for example, provisional, preaccreditation, continuing.

No allied health accrediting agency provides information about those standards that a program met, met only partially, or did not meet at the time of its accreditation review. Yet most accredited programs have deficiencies that are identified during the accreditation process. Would accreditation be of more value to the public if information on the level of compliance with standards were available? Does the public possess the sophistication necessary to understand and interpret what was meant by a judgment of partial compliance or not met? Would other competitive educational programs abuse information intended for program improvement in negative marketing?

Of course, individual programs have significant freedom to publish information about their accreditation. Major activities that programs undertake during the process of creating their self-studies yield excellent information about the quality of the program. Information from site team reports can also be used, in whole or in part, to inform the public about various strengths of the program as well as what needs to be reviewed and addressed for improving quality in the future.

It is likely debates will continue about how the public can best be served through accreditation. The accreditation process for each program produces a vast amount of information to address the question of quality yet the public wants to know whether the program is accredited or not. In the information age, will this continue to satisfy the need to know and the demand to know more?

### Rating Scales in Accreditation

Closely aligned to the issue of public information on accreditation is the use of rating scales in accreditation. College and university faculty and administrators await each year's publication of popular magazine rankings of their institutions and programs, and books are published with frequency about the so-called best colleges and universities or those that offer the most value for the cost. Institutions and programs with high marks eagerly broadcast their rankings as proof to the public of their high quality. They also use the rankings for other purposes, such as fund-raising.

Most college and university administrators, even those in institutions and programs at the top of these lists, concede the rankings do not differentiate quality but rather demonstrate unique strengths and characteristics. Near unanimous agreement exists that this range of differences is the fundamental strength of the American higher education system. Many will also acknowledge that the methodologies employed by the ratings systems are faulty at worst and questionable at best.

On the other hand, one might argue accreditation is an intense process that produces a judgment about the quality of a program based on a clear set of standards that all similar programs must meet. Yet under current practice this lengthy, in-depth assessment process essentially yields only one public result: thumbs-up or thumbs-down; accredited or not accredited. What might result from an accreditation process that used a ranking system in its accreditation decisions? Would institutions strive harder to achieve five stars, for example, than to achieve three stars? What inferences about quality would the students and the public make about programs with higher or lower rankings? Other alternative ranking systems have been suggested. To date, however, the consensus seems to be that the potential misuses of accreditation ranking systems outweigh the potential benefits. Nonetheless, accreditation strategists should continue to explore positive applications of rating systems in accreditation that maximize the benefit of the substantial resources that are invested in a program's accreditation by both institutions and agencies.

## Increasing Value and Reducing Costs

The costs of accreditation, both direct and indirect, in schools of allied health are significant budgetary expenses. Schools with many programs may have more than one site visit annually with associated high expenses for each. It is not unusual for a faculty member's responsibilities in each program to be partially reassigned during the period of accreditation preparation in order to provide leadership and conduct the necessary activities required for a comprehensive self-study process. Numerous meetings of faculty, students, advisory committees, and school and university officials accumulate costs. Finally, development and printing of the self-study adds further expense. For programs in which continuous planning and evaluation are well structured and part of ongoing academic management, the cost of accreditation itself will be less, but even in such instances accreditation adds expenses that would not otherwise be necessary.

The question, however, is not cost but value. Are the outcomes of accreditation equal to or greater than its cost? Also, can costs be reduced while maintaining or improving outcomes?

Among allied health educators, the response to the question of value would be nearly universal, for without accreditation, many program graduates would be unable to sit for examinations that lead to professional licensure/registration/certification. In these situations, the value is inescapably high.

Would leaders of programs whose graduates do not need such credentials feel the same about the value of specialized accreditation? The belief that accreditation has value is firmly entrenched in higher education. Even where it is truly voluntary, most programs seek to be accredited as evidence to colleagues, applicants and their parents, and the broader public—including trustees and advisory committee members—that the program's quality is recognized through the accreditation process. This confidence, however, does not infer that improvements are unneeded, and among both institutional and programmatic accrediting agencies ideas are being developed and tested to streamline the process to reduce costs and increase value, including:

- More focused/less open-ended, briefer self-study reports that concentrate on measurement of outcomes data and their interpretation
- Coordination of two or more accreditation site visit teams to reduce redundancy and take advantage of their expertise
- Self-study processes that are designed to address specific needs of individual programs
- Actions of accrediting agencies based on annual reporting of outcomes and other data that address quality indicators
- Reduction of the number of standards to be assessed
- Fewer members of site visit teams
- Site visit reports that follow standard format and include information which programs can use for continuous improvement
- Greater use of electronic communications to expedite all steps in the accreditation process

As innovations across many accrediting agencies demonstrate they reduce costs, maintain or increase the value of various aspects of the process, and gain acceptance, many more ideas will be developed and tested.

### *Increasing Predictability in the Accreditation Process*

Peer judgment about a program's quality will continue to dominate accreditation decision-making. Yet this particular strength in the American system of education is also its greatest potential weakness, for peers bring to their decision making many values, biases, and prejudices. Although all who participate in decision making are cautioned that accreditation judgments must be driven by standards, not by individual preferences, a system so highly dependent on people—and so many of them—will inevitably suffer from variability. In allied health, the sheer number of programs, sets of standards, accrediting agencies, site visitors, and boards dramatically diminishes the likelihood that a program's administrator can predict the outcomes from one accreditation to the next, for the same program or from program to program.

Why is predictability important? Academic administrators continually make decisions about the allocations of scarce resources. Among the primary considerations in those decisions is to ensure that a program's accreditation remains secure. Consequently, it is imperative they be able to predict, within a limited tolerance, of course, the effect those decisions may have on the program's accreditation status. For example, if a standard requires that the program have sufficient faculty to implement the curriculum, the administrator must be able to predict that maintaining the same number of faculty will not jeopardize the program's accreditation, assuming other factors such as the number of students remain relatively constant.

Predictability also pertains across programs. If the same degree program is accredited at institutions A, B, and C, the public should be reasonably confident that all three met the same set of standards in a reliable and predictable way. Parents and students often use accreditation status as their minimal criterion when considering applying to a program. This status should reassure them that all three have passed the same test.

The most significant threats to predictability in accreditation are differences among site-visit teams. Standards are stated in general terms to provide both academic staff and site visitors room to make judgments. However, individual site visitors as well as site teams can and do interpret a program's level of compliance with standards with rather dramatic variations. These divergences have diminished credibility in the accreditation process more than any other single issue academic program leaders have experienced.

What can be done to enhance predictability and reliability? As noted earlier, many accrediting agencies have implemented site visitor training programs to increase the capability of these volunteers. Through role-playing, case studies, simulation activities, and other techniques, trainees learn how to seek and identify information and data that address the standards while recognizing and minimizing the effect of their personal values in how the standards are interpreted. A number of agencies also emphasize that one of the most critical outcomes of the accreditation process is program improvement for the future, not negative sanctions for events of the past. They encourage looking at trends over time and the capability of the program to plan for the future. As programs demand more accountability from accrediting agencies whose resources they provide, new means of reducing the vagaries that accompany the accreditation process will be studied and implemented.

### Encouraging Innovation

An examination of allied health accrediting agencies would reveal that their approaches to the task are more alike than different. Yet the programs being accredited, even by a single agency, exhibit many differences. In their zeal to ensure minimal levels of quality, accrediting agencies must accord equal fervor to encouraging academic diversity.

Accreditation standards, by and large, do not promote innovation. Built into the standards are many assumptions about the conditions that must be present to achieve certain outcomes. However, it is a well-established fact that students have varying learning styles and, whether provided as part of the instructional program or not, they discover alternative approaches to their own success. Many routes lead to the same place. In this respect, accreditation should serve as a primary energizer for educational innovation. To do so will require that accreditation's focus remain squarely on educational outcomes; inputs, structure, and process are variables to be manipulated to produce outcomes. Many programs are demonstrating that innovations in these variables can result in great gains in outcomes.

Accrediting agencies should undergird innovation at the program level by being innovative, learning organizations themselves. All strategies should be questioned, and new approaches must be tested to determine how better results can be achieved. The entire accreditation system, at program and agency levels, should be continuously improving itself through innovation.

## CONCLUSION

Accreditation has become a pervasive feature in the life of the nation's allied health schools. Unlike their sister health profession schools that deal with a single accrediting agency, allied health schools—depending on the number of programs in them—must manage multiple accreditations from many different agencies. Even small programs with only a few students have independent accreditations. Without question, accreditation in allied health schools and programs encompasses a large portion of academic life.

The universal acceptance and support in American society for accreditation demonstrates the confidence the public and professional educators have in the system. Although the public understands little about accreditation, it has been persuaded that the imprimatur accreditation represents is essential. Professional educators who admit the accreditation system has its flaws nonetheless support it enthusiastically for a host of reasons. Primary among those reasons is maintaining nongovernment control over quality in American higher education.

Although the purpose of accreditation was singular and straightforward at its inception, a century later it has become—intentionally in some cases and accidentally perhaps in others—the means by which many goals may be accomplished. Some of these are admirable; others questionable, at least as objectives of accreditation. Accrediting agencies' close relationship with their professional organizations blurs their claims of independence and raises questions about whether accreditation is used for professional aggrandizement.

Over the past quarter century, the acceleration of change in American higher education has been extraordinary. This period has also marked an era of phenomenal change in allied health—new professions, advanced degree levels, expansion and development of new schools, parity of faculty in the academy, sophistication of research, etc. Throughout this period, however, accreditation remained much the same—until it was challenged by distance learning. Standards developed for campus-based programs suddenly could not be directly translated for virtual programs. Fortunately, as accrediting agencies, educators, and others collaborated to address the need for creativity in accreditation to meet new structural demands, the door also opened to the potential for other innovations to address a range of traditional and nonconventional educational practices.

Other movements in higher education were also fomenting during this time. Accountability mushroomed as a theme with its foundation in outcomes assessment. Nontraditional students were flooding college classrooms—both on campus and through virtual attendance. Globalization was expanding with more American students studying abroad and more international students attending U.S. schools. These and other trends raised challenges for accrediting agencies. While problems in all of these dimensions were being addressed, many accrediting agencies became more adaptive, flexible, and responsive. Successes in one agency are being studied by other agencies; in some cases, successful programs are being adopted by others.

Accreditation of allied health programs will continue to be at the heart of allied health education. It is a major tool for improving the quality of education for allied health practitioners.

## BIBLIOGRAPHY

American Medical Association (2001-2002). *Health professions career and education directory,* Twenty-ninth edition. Chicago: Author.

Burrows, W. R., and Hedrick, H. L. (1988). Allied health education and accreditation. *JAMA: Journal of the American Medical Association, 260* (8), 1113-1119.

Center for Collaborative Research, College of Health Professions, Thomas Jefferson University (1999). *Allied health accreditation project: Final report to the Commission on Accreditation of Allied Health Educational Programs and the Bureau of Health Professions Health Resources and Services Administration.* (RFQ No. 98-BHPR-E060981 MJS). Philadelphia: Thomas Jefferson University.

Commission on Accreditation of Allied Health Education Programs (2001). Retrieved from the World Wide Web November 2001: <http://www.caahep.org>.

Committee on Organizational Effectiveness and Future Directions, North Central Association of Colleges and Schools, Commission on Institutions of Higher Education (1998). *Effective collaboration for the twenty-first century: The commission and its stakeholders.* Chicago: Author.

Council for Higher Education Accreditation (2001). Retrieved from the World Wide Web November 2001: <http://www.chea.org>.

Dill, W. R. (1998). Specialized accreditation: An idea whose time has come? Or gone? *Change* (July/August), pp. 18-25.

Ewell, P. T. (1992). *Outcomes assessment, institutional effectiveness, and accreditation: A conceptual exploration.* (Resource paper). Washington, DC: Council on Postsecondary Accreditation.

Farber, N. E., McTernan, E. J., and Hawkins, R. O. Jr. (Eds.) (1989). *Allied health education: Concepts, organization, and administration.* Springfield, IL: Charles C Thomas.

Fauser, J. E. (1989). Accreditation. In Farber, N. E., McTernan, E. J., and Hawkins, R. O. Jr. (Eds), *Allied Health Education: Concepts, organization, and administration.* Springfield, IL: Charles C Thomas.

Gelmon, S. B., O'Neil, E. H., Kimmey, J. R., and the Task Force on Accreditation of Health Professions Education (1999). *Strategies for change and improvement.* San Francisco: University of California at San Francisco, Center for the Health Professions.

Graham, P. A., Lyman, R. W., and Trow, M. (1995). *Accountability of colleges and universities: An essay.* New York: Columbia University.

Kassebaum, D. G. (1998). Achieving better institutional self-study. *Academic Medicine, 73* (9), 925-927.

Kassebaum, D. G., Cutler, E. R., and Eaglen, R. H. (1997). The influence of accreditation on educational change in U.S. medical schools. *Academic Medicine, 72,* 1128-1133.

North Central Association of Colleges and Schools, Commission on Institutions of Higher Education (1994). *Handbook of accreditation: 1994-96.* Chicago: Author.

O'Neil, E. H. (1994). Critical challenges facing allied health accreditation: Pew Health Professions Commission's recommendations. *Journal of Allied Health, 23* (1), 15-17.

Robiner, W. N., Langer, S., Howe, R., Ziegler, R., and Erlandson, J. V. (1999). Time to rethink accreditation criteria for programs that train health professionals. *Academic Medicine, 74* (2), 97-100.

Rodenhouse, M. P. (Ed.). (1999). *Higher education directory,* Seventeenth edition. Falls Church, VA: Higher Education Publications.

Ruben, B. D. (1995). The quality approach in higher education: Context and concepts for change. In B. D. Ruben (Ed.), *Quality in Higher Education* (pp. 1-34). New Brunswick, NJ: Transaction Publishers.

Simmons, H. L. (1994). Critical challenges facing allied health accreditation: Pressures on accrediting bodies. *Journal of Allied Health, 23* (1), 23-27.

Simpson, D. E., Golden, D. L., Rehm, J. M., Kochar, M. S., and Simons, K. B. (1998). The costs versus the perceived benefits of an LCME institutional self-study. *Academic Medicine, 73,* 1009-1012.

Terenzini, P. T. (1989). Assessment with open eyes: Pitfalls in studying student outcomes. *Journal of Higher Education, 60* (6), 644-664.

Van Kollenburg, S. E. (Ed.) (1999). *A collection of papers on self-study and institutional improvement.* Chicago: North Central Association of Colleges and Schools, Commission on Institutions of Higher Education.

Weithaus, B. (1993). New directions for allied health education accreditation. *Journal of Allied Health, 22* (3), 239-247.

Willis, C. R. (1994). The cost of accreditation to educational institutions. *Journal of Allied Health, 23* (1), 39-41.

Chapter 12

# Allied Health Education
# in a Global Community

Cheryl T. Samuels

## *INTRODUCTION*

Several months ago, Chira Banda, an east African immigrant, severely injured her back in an automobile accident. She currently receives physical therapy treatment at a local clinic twice a week and the muscle spasms in her back are improving. Ms. Banda's therapist noticed a red string tied around her waist, but she has been reluctant to inquire about its purpose.

Like many immigrants to the United States, Ms. Banda has her own beliefs and practices about healing and restoration of health. It is common practice among some east African women to wear strings around their waists to promote healing. Practices such as wearing beads or rosaries, or carrying certain healing stones, usually indicate a connection with the spiritual and/or religious beliefs of members of that community. These practices have a long tradition and the impact of these beliefs and practices on compliance with more traditional Western therapies and behaviors needs to be understood by health care providers.

Understanding, also known as cultural competence, is becoming increasingly more important for allied health providers in the United States, particularly since they are practicing in a global community that has greater racial and ethnic diversity than in the past. Consequently, health care providers must consider cultural beliefs and practices, their influence on health and healing, and how non-Western alternative or complementary health approaches can be integrated with conventional forms of health care. This chapter provides information about the increasing racial and cultural diversity in the United States and the resulting trends that are shaping the growing interest in complementary and alternative approaches (CAAs) to health care. The chapter also includes a discussion of these influences on allied health education and practice, and suggests how allied health professionals can further their knowledge and experience to become culturally competent in order to work more effectively in a global community.

## OVERVIEW OF RACE AND ORIGIN
## OF THE U.S. POPULATION

U.S. Census data indicate there is an increasing racial and ethnic diversity of the U.S. population. Table 12.1 from the 2000 U.S. Census shows the distribution by race, with a specific ethnic category for individuals of Hispanic or Latino origin. The figures indicate that 75 percent of the U.S. population is white and 12.5 percent is Hispanic or Latino. The 75 percent who reported they are white includes 48 percent of the Hispanic or Latino population who also reported they are white. *White* refers to people having origins in Europe, the Middle East, or North Africa. It is clear that even in this grouping there is considerable ethnic diversity. The black or African-American race comprises 12.3 percent of the U.S. population. The Census indicates there have been significant increases in population among Asians (3.6

TABLE 12.1. Population by Race and Hispanic Origin for the United States, 2000

| Race and Hispanic or Latino | Number | Percent of Total Population |
|---|---|---|
| *Race* | | |
| Total population | 281,421,906 | 100.0 |
| One race | 274,595,678 | 97.6 |
| White | 211,460,626 | 75.1 |
| Black or African American | 34,658,190 | 12.3 |
| American Indian and Alaska Native | 2,475,956 | 0.9 |
| Asian | 10,242,998 | 3.6 |
| Native Hawaiian and Other Pacific Islander | 398,835 | 0.1 |
| Some other race | 15,359,073 | 5.5 |
| Two or more races | 6,826,228 | 2.4 |
| *Hispanic or Latino* | | |
| Total population | 281,421,906 | 100.0 |
| Hispanic or Latino | 35,305,818 | 12.5 |
| Not Hispanic or Latino | 246,116,088 | 87.5 |

*Source:* U.S. Census Bureau (2000a), Census 2000 Redistricting (Public Law 94-171) Summary File, Tables PL1 and PL2.

percent), "some other race" (5.5 percent), and "two or more races" (2.4 percent). Asians include people with origins in the Far East, Southeast Asia, or the Indian subcontinent. The "some other race" category is composed primarily of Hispanics, since 42 percent of Hispanics reported themselves as "some other race." The "two or more races" category is predominately people of two races with the most common being "white and some other race." American Indians and Alaska Natives remain slightly below 1 percent of the reported population.

Diversity characteristics vary dramatically across the United States, particularly in the four most populous states: California, Texas, Florida, and New York. In California, Hispanics or Latinos comprise 32.4 percent of the population, while Asians constitute 10.9 percent. In Florida, Hispanics or Latinos represent 16.8 percent of the state's inhabitants, and black or African Americans represent 14.6 percent. In New York, Hispanics or Latinos comprise 15 percent; blacks or African Americans, 15.9 percent; Asians, 5.5 percent; and "two or more races," 3 percent (U.S. Census, 2000i). Even the traditionally white Upper Midwest is becoming more diverse as immigrants from Cambodia, Vietnam, and Somalia, for example, are brought to these communities by church groups.

This diversity is expected to increase significantly. The fastest-growing population, those of Hispanic or Latino origin, increased 60 percent during the 1990s (O'Brien, 2001). It is anticipated this growth rate will continue well into the future, particularly with the influx of legal and illegal immigrants and high birth rates among those of Hispanic or Latino origin. In addition, the foreign-born population is increasing at a rate about four times faster than that of the general population. Based on immigration and birth rates, the Immigration Public Policy Center has projected what the race and ethnic origin of the U.S. population will be in 2050 (see Table 12.2). In 1995, based on current trends, their total population estimate for 2050 was revised to 394 million. The center projects those of Hispanic or Latino origin, who constituted 12.5 percent of the population in the 2000 census, will increase to 21 percent of the U.S. population in 2050. As suggested by 2000 census data by state, those percentages will continue to vary across the country in the years ahead. Table 12.3 lists population projections for California, the most populous state, in the year 2025. The percentage of white Californians is expected to decrease from 52.6 percent in 1995 to 33.7 percent in 2025. The percentage of African Americans in California is expected to decrease slightly while the percentage of Hispanics and Asians and Pacific Islanders is projected to increase to 43 percent and 17.4 percent respectively (Cerritos College Databook, 2000).

TABLE 12.2. U.S. Population in Millions (Percent)

| Group | Actual 1992 | | Projection 2050 | |
|---|---|---|---|---|
| U.S. Total | 258 | | 383 * | |
| White (non-Hispanic) | 191 | (75%) | 202 | (53%) |
| Black | 32 | (12%) | 62 | (16%) |
| Hispanic | 24 | (9%) | 81 | (21%) |
| Asian | 9 | (3%) | 41 | (11%) |
| Indian | 2.2 | (0.8%) | 4.6 | (1.2%) |

*In 1995, projection modified to 394 million.

*Source:* Immigration Public Policy Center (Data: Census Report, December 1992).

TABLE 12.3. Population Projections for California

| Group | Actual 1995 (Percent) | Projected 2025 (Percent) |
|---|---|---|
| White | 52.6 | 33.7 |
| African American | 6.9 | 5.4 |
| Hispanic | 29.1 | 43.1 |
| Asian and Pacific Islanders | 10.7 | 17.4 |

*Source:* Cerritos College Databook, 2000.

## CULTURAL COMPETENCE IN A GLOBAL COMMUNITY

With such increasing diversity, allied health professionals must be prepared to work with patients' beliefs, rather than against them, and bridge cultural gaps if improved health outcomes for patients/clients and their families are to be achieved. The following seven domains of cultural competence, as adapted from *Cultural Competence: A Journey* (BPHC, 2001), provide guidance for practitioners, educators, and students who wish to improve their effectiveness in providing care to patients from different cultural backgrounds and ethnic origins.

1. *Values and attitudes:* Be aware that beliefs may influence the way a patient responds to health, illness, and death. For example, religious beliefs may interfere with compliance with treatments since the per-

son believes that God controls all. In this context it may be necessary to work with the patient and family, and possibly the priest or healer, to partner with the patient in using his or her faith to support the treatment and healing process. In addition, the use of role models in the community who have been successfully treated for the same condition can be helpful in overcoming a patient's fatalistic attitude.

2. *Communication styles:* Sensitivity is key to understanding and being understood. In Latino cultures, for example, relationships between people are very important. Latinos see health care providers as authority figures and may not want to question their approach. Active steps to gain their trust and engage the patient and family in the treatment planning process is important to successful outcomes. Bilingual staff or volunteer interpreters can be essential to understanding a person's health care needs and priorities.

3. *Family/community participation:* Many non-Western cultures are very family and community oriented. Therefore, understanding the roles and status of various members of the family and community and knowing how to best include their participation in the planning and treatment process may be very important to the healing process.

4. *Physical environment:* Office space should reflect the cultural identities, including language, of the community members it serves. Patients/clients should feel their cultural heritage and language are valued.

5. *Policies and procedures:* These should be conveyed in a way that reflects an understanding of patients' language and differences in approaches to health and disease. For example, understanding the roles of women, men, and parents in the culture and understanding who needs to be involved in decision making about the use of contraception or decisions about children is very important.

6. *Population-based clinical practice:* Providers need to understand the importance of their own and others' worldviews and sociopolitical influences and be able to show respect for views that are different from their own.

7. *Training and professional development:* Providers need to value cultural competence in their co-workers and recognize the need to include cultural competence training and professional development for health care professionals at all levels.

An instrument such as the self-assessment checklist developed by Goode (2000) is an excellent way for students and practitioners to heighten their own awareness and sensitivity to cultural diversity and improve cultural competence.

## TRENDS SHAPING USE OF COMPLEMENTARY
## AND ALTERNATIVE APPROACHES

Certainly, racial and cultural diversity are major factors that have influenced the growth of CAAs. People from non-Western cultures often use behavioral and dietary practices and home remedies such as homeopathy, herbal preparations, and yoga that are now seen in this country as complementary or alternative approaches to medicine. They may seek care from a healer in their community prior to seeing a health care provider with a Western educational background.

The aging of the population is another major trend that influences diversity and the use of CAAs. Thirty percent of the population is now in the age thirty-five to fifty-four age group, and 14 percent are already over the age of sixty-two (U.S. Census, 2000c). Aging baby boomers who were born between 1946 and 1962 expect to live longer and experience fewer years of disabling disease later in life. Therefore, aging and its effects will become an even greater focus over the next ten to twenty years, as represented by the Healthy People 2010 goal of improving quality of life through the control of arthritis, osteoporosis, low back pain, disabilities, and various secondary health conditions (Satcher, 2000, p. 23).

Many other factors influence people of all ethnic and cultural backgrounds to explore CAAs, often as an adjunct to more conventional therapy. Health information abounds in the popular press and on the Internet and increasingly people are educating themselves about ways to improve their quality of life, health, and wellness. More and more, people are turning to CAAs as their dissatisfaction with conventional medicine grows. In an often-quoted study in the *New England Journal of Medicine,* David Eisenberg et al. (1993) found that one in three people surveyed used some form of unconventional therapy in the past year, primarily for chronic conditions. In addition, the value they placed on these approaches is indicated by the fact that most of them paid for these services out of pocket. Another key study by Dean Ornish et al. (1990), published in *The Lancet,* has influenced attitudes toward conventional therapies. That study of twenty-eight patients with coronary heart disease found that the combination of a low-fat vegetarian diet, smoking cessation, stress-management training, moderate exercise, and a support group actually reversed coronary lesions after one year. In contrast, the size of coronary lesions continued to progress for those in the control group who were not asked to make any lifestyle changes during the same time period.

Since the early 1990s, more attention has been given to the study of the impact of lifestyle changes and CAAs on health. In 1992, Congress created the Office of Complementary and Alternative Medicine within the National Institutes of Health. Based on heightened consumer interest and encouraging results from various research studies, support for that office has grown considerably. It has since become a center and has an annual budget of more than $80 million.

Although care systems such as traditional Chinese medicine, homeopathy, and Ayurveda have been practiced for hundreds of years, the medical profession has remained skeptical about the efficacy of many of these techniques. However, studies such as those sponsored by the Center for Complementary and Alternative Medicine and other researchers are successfully distinguishing what works from what does not (Pew Health Professions Commission, 1998). Consequently, an increasing number of both consumers and health care practitioners now embrace these practices, often in conjunction with more conventional therapies, to support health, prevent disease, and manage chronic conditions, particularly those for which conventional modalities remain ineffective.

In response to these trends, there has been a dramatic growth in the number of complementary and alternative health providers. The Institute for Alternative Futures (1998) study projects that by 2010 the number of providers, including physicians, trained in Oriental medicine will swell to 24,000 and the number of chiropractors will double to 103,000. Insurance companies are also seeing value in many of the CAAs. Ziegler (1997) reported on a study that found regular use of mind-body therapies can cut health care costs by 33 percent. In the foreword to a new textbook, *Complementary and Alternative Medicine: A Research-Based Approach* (Freeman and Lawlis, 2001), John Weeks states that approximately two-thirds of health maintenance organizations currently offer some coverage for complementary and alternative medicine (CAM). In addition, integrative clinics, in which CAM and conventional providers work side by side, are springing up across the United States. Weeks also indicates that by 1997, seventy-five medical schools were offering education in CAM compared to a few years prior, when only a handful included this information in their curricula.

To further support the trend toward complementary and alternative medicine, therapeutic and preventive advances that advocate personalized health care are also being developed (Institute for Alternative Futures, 1998). Consumers will increasingly have access to effective self-care tools, such as biomonitors and other diagnostic and screening devices, that will enable them to monitor and treat some conditions in their own homes. Personalized health care can be further enhanced by CAAs, such as Oriental medicine and Ayurveda, both of which employ diagnostic and therapeutic systems based on individual differences, treating the person as a whole, and utilizing mind-body connections. The uniqueness of the individual is also recognized in the developing field of genomics, which identifies genes most relevant to the treatment of certain diseases.

The Institute for Alternative Futures (1998) concludes that combined, these trends will lead to managed care in 2010 that is far more effective, prevention-oriented, and customized than at present. By 2010, a major source of competition for managed care will be self-managed care, as some families and individuals choose to manage their own care, using deductible catastrophic insurance only as a backup. Consumers seeking prevention and wellness will continue to go beyond what conventional medical care or medical care coverage provides.

## IMPLICATIONS FOR EDUCATION AND PRACTICE

The convergence of increased population diversity and increased demand and use of CAAs in the global community should have a major impact on the form and substance of allied health education at all levels. As recommended in the National Commission on Allied Health's report on the future of allied health (USDHHS, 1999, p. 20), efforts must continue to focus on recruiting health professions students who represent the disadvantaged, the disabled, and cultural and racial minorities. The benefits of this approach are numerous. According to the Pew report of 1998, students who come from underserved neighborhoods are more likely to return to those neighborhoods to practice. In California, for example, the Latino and African-American communities lack an adequate number of physicians. Furthermore, students from minority cultures who have grown up with the language and cultural mores of a particular group can offer a more complete and effective kind of care to clients/patients from that group (Pew Health Professions Commission, 1998, p. 26). Diversity among allied health students and practitioners allows students to learn firsthand from one another. Openness to learning about different cultures and belief systems can positively influence students' and practitioners' approaches to health behaviors and practices that promote health while respecting cultural differences.

Currently, diversity in the health professions does not begin to match the diversity in the population. Although some progress has been made, on average, minority groups are not represented in the ranks of the allied health fields in the same percentages as they are represented in the national population (USDHHS, 1999, p. 20). Since minority students remain underrepresented in allied health programs, this trend seems destined to continue as the country becomes more diverse, with unfortunate implications for those diverse populations (Pew Health Professions Commission, 1998, p. 22).

Commitments of both resources and energy must be made at all levels in private and public sectors if Healthy People 2010's goal of eliminating disparities in health care, particularly among different racial and ethnic groups, is to be realized (Satcher, 2000, p. 23). Allied health and other educational communities that train health care providers must work with government and private agencies to recruit and retain more workers, particularly those from minority groups who are interested in practicing in underserved areas. The Commission on Allied Health's report (USDHHS, 1999, p. 19) recommends that recruitment of students in allied health professions should begin before high school. These efforts will be facilitated by partnerships among the elementary and high school system, higher education, and the health care industry. Employers and educators should consider offering incentives such as paid leave or internship credit to employees or students who are willing to serve as role models and actively work to recruit and retain a diverse allied health workforce. Role models from various cultural backgrounds are an important component if recruitment and retention efforts are to be successful.

### *Educational Outcomes*

Allied health educational programs must require their students and graduates to demonstrate a culturally sensitive client/patient relationship that emphasizes individualized health care. Patients today demand a collaborative relationship with care providers and expect providers to be sensitive to cultural, spiritual, and emotional aspects of patient health. Therefore, the educational environment must teach and expect students to demonstrate these values and behaviors. The health care system must be able to evaluate and reward these behaviors not only in health care settings within the community but also in classrooms, laboratories, and informal settings. Opportunities to acquire and continually improve effective communication skills are essential. This can be accomplished through interviewing, listening, writing, teaching, learning, presenting, and practicing conflict-resolution skills. Students should learn to model respectful, caring, and compassionate behavior in all interactions with other students, staff, patients, and the community (Pew Health Professions Commission, 1998, p. 36).

In addition to focusing on prevention and wellness care and public health, graduates of allied health programs need to learn about forms of complementary care and how these approaches are commonly integrated into the health care system. The health care curriculum must reinforce the view that clients/patients are complex individuals who need and deserve holistic care. Students need to be prepared to answer patients' questions about CAAs and be able to suggest additional resources and referral information. Table 12.4 includes basic information about the most commonly practiced medical or health-oriented philosophies. The National Center for Complementary and Alternative Medicine (NCCAM) Web site <http://nccam. nih.gov> is also an excellent source of information for both the practitioner and the consumer. This resource outlines the major domains of CAM and provides general facts about certain CAAs, including information about cancer and dietary supplements. The NCCAM Web site also provides access to PubMed, a database which allows a person to easily find journal citations related to CAM. This is particularly helpful for allied health students and graduates who need to remain current on the most recent research relevant to their practice discipline.

By integrating CAAs throughout the curriculum, allied health programs can also focus on the belief systems that underlie CAAs. This allows the program to incorporate knowledge and principles of a wide range of cultural values, beliefs, and customs, with the expected outcome being that practitioners will provide culturally sensitive care to a diverse society (Pew Health Professions Commission, 1998, pp. 36, 37). As recommended in the Pew report, the education of health care providers must introduce them to nontraditional, alternative, and complementary health practices they may encounter in clinical practice. Health care providers should then consider these CAAs in the context of cultural values and beliefs. The report, *Building the Future of Allied Health* (USDHHS, 1999, p. 20), supports the expanding role of allied health providers with the overarching goal being to prepare allied health professionals to provide a wide range of services, optimize access to needed services, provide positive clinical outcomes, and maintain cost effectiveness.

### Educational Strategies

Several strategies can assist students and practitioners in achieving the educational outcomes discussed in the previous section. One of the most essential is to structure multiple experiences throughout the curriculum that allow students to interact with culturally different individuals, families, and communities, with a special focus on local populations. Public service activities, even prior to enrolling in an allied health program, can be a positive force for both a lasting commitment to public service and a better under-

TABLE 12.4. A Summary of Medical Philosophies

| Philosophy/Proponent | Summary |
|---|---|
| 1. Allopathic Medicine<br>William Osler, MD | This system of medical practice combats disease through treatments that produce effects different from those produced by the disease treated. An allopath would treat an inflammation or infection with an anti-inflammatory (aspirin) or anti-infective (penicillin). The cause of most disease is believed to be physical. Treatment is generally restricted to surgery, radiation, and pharmaceuticals. |
| 2. Biomolecular Medicine<br>Alan Gaby, MD | This is also called nutritional, orthomolecular, or functional medicine. It is the field of health care that employs assessment and early intervention to improve physiological, emotional/cognitive, and physical function. It uses applied nutritional science to a spectrum of therapeutic biological modifiers such as dietary nutrients and supplements, phytochemicals, and nutrient medicinal foods. |
| 3. Botanical Medicine<br>Andrew Weil, MD | This is the philosophy of using plant material as medicinal agents to heal disease and prevent illness. Approximately 25 percent of all prescriptions contain ingredients isolated from plants. |
| 4. Environmental Medicine<br>Doris Rapp, MD | This medical philosophy (also called clinical ecology) deals with environmental hazards including chemicals, ionizing radiation, air pollution, sensitizing substances, social and work settings, and communicable disease. Environmental illness is usually a polysymptomatic, multisystem, chronic disorder manifested by adverse reactions to environmental excitants (foods, inhalants, chemicals) as they are modified by individual susceptibility in terms of specific adaptation. In other words, there are environmental substances (excitants) present in our air, water, food, drugs, and habitat, and we all react to them biochemically in an entirely individual manner. For a certain percentage of Americans, the manner in which they react causes illness. Environmental medicine physicians also frequently work with patients who have chronic fatigue syndrome, systemic candidiasis, and ordinary allergies. As opposed to ordinary allergies, environmentally ill people respond to toxins in the environment through pathways not necessarily mediated by the immune system. Environmental illness is a toxic, but not always immunological, reaction to foreign substances. |

TABLE 12.4 *(continued)*

---

5. Ethnomedicine

Ayurvedic Medicine
Deepak Chopra, MD

This is a branch of traditional Indian medicine. Ayurvedic is etymologically derived from Sanskrit roots, in which *ayus* means "life" and *veda* means "knowledge" or "science." It is translated as "the science of life." Disease is seen as an imbalance in the life force *(prana),* or it may be karmically preordained. Central to Ayurvedic diagnosis and treatment is the principle of biological individuality. It emphasizes host factors as the primary factor in the etiology of disease. It places importance on mental and emotional factors, which it sees as critical to the development of these imbalances. Three irreducible principles (called *doshas*) regulate the different functions of mind and body. They are *Vata, Pitta,* and *Kapha.* The proportion in each person determines the psychophysiological type of that person. Only its yogic exercises and meditation practices are well known in the United States.

Native American
Medicine
Lewis Mehl, MD

Native American medicine and spirituality come together to form the basis of healing and health. Relationship with the Creator begins early, and it comes from an inner guidance and leadership. Everyone is connected to the Creator and has some sort of direct relationship. It involves a respect for all of God's creations including plants, animals, and humans. Earth, air, fire, and water are important energies involved with Native American medicine and ceremonies. Disease is caused by some disharmony in the cosmic order as well as by hexing, breaking a taboo, fright, or soul loss.

Traditional Chinese
Medicine (TCM)

This is an ancient method of health care that combines the use of medicinal herbs, acupuncture, food therapy, massage, and therapeutic exercise. TCM looks for underlying causes of imbalances and patterns of disharmony in the body, and it views each patient as unique. A diagnosis might include describing the body in terms of the elements—wind, heat, cold, dry, damp. Yin is used to refer to the tissue of the organ and yang refers to its activity. TCM works with *qi,* the life force that is all inclusive of the many types of energy within the body and flows through the body in pathways called meridians. For diagnosis, the TCM practitioner obtains a good history from the patient and performs at least four methods of investigation: inspection of the complexion, general demeanor, body language, and tongue.

---

| | |
|---|---|
| 6. Fitness/Exercise Medicine Ken Cooper, MD | This philosophy employs the use of aerobic and anaerobic methods to help an individual become well adapted to his or her environment and be able to respond to its changing demands. Aerobic exercise is an activity that increases the heart and respiratory rate so extra oxygen is needed. Anaerobic exercises are those in which increased oxygen is not needed. These include stretching, muscle toning, muscle building, and activities designed to improve balance, flexibility, agility, and coordination. |
| 7. Homeopathic/Energy Medicine Norm Shealey, MD | This is an area of medical practice that involves subtle or very low intensity nonmaterial stimuli. Examples include healer interventions, homeopathy, electromagnetic therapies, Reiki, therapeutic touch, Jin Shin Jyutsu, acupuncture, light and color techniques, Qi Gong, and tai chi. |
| Homeopathy | Homeopathy is a natural pharmaceutical science that uses microdoses of substances to stimulate the body's own immune defense systems. Substances from the mineral, plant, and animal world are used for treatment based on data taken from controlled studies in toxicology. The two guiding principles of homeopathy are the Law of Similars (like cures like) and the Law of the Infinitesimal Dose (the most potent remedies are those in the greatest dilution). The belief is that remedies retain their effect because of electromagnetic frequency imprinting. The cardinal doctrine of homeopathy is that there is a vital force in the body that strives for health. Disease or disruption of this force cannot be classified but is unique to each person. |
| Acupuncture | Acupuncture is based on a philosophy that a cycle of energy flowing through the body controls health. Pain and disease develop when there is a disturbance in that flow. Needles inserted at certain points in the body can remedy that imbalance or disturbance and can effect a therapeutic response elsewhere in the body. |
| 8. Manual Medicine John Upledger, DO | This philosophy believes that improving the structure and functioning of the human body will improve health and treat many diseases. |
| Bodywork | Bodywork includes therapies such as massage, deep tissue manipulation, movement awareness, and energy balancing. Principles include alteration of muscle and tissue through pressure or deep friction, movement, education and self-awareness, breathing, and emotional expression. Some of the popular types of bodywork are massage, Alexan- |

TABLE 12.4 *(continued)*

|  |  |
|---|---|
|  | der technique, Feldenkrais method, Rolfing, Aston-Patterning, Hellerwork, Trager approach, and Bonnie Prudden myotherapy. |
| Chiropractic | Chiropractic is based on the theory that we have an innate intelligence flowing through the central nervous system to regulate bodily functions. There must be a balance between the central, peripheral, and autonomic nervous systems, which are all intimately related to the spinal column. Subluxations between vertebrae can cause compression of the spinal cord of nerve roots, which can then cause disease in any part of the body. Chiropractic centers on removing obstructions to nervous system flow through spinal adjustments. |
| Osteopathy | Osteopathy centers on the musculoskeletal components of health and illness since that system uses most of the body's energy. It is based on the interrelationship of structure and function. Tension, restriction, or inefficiency in the musculoskeletal system can waste energy, which can lead to a wide variety of health problems. Osteopaths use mobilization, articulation, release methods, soft tissue techniques, muscle relaxation, and cranial sacral manipulation. |
| 9. Mind/Body Medicine (Psychoneuroimmunology) Herbert Benson, MD | This philosophy is based on the belief that our psychological and emotional components influence our physical health. Stress, coping skills, personality traits, social connectedness, and self-esteem all correlate with susceptibility and resistance to physical illness. Some of the approaches used include art therapy, bioenergetics, guided imagery (visualization), dance and movement therapy, dream work, focusing, Gestalt therapy, hypnotherapy, journaling, Jungian analysis, neurolinguistic programming, postural integration, primary therapy, psychodrama, psychosynthesis, rational emotive therapy, reality therapy, rebirthing, Reichian analysis, and transactional analysis. |
| 10. Naturopathic Medicine Michael Murray, ND | This is a distinct system of healing. It is a philosophy, science, art, and practice that seeks to promote health through education and the rational use of natural agents. Its principles are based on the concept that the body is a self-healing organism. It centers on six basic principles: (1) the healing power of nature; (2) treat the cause, not the effect; (3) first, do no harm; (4) treat the whole person; (5) the physician is a teacher; and (6) prevention is the best cure. Many different modalities |

|  |  |
|---|---|
|  | are used including nutritional therapy, herbs, homeopathy, acupuncture, hydrotherapy, bodywork, counseling, and lifestyle modification. |
| 11. Spiritual Medicine<br>Larry Dossey, MD | This philosophy refers to the wholeness and unity of our personal existence and to the integration of the many dimensions that make up that wholeness. That includes the biological, physical, intellectual, and religious dimensions. It encompasses our feelings, relationships, attitudes, values, goals, ethical principles and behavior, religious beliefs, and all that makes us fully human. Spiritual healing is rooted in the belief that there is a supreme being or universal energy at work in the world. Health and illness can be influenced by our connection with that being or energy. This supreme being or energy is known by various names including God, Goddess, Allah, Krishna, Brahman, the Tao, the Universal Mind, the Almighty, the One, chi, prana, the Great Spirit, love, the Life Force, and the Absolute. Prayer is most important in spiritual medicine. Prayer can be defined as asking something for one's self or for others. Prayer, of course, can also be for confession, lamentation, adoration, invocation, and thanksgiving. Prayer is nonlocal, meaning it is infinite in time and space. Prayer is not sending energy and, since nothing is sent, the Divine factor in prayer is internal, not external, to everyone. In essence, all spiritual healing is a form of self-healing, since it is believed that God is present to some degree in all individuals. Spiritual medicine includes a belief structure, a sense of meaning in one's life, a sense of connection and belonging, and religious views and traditions. |

*Source:* Permission to reprint courtesy of Bill Manahan, MD.

standing of the needs of various population groups and the cultural influences that affect health attitudes and behaviors. National service could play an even greater role in meeting Healthy People 2010's goals if programs that forgave debt were extended to more health professional graduates (Pew Health Professions Commission, 1998, p. 28). The Pew report further recommends that professional associations actively incorporate public service into regulation and professional development activity.

Clearly, public service initiatives in addition to program-based clinical and community experiences, should provide students a variety of experiences. Students should have the opportunity to meet with clients/patients on a one-on-one basis, work in a group setting for educational sessions, and work with teams of community members and providers to assess, plan, and implement population-based screening and intervention programs. Students also need to work with patients and families in situations in which ethical issues arise, such as end-of-life decisions, allocation of scarce resources, patient confidentiality, and patient/family choices that might conflict with those of providers or with social norms (Pew Health Professions Commission, 1998, p. 38). During these experiences, each student should be expected to keep a journal that charts his or her personal journey toward becoming a person who addresses people from a holistic perspective, who values diversity, and who understands its impact on health behaviors and attitudes and therefore is able to provide culturally sensitive care. These behaviors can be further strengthened by providing experiences for students to work in interdisciplinary teams where they can learn to collaborate and appreciate one another's unique and collective capabilities and contributions to the team (Pew Health Professions Commission, 1998, p. 51).

The benefits of providing opportunities for students and practitioners to examine their own values and attitudes and to discuss their experiences with persons of diverse backgrounds in a safe, trusting classroom setting, can have a positive impact for each person (Fellman, 1996). Appel et al.'s 1996 review of the literature, *The Impact of Diversity on Students,* found that student participation in diversity is related to changes in attitudes, openness to differences, and commitments to social justice. Equally important, such participation is increasingly related to satisfaction, academic success, and cognitive development.

Study abroad experiences can also be enriching and provide unique opportunities for personal and professional growth for both students and faculty. Cross-cultural experiences can be structured to enable students and faculty to observe different care delivery systems. For example, in northern India, one can observe three distinctly different systems of care: Western or allopathic systems, homeopathic systems, and Ayurveda systems, which have a long-standing tradition in India and Tibet. Integration of study abroad experiences into health education programs can greatly enrich the learning experience and, in fact, be life-changing for many people. However, careful and detailed planning is necessary. Iammarino and O'Rourke (1999) provide practical suggestions for the design and implementation of study abroad programs.

New international study opportunities have developed in recent years. Consortiums of health education programs now exist in Europe and North America (Kraemer, 1998). In 1990, the Consortium of Institutes of Higher Education in Health and Rehabilitation in Europe (COHEHRE), was established to promote international cooperation through exchange of students and faculty. Today, institutions from Middle Eastern and European countries are members. In 1993, the North American Consortium for Nursing and Allied Health (NACNAH), a framework for a formal U.S.-European consortium based on the COHEHRE model, was launched. Kraemer (1998) states that by bringing together multiple institutions with common purposes but with different cultural environments, all programs have been able to identify ways of participating collectively and individually. Areas of mutual interest include student exchanges and study tours, faculty/staff exchanges, technology exchanges, and joint research projects. Kraemer's discussion of barriers and rewards is a useful reference for those who wish to participate in international initiatives.

## *SUMMARY*

- The U.S. population is increasingly becoming racially and ethnically diverse, and this trend will continue. Consequently, health care providers are practicing in communities that reflect a more global society.
- Students and practitioners must develop and value cultural competence in order to achieve successful outcomes with clients/patients from various cultures.
- With increasing diversity among people living in the United States, alternative and complementary approaches are becoming mainstream. These approaches are being integrated with or substituted for more conventional medical treatments.
- Education of health professionals must involve more clinical and community-based experiences at home and abroad, if possible, to ensure students have an opportunity to interact with persons from diverse cultural and ethnic backgrounds and with those who are using, or want to explore, alternative approaches to health promotion and/or disease treatment.
- Educators and employers must partner to recruit and retain students and graduates from underrepresented groups to ensure the population of providers reflects the diversity in the United States.
- Education of health professionals must encourage lifelong learning and public service so graduates can effectively contribute their expertise to promote good health and quality of life.

## BIBLIOGRAPHY

Appel, M., Cartwright, D., Smith, D., and Wolf, L. (1996). *The Impact of Diversity on Students: A Preliminary Review of the Research Literature*. Washington, DC: Association of American Colleges and Universities.

Bureau of Primary Health Care (BPHC) (2001). *Cultural Competence: A Journey.* Retrieved from the World Wide Web: <http://www.bphc.hrsa.gov/culturalcompetence/Default.htm>.

Cerritos College Databook (2000). *California's Projected Demographics* (pp. 1-2). Retrieved from the World Wide Web: <http://www3.cerritos.edu/databook/zdata/Databook/8cafut.html>.

Eisenberg, D., Kessler, R., Foster, C., Norlock, F., Calkins, D., and Delbanco, T. (1993). Unconventional Medicine in the United States: Prevalence, Costs, and Patterns of Use. *The New England Journal of Medicine* 328(4):246-252.

Fellman, A. (1996). *Ourselves as Students: Multicultural Voices in the Classroom.* Carbondale, IL: Southern Illinois University Press.

Freeman, L.W., and Lawlis, G.F., (Eds.) (2001). *Complementary and Alternative Medicine: A Research-Based Approach.* St. Louis, MO: Mosby, Inc.

Goode, T. (2000). Cultural Competence Self-Test. Retrieved from the World Wide Web: <http://www.aafp.org/fpm/2001000/58cult.html>.

Iammarino, N.K. and O'Rourke, T.W. (1999). Planning and Implementing an International Travel/Study Course Experience for Health Professionals and Students. *Journal of Health Education* 39(3):166-172.

Independence Institute (2000). *Immigration Public Policy Center* (pp. 1-5). Retrieved from the World Wide Web: <http://i2i.org/failsafe.ippc.htm>.

Institute for Alternative Futures (1998). *The Future of Complementary and Alternative Approaches (CAAs) in US Health Care* (p. 3). Alexandria, VA: NCMIC Insurance Company.

Kraemer, L.G. (1998). Transatlantic Cooperation: Using a Consortial Approach to Enhance Health Professions Education and Practice. *Journal of Allied Health* 27(1):19-24.

National Center for Complementary and Alternative Medicine (2001a). *Complementary and Alternative Medicine Fact Sheets* (pp. 1-3). Retrieved from the World Wide Web: <http://nccam.nih.gov>.

National Center for Complementary and Alternative Medicine (2001b). *Major Domains of Complementary and Alternative Medicine* (pp. 1-3). Retrieved from the World Wide Web: <http://nccam.nih.gov>.

NIH Office of Alternative Medicine (NIHOAM) (1995). *Classification of Alternative Medical Practices.* Bethesda, MD: NIHOAM (p. 1).

O'Brien, J. (2001). U.S. Mayor Article, Washington Outlook. *Census Shows Hispanics Now Largest Ethnic Minority Other Surveys: Latino Population Increases Will Continue* (pp. 1-2). Retrieved from the World Wide Web: <http://www.usmayors.org/uscm/us_mayor_newspaper/documents/04_16_01/census.asp>.

Ornish, D., Brown, S., Scherwitz, L., Billings, J., Armstrong, W., Ports, T., McLanahan, S., Kirkeeide, R., Brand, R., and Gould, K. (1990). Medical Science: Can Lifestyle Changes Reverse Coronary Heart Disease? The Lifestyle Heart Trial. *The Lancet* 336:129-133.

Pew Health Professions Commission (PHPC) (1998). *Recreating Health Professional Practice for a New Century: The Fourth Report of the Pew Health Professions Commission.* San Francisco, CA: PHPC (p. 24).

Satcher, D. (2000). Health for All: Pipe Dream or Possibility? In Osterweis, M. and Holmes, D. (Eds.), *Global Dimensions of Domestic Health Issues.* Washington, DC: Association of Academic Health Centers (p. 23).

U.S. Census Bureau (2000a). *Overview of Race and Hispanic Origin.* (pp. 1-11). Retrieved from the World Wide Web: <http://usinfo.state.gov/topical/global/immigration/01031201.htm>.

U.S. Census Bureau (2000b). *Population Change and Distribution.* (pp. 1-7). Retrieved from the World Wide Web: <http://www.census.gov/population/www/cen2000/briefs.html>.

U.S. Census Bureau (2000c). *Profiles of General Demographic Characteristics: 2000 Census of Population and Housing.* (pp. 1-5). Retrieved from the World Wide Web: <http://www.census.gov/prod/cen2000>.

U.S. Census Bureau (2000d). *QT-01. Profile of General Demographic Characteristics: 2000. Geographic Area: United States.* (pp. 1-3). Retrieved from the World Wide Web: <http://www.census.gov/prod/cen2000>.

U.S. Census Bureau (2000e). *QT-03. Profile of Selected Economic Characteristics: 2000. Geographic Area: United States.* (pp.1-3). Retrieved from the World Wide Web: <http://www.census.gov/prod/cen2000>.

U.S. Census Bureau (2000f). *QT-P3. Race and Hispanic or Latino: 2000. Geographic Area: California.* (pp. 1-2). Retrieved from the World Wide Web: <http://www.census.gov/census2000/states/ca.html>.

U.S. Census Bureau (2000g). *QT-P3. Race and Hispanic or Latino: 2000. Geographic Area: Florida.* (pp. 1-2). Retrieved from the World Wide Web: <http://www.census.gov/census2000/states/fl.html>.

U.S. Census Bureau (2000h). *QT-P3. Race and Hispanic or Latino: 2000. Geographic Area: Iowa.* (pp. 1-2). Retrieved from the World Wide Web: <http://www.census.gov/census2000/states/ia.html>.

U.S. Census Bureau (2000i). *QT-P3. Race and Hispanic or Latino: 2000. Geographic Area: New York.* (pp. 1-2). Retrieved from the World Wide Web: <http://www.census.gov/census2000/states/ny.html>.

U.S. Census Bureau (2000j). *State and County QuickFacts: Virginia.* (pp. 1-2). Retrieved from the World Wide Web: <http://quickfacts.census.gov/qfd/states/51000.html>.

U.S. Department of Health and Human Services (USDHHS) (1999). *Building the Future of Allied Health: Report of the Implementation Task Force of the National Commission on Allied Health.* Rockville, MD: USDHHS.

Ziegler, J. (1997). The Mind, the Body and the Benefits Budget. *Business and Health.* (pp. 23-28).

Chapter 13

# Genomics, Proteomics, and Allied Health

Thomas W. Elwood

As the radius of knowledge gets longer,
the circumference of the unknown expands even more.

Anonymous

## *INTRODUCTION*

Gregor Mendel, an Austrian monk who belonged to the Augustinian religious order, is credited as the father of genetics. He conducted pea-breeding experiments between 1860 and 1865 that demonstrated how physical traits such as height and color are passed from one generation to the next through genes. Unfortunately, Mendel died in 1884 and the significance of his efforts went unrecognized and unappreciated until the early 1900s when the results of his work were confirmed by independent investigators.

During the first half of the twentieth century, researchers such as James Neel at the University of Michigan's Heredity Clinic were involved in estimating mutation rates. These initial formal studies of many diseases later featured prominently in the first gene mapping successes in human genetics.[1]

Perhaps the most significant milestone in the blossoming field of genetics occurred with the publication of an article of fewer than 900 words in the April 2, 1953, issue of *Nature* by British scientist Francis Crick and his American colleague James Watson. Titled, "A Structure for Deoxyribose Nucleic Acid," the article was free of jargon and hyperbole. Crick and Watson's simple, understated prose unleashed a major chain of events in the scientific world. Their opening words follow:

> We wish to suggest a structure for the salt of deoxyribose nucleic acid (D.N.A.). This structure has novel features which are of considerable biological interest.

Several paragraphs later, they concluded:

> It has not escaped our notice that the specific pairing we have postulated immediately suggests a possible copying mechanism for the genetic material.[2]

Another breakthrough occurred in 1956, when it was established that for human beings the correct diploid chromosome number is forty-six. Previously, it was erroneously believed that forty-eight chromosomes characterized our species. McKusick noted that

> the advance was significant to medicine, not because of the specific numerology but because of the associated simple improvements in technique that made chromosome analysis feasible in the study of disease and in clinical diagnosis. [3]

From 1956 until the present, great strides have been made and are expected to continue to be made at a dizzying pace. An event observed by television viewers around the globe occurred on June 26, 2000, when Francis Collins, Director of the National Human Genome Research Institute at the National Institutes of Health (NIH), and J. Craig Venter, Founder and President of Celera Genomics, appeared at the White House to announce completion of initial and public drafts of the human genome sequence. The first draft of the sequence was published in the following year. The expected completion date is 2003.

Meanwhile, on almost a daily basis, items are reported in the media that describe various developments stemming from research efforts to link particular genes with the onset of disease as well as with attempts to cure certain conditions. An example of a widely reported incident involved Jesse Gelsinger, a teenager who died in a gene therapy clinical trial at the University of Pennsylvania in Philadelphia. A viral vector that was used in his treatment resulted in an immune response that proved fatal. The episode resulted in congressional hearings.

## OVERVIEW

This chapter will deal with some of the implications of genomics and proteomics for allied health. Before proceeding, it will be useful to clarify terminology and provide a basis for the material that follows. *Genetics* involves the study of how human characteristics are inherited from one's parents. These attributes range anywhere from hair color and texture to one's susceptibility to diseases such as cancer. A *genome* is an entire system of genes, and *genomics* is the study of how genes interact and influence the biology and physical characteristics of living things. The gene's role is to synthesize proteins, and *proteomics* entails cataloging the identity and function of all the proteins in living organisms. As Service indicated,

> whereas genes remain essentially unchanged through life, proteins are constantly changing, depending on the tissues they're in, a person's age, and even what someone ate for breakfast. In genomics, the end point is well defined: the full sequence of an organism's DNA. With proteomics that's completely different. It's an attempt to capture the dynamics of a living system.[4]

DNA is the chemical inside the gene that carries the instructions for producing living organisms. DNA consists of lengthy, twisting molecules organized in a form often referred to as the double helix. The ladderlike arrangement of a DNA molecule consists of sugars, phosphates, and four nucleotide bases: adenine (A), thymine (T), cytosine (C), and guanine (G). The genetic code is specified by the order of some three billion nucleotide bases that would fill 150,000 pages of a telephone book with arrangements of these four letters. Amazingly, this phenomenon is equivalent to having an encyclopedia containing an alphabet of only four letters that are employed to make a total of sixty-four different three-letter words (codons). If placed in an edition of *The New York Times,* that issue of the newspaper would amount to an estimated 75,490 pages.[5]

Each gene possesses a unique sequence of base pairs. These base sequences enabled researchers to locate the position of genes on chromosomes and to construct a map of the entire human genome. Prior to completion of the human genome project, it was believed that members of our species each possessed approximately 100,000 genes. As of early 2002, that figure is more conservatively stated as 30,000 to 40,000 genes.

Apart from reproductive cells, each cell of the human body contains twenty-three pairs of chromosomes. Each one is a unit of compressed and twisted DNA. Every strand of DNA is a huge natural polymer of repeating nucleotides, embodying a code of the four characters (As, Ts, Cs, and Gs) that provide the blueprint for human life. The sequence of bases on a DNA strand is the recipe for encoding proteins. The strands are linked by hydrogen bonds between adenine and thymine (A—T) and between cytosine and guanine (C—G). Each linkage forms a base pair, with approximately three billion base pairs constituting the human genome. An easy way of remembering the four bases is to construct the following phrase from the initial letter of each nucleotide:

And
This
Creates
Genetics

Human beings tend to pride themselves on their uniqueness not only among themselves but also in relation to the animal kingdom as a whole. DNA sequences in humans, however, are 99.9 percent identical. Significantly, it is that 0.1 percent of variation that is expected to provide clues to genetic risk for common illnesses. Meanwhile, humans and chimpanzees are more than 98.5 percent identical at the DNA level. Perhaps even more humbling is the fact that only 300 human genes have no counterpart in the mouse genome.

During his remarks on June 26, 2000, President William Clinton referred to the human genome as the "Book of Life." To take that analogy a little further, the book may be viewed as consisting of twenty-three chapters (the chromosomes) containing thousands of stories (the genes), which in turn consist of paragraphs (exons) made up of words (codons) that consist of letters (nucleotide bases). The important sections of a gene are called exons, in which the instructions for making proteins reside. Longer sections are interspersed with "extra" or "nonsense" DNA. These sections are called introns. Genes also involve regulatory sequences that determine when, where, and which proteins are made and in what amounts.

If these sequences have extra bases, incorrectly ordered bases, or missing bases, the cell could make either a wrong protein or too much or too little of the correct one. Such miscalculations may result in disease. For example, a single misplaced base can cause sickle-cell anemia. Marshall indicated that

> people who inherit the mutation from both parents produce an abnormal hemoglobin that forms a polymeric fiber, making red blood cells rigid and sticky. Because having a single copy can help protect against malaria, the gene occurs widely in tropical regions. But having two copies causes red blood cells to form clumps and block circulation, damaging organs. Roughly one in 13 African Americans carries the gene, and about 72,000 people in the United States have the disease, which can be fatal.[6]

The genome may resemble a book in certain respects, but it lacks capital letters and punctuation, there are no breaks between words, sentences, or paragraphs, and there can be huge strings of nonsense letters that are scattered both between and within sentences. Consider the following cluster of letters:

wmtjchfpqicthepurmnswuchaptersapzmeirofdiskl
plwmqisxnfpthislaquwrcnslgptbooklqazpiuytwha
veiwmskdjywnaxmwklotcjelhsxpoflwamnzakjshd
pqofoodwieurypqnxiwmfactsomzjyslewnvqpcmei

Buried within this cluster is the message, "The chapters of this book have a lot of food facts." I did not intend to write food facts, but that is the mutation that occurred when a finger struck the letter f on the keyboard instead of the letter g. The mistake results in an entirely different meaning than the one intended originally. This example may appear somewhat silly, but consider the following sequence offered by Davies:

ACTAGCAACCTCAAACAGACACC**ATG**GTGCACCTGACTCC

TGAGGAGAAGTCTGCCGTT . . . GCCCACAAGTATCAC**TAA**

AAGCTCGCTTTC

ATG is a marker to start protein synthesis for hemoglobin while the marker TAA sends a signal to stop. In the sequence below, each triplet of letters furnishes the code for a specific amino acid. In this instance, **GAG** codes for glutamic acid while **GTG** codes for valine. Coding for **GAG** produces the malformed hemoglobin protein that results in sickle-cell anemia.[7]

ATG GTG CAC CTG ACT CCT GAG GAG AAG TCT

Readers with an interest in the themes of the driving force of medical research agendas, the potency of racial stereotypes, and the power of social circumstances to dictate patterns of diagnosis and treatment may find it worthwhile to obtain a copy of a book titled, *Dying in the City of the Blues: Sickle Cell Anemia and the Politics of Race and Health* by Keith Wailoo (Chapel Hill: University of North Carolina, 2001).

## ROLE OF GENETICS IN HEALTH CARE

Guttmacher stated that prior to the sequencing of the human genome, genetics played a relatively small role in medicine. The emphasis used to be on relatively rare conditions involving an extra or missing chromosome or part of a chromosome, as in the case of Down syndrome, or when mutation of a single gene occurs, such as in cystic fibrosis. Only a limited group of health professional specialists was involved in treating these conditions, often in tertiary care centers.[8]

As of early 2002, however, more than 5,000 distinct genetic disorders have been identified and the focus has been expanded to include polygenic disorders such as diabetes and cardiovascular conditions in which several different genes may be implicated. Unraveling the genome also offers the potential to obtain a better understanding of nongenetic factors. Increasingly, health care will place an emphasis on health maintenance instead of on disease treatment. Following is a list of the leading causes of mortality in the United States in 1999.

1. Diseases of the heart (30.3 percent of deaths)
2. Malignant neoplasms (23.0 percent)
3. Cerebrovascular diseases (7.0 percent)
4. Chronic lower respiratory disease (5.2 percent)
5. Accidents or unintentional injuries (4.1 percent)
6. Diabetes mellitus (2.9 percent)
7. Influenza and pneumonias (2.7 percent)
8. Alzheimer's disease (2.8 percent)
9. Nephritis, nephrotic syndrome, and nephrosis (1.5 percent)
10. Septicemia (1.3 percent)
11. All other causes (20.2 percent)

One or more genes are directly implicated in the top nine causes of mortality except for injuries.[9] Even then, it is still possible that genetic factors may play a role in causing balance problems that result in falls or in sleep disorders that lead drivers to doze at the wheel.

Collins and Guttmacher point out:

> once hereditary contributions to disease are identified, it is potentially only a short step to the possibility of predictive diagnostics, as exemplified by the case of hereditary nonpolyposis colorectal cancer. However, before moving such diagnostic tests into mainstream medicine, it is critical to collect data about their clinical validity and utility. Premature introduction of predictive tests, before the value of the information has been established, actually could be quite harmful. Concerns about adequate oversight of this process have been recently addressed by the Secretary's Advisory Committee on Genetic Testing, which has urged more direct Food and Drug Administration oversight of genetic

tests, particularly when they are being proposed for predictive purposes in currently healthy individuals.[10]

Meanwhile, in many states activist parents are expressing dissatisfaction with public health officials who are viewed as moving too slowly in making tandem mass spectrometry accessible, a kind of technology aimed at screening newborns for several inherited diseases.[11]

Clearly, many benefits are derived from gene testing. Apart from the discomfort of having a blood sample taken, there usually is little personal risk. A negative result can cause a tremendous sense of relief and may eliminate the need for frequent checkups and tests that are routine in families with a high risk of cancer. Even a positive result can relieve uncertainty and allow a person to make informed decisions about the future. A positive result also affords an opportunity for a person to take steps, such as losing weight, trying to reduce stress, or stopping the use of tobacco products, to reduce risk before disease can develop.

Gene testing offers several benefits. Retinoblastoma testing provides a good example of the value of administering this procedure. This condition occurs in early childhood and affects about one youngster in 20,000. The tumor develops from the immature retina, the part of the eye responsible for detecting light and color. Retinoblastoma occurs in both hereditary and nonhereditary forms. In the hereditary form, multiple tumors are found in both eyes; in the nonhereditary form only one eye is affected and by only one tumor. Untreated, the result is usually fatal, but early diagnosis and treatment can produce a survival rate higher than 90 percent.

Yet many concerns are associated with genetic testing. Some procedures may not be cost-effective. For example, women who have the factor V Leiden allele who use oral contraceptives are at increased risk for venous thrombosis, a condition that could prove fatal. Yet it would be difficult to justify testing every woman for the presence of this genetic factor as a prerequisite for prescribing oral contraception. Tests currently are available for more than 500 genetic diseases and some of these diagnostics can cost more than $1,000.

The situation is complicated by the fact that many polygenic conditions are influenced by environmental factors such as diet and tobacco smoking. Some disorders that occur in families can be traced to shared environmental exposures, such as too much sunlight, rather than any inherited susceptibility. Furthermore, some mutations that are detected by a positive test may never lead to disease. In addition, because existing tests are geared to detect only the more common mutations in a gene, some disease-causing mutations may escape detection, creating a false sense of assurance.

## *ETHICAL, LEGAL, AND SOCIAL ISSUES*

Because gene test results hold a wealth of information, confidentiality is a major concern. Individuals have been denied health insurance, have lost jobs or promotions, and even have been denied the opportunity to adopt children because of their gene status. Perhaps the most serious limitation of gene testing is that test information is not matched by appropriate diagnostics and therapies. For example, Huntington's disease is an extremely debilitating and ultimately fatal condition. A question worth pondering is who really would want to know many years before its onset that a fatal disease will occur and be cognizant that no treatment of any kind is available?

Many related questions remain unresolved and will continue to attract the attention of health policymakers. When the Human Genome Research Project was started at the NIH in the early 1990s, funding was set aside to study the ethical, legal, and social implications (ELSI) of unraveling the genome's mysteries. The following issues need to be addressed:

- Who should have access to genetic information?
- Should there be an obligation to inform spouses and children of test results?
- Should the government be able to mandate individual or community-wide screening?
- Should release of records to employers be a condition for employment?
- Should insurance companies use information to determine risk?
- Should tests be covered by insurance?
- When does a genetic condition qualify for protection by the Americans with Disabilities Act?
- Will persons who have low income or no income have access to tests?
- Will incarcerated criminals have access to tests?
- Should designing of perfect babies be allowed to occur so that those who can afford to do so may attempt to produce children who are gifted in a variety of intellectual, artistic, and athletic ways?
- If it subsequently is shown that the divorced spouse of a woman with a severely handicapped child was not the one who impregnated her, should he be compelled to pay child support to cover the child's treatment costs?

Because gene tests reveal information not only about the individual, but also about relatives and future offspring, the results can challenge family and other personal relationships. With whom should a person share test results? Do other family members really want to know if they are at risk for a condition that cannot be treated?

Apart from subsidizing research, the federal government increasingly is being drawn into related aspects of debates involving the human genome. President William Clinton issued an executive order on February 8, 2000, prohibiting agencies from using protected genetic information as a basis for employment decisions. Burlington Northern Santa Fe Railway was found in violation of the Americans with Disabilities Act in February 2001 for genetic testing on chromosome 17 in relation to carpal tunnel syndrome. Toxic tort lawsuits are expected to increase based on a claim that a commercial product such as a vaccine or a drug aimed at preventing or treating one disease poses additional risks to individuals with specific genetic susceptibilities.

For example, a vaccine for Lyme disease is implicated in the cause of crippling arthritis. Defendants in these cases, such as drug, cosmetic, and chemical companies, can be expected to counter with the claim that any adverse reaction which may ensue is caused by a rare susceptibility in a person's genes. In December 2000, the National Institute of Environmental Health Sciences (NIEHS) established five National Centers for Toxicogenomics to learn more about the relationship between genes and environmental factors.

During the first session of the 107th Congress in 2001, bills were introduced in both the House of Representatives (HR 602) and the Senate (SR 318) to prohibit genetic discrimination. Proposed legislation in the form of HR 1644 and SR 790 were introduced in the same session to ban human cloning. In January 2002, SR 1893 was introduced in the second session to prohibit human cloning, whereas SR 1899 was introduced to ban human cloning and protect stem cell research. Advocates of cloning often make a distinction between reproductive cloning and therapeutic cloning. The former involves creating a person who is a genetically identical copy of another person. The latter is designed to create new tissue to replace diseased cells and organs.

The continuation of efforts to examine the potential of stem cells in the treatment of disease has many supporters on Capitol Hill. Theoretically, stem cells from embryos can be grown into any kind of human tissue such as heart, blood, pancreas, nerve, muscle, cartilage, skin, and bone cells. In vitro fertilization is employed by uniting donor DNA with an unfertilized egg to start the growth of an embryo. By the fifth or sixth day, a trophoblast consisting of an outer ring of cells that will form the placenta has developed; inside, the growing embryo mass contains stem cells. This inner cell mass then is separated and the stem cells are cultivated to make colonies of cells, each of which has the potential to grow into different kinds of tissue. These specialized cells then could be grown into tissues that can be transplanted to patients.

In the summer of 2001, President George W. Bush announced a decision to allow federal funding of limited research using embryonic stem cells. Federal support of research using existing embryonic stem cells will be permitted, but the funding cannot be used to develop new lines of stem cells. Following this decision, a controversy arose over the number of existing stem cell lines that are available and the degree to which they are accessible to researchers.

Many states already have banned human cloning and they continue to provide another arena in which action is ongoing for related cases. For example, in Massachusetts a dispute arose over the issue of whose names should be listed as parents on a child's birth certificate. The case, which involves a couple and an unrelated woman who was paid to carry the embryo and deliver a pair of twins, went to the commonwealth's Supreme Judicial Court. The question before the judges is whether the genetic mother can and should replace the birth mother on the babies' birth certificates. If not, the genetic mother would have to go to court to adopt her children legally from the woman who gave birth to them.[12]

## *PHARMACOGENOMICS*

Phillips et al. assert that

> several highly publicized reports and policy initiatives have urged greater efforts to reduce the rate of adverse events in medical care. Pharmaceutical agents are one of the most commonly identified causes of adverse events, resulting in significant patient morbidity, mortality, and excess medical care costs. A widely cited meta-analysis estimated that more than two million hospitalized patients have severe adverse drug reactions (ADRs) annually in the United States even when drugs are appropriately prescribed and administered, and that ADRs ranked between the fourth and sixth leading cause of death in the United States in 1994. One possible cause of ADRs is genetic variation in how individuals metabolize drugs.[13]

In most cases, two individuals diagnosed with the same condition may be prescribed identical drugs in the same dosages. Pharmacogenomics holds the promise of changing this one-drug-fits-all approach. Individualized medication based on genetically determined variation in effectiveness and adverse side effects provides an opportunity to predict responsiveness to drug interventions. The potential also may exist for the development of new medications.

## *The Role of the Health Professions*

The transition from genetics to genomics has resulted in a change from having only a small number of health specialists involved in patient care to a much larger and more diverse group of practitioners. As popular magazines, television news, and special sections of major newspapers furnish descriptions of every theoretical and actual breakthrough in the genetic aspects of diagnosing and treating disease, the public's appetite for additional information becomes increasingly whetted. The result is that all kinds of health professionals may be asked to answer questions about genetic tests and disease risks.

The National Coalition for Health Professional Education in Genetics (NCHPEG) was formed in 1996 in response to this situation. Partial funding was obtained from the Department of Energy and The Robert Wood Johnson Foundation to launch the coalition. More than 100 diverse health professional organizations constitute its membership. The organization's role is to identify core competencies in the health professions and integrate genetics into continuing education, licensure, and certification exams.

Core competencies have been developed and arranged into the overall areas of knowledge, attitudes, and skills health professionals should have regarding genetics. The knowledge section consists of seventeen different items such as possessing a basic genetics terminology, understanding the role of genetics in health and disease, and knowing the indications for testing and interventions. The attitudes section is made up of ten items such as being able to appreciate the sensitivity of genetic information, the need for privacy and confidentiality, and being able to recognize the limits of one's own genetics expertise. The skills section covers seventeen items, including the ability to identify clients who would benefit from genetic services, being able to seek assistance from and refer to appropriate sources, and being able to use new technologies to obtain current, credible information.

Not all health professionals must be versed in the forty-four different competencies. Steps already are being taken to determine which competencies are appropriate for each profession. A significant move in the direction of ascertaining the role of allied health in this regard occurred with the funding of a project by the Bureau of Health Professions. Under the direction of David D. Gale, Dean of the College of Health Sciences at Eastern Kentucky University, efforts began in November 2000 to examine how genetics should be incorporated into the following professions:

Clinical laboratory science
Dietetics

Occupational therapy
Physical therapy
Physician assistant
Radiologic technology
Respiratory therapy
Speech-language pathology

Individuals representing these professions met over the course of one year to consider which aspects of genetics should be emphasized, whether new academic courses need to be offered, and whether existing courses should be supplemented with information about genetics. Other considerations involve the preparation of texts, Web-based information, case studies, and continuing education courses. A relevant question is what should be done at both preservice and inservice levels of education? One outcome of the project is a set of documents that will be published on the NCHPEG Web site to provide strategies and concrete examples on how to infuse genomics into the curricula of different academic programs. This material will also be available in CD-ROM format.

The needs of both current and future students as well as those individuals already in practice should be addressed. A challenge for each profession is to see how advances translate into current patterns of health care. The process of adopting any curricular innovations may have to be implemented in different ways by each group. Examples of necessary steps to take include making presentations to a professional association's board of directors, publishing articles in journals and making speeches at annual conferences to stimulate interest, and influencing accreditation, licensing, and credentialing agencies to accept proposed changes in the curriculum.

Much research remains to be carried out and not all of it will be in laboratories. Although major emphasis will be placed on learning more about the human genome, particularly about the prevalence of gene variants and the magnitude of risk associated with such variants, genetic tests and interventions should undergo evaluation. In addition to studying interactions between gene variants and the environment, attention must also be paid to conducting population-based studies.

The perceptions of both the health professions community and the general public should be taken into account regarding gene testing, gene therapy, and the extent to which genomics is viewed as a specialty area reserved for a small number of specialists who treat rare disorders. Information and communication needs of both health professionals and laypersons must be assessed and met. Another fruitful line of investigations will be to examine how different health systems such as managed care organizations affect the provision of genetic tests and prevention/treatment services.

## *CONCLUSION*

McKusick stated the estimated 30,000 to 40,000 human genes encode more than ten times that number of proteins.

This disparity has resulted in a partial shift of focus from the gene to proteins and from genomics to proteomics. The availability of the human genome sequence and information on proteomics related to the sequence is likely to change medicine in many ways. It will influence reproductive medicine, for example, pemitting ever more specific diagnoses at earlier stages. [14]

Just as genomics and proteomics will continue to evolve, health professionals will have to adapt accordingly and not simply rely on dogmatic thinking often used in the past. In many instances, roles have yet to be clearly defined and it remains unclear what members of various professions will need to know about these areas in order to function effectively in this new milieu. The situation will be further complicated by the fact that changes will continue to occur which may pose new educational challenges as well as provide new opportunities.

## REFERENCE NOTES

1. Weiss, K.M. and Schull, W.J. (2002). Perspectives Fulfilled: The Work and Thought of J.V. Neel (1915-2000). *Perspectives in Biology and Medicine,* 45(1): 46-64.

2. Crick, F. and Watson, J.A. (1953). Structure for Deoxyribose Nucleic Acid. *Nature,* (April 2): 737.

3. McKusick, V. (2001). The Anatomy of the Human Genome: A Neo-Vesalian Basis for Medicine in the 21st Century. *JAMA,* 286(18): 2289.

4. Service, R. (2001). High-Speed Biologists Search for Gold in Proteins. *Science,* 294: 2074-2075.

5. Wade, N. (2001). Analysis of Human Genome Discovers Far Fewer Genes. *The New York Times.* (February 11, 2001). Retrieved from the World Wide Web: <http://www.nytimes.com>.

6. Marshall, E. (2001). Gene Gemisch Cures Sickle Cell in Mice. *Science,* 294 (December 14), p. 2268.

7. Davies, K. (2001). *Cracking the Genome: Inside the Race to Unlock Human DNA.* New York: The Free Press, pp. 38-39.

8. Guttmacher, A. (2001). Plenary Session Address. Association of Schools of Allied Health Professions Annual Conference. Norfolk, VA, October 8.

9. National Center for Health Statistics. Deaths: Leading Causes for 1999. *National Vital Statistics Report.* 49(11); 88 pp.: 2001, p. 8.

10. Collins, F. and Guttmacher, A. (2001). Genetics Moves into the Medical Mainstream. *JAMA,* 286(18): 2322.

11. Marshall, E. (2001). Fast Technology Drives New World of Newborn Screening. *Science,* 294: 2272-2274.

12. Ferdinand, P. (2001). Massachusetts Tests Legal Standing of Surrogate, Genetic Mothers. *The Washington Post.* September 6, p. A06.

13. Phillips, K., Veenstra, D.L., Oren, E., Lee, J.K., Sadee, W. (2001). Potential Role of Pharmacogenomics in Reducing Adverse Drug Reactions: A Systematic Review. *JAMA,* 286(18): 2270.

14. McKusick, Anatomy of the Human Genome, p. 2294.

## RESOURCES ON THE WORLD WIDE WEB

Centers for Disease Control and Prevention (CDC), Office of Genetics and Disease Prevention, <www.cdc.gov/genetics>.

Federal Legislation, <http://thomas.loc.gov/>.

Genomic and Genetic Resources at the National Human Genome Research Institute, <http://www.nhgri.nih.gov/Data/>.

National Coalition for Health Professional Education in Genetics (NCHPEG), <http://www.nchpeg.org/>.

Online Mendelian Inheritance in Man (a catalogue of human genes and genetic disorders), <http://www.ncbi.nlm.nih.gov/omim/>.

TREEBuilder (a consumer-oriented tool for recording a family medical history and drawing a multigenerational pedigree), <www.genetichealth.com>.

Chapter 14

# Interprofessional Collaborative Alliances

Lorna Hayward
Rosanna DeMarco
M. Marcia Lynch

## *INTRODUCTION*

The information presented in this chapter has broad implications and pragmatic value for students enrolled in programs of nursing and in the allied health professions of physical therapy, nursing, respiratory therapy, speech and language pathology, occupational therapy, cardiopulmonary sciences, and exercise physiology. However, this chapter is also designed for use by a diverse professional audience including novice allied health practitioners, managers, faculty, and policymakers. It is important to realize that collaborative skills learned and practiced in the classroom are transferable to clinical practice and any work environment. This is true because the principles of collaboration, whether used in the classroom, in the clinical setting, or with an interdisciplinary team in academia, follow the same theoretical framework.

The purpose of this chapter is to provide the reader with an appreciation for the necessity and value of collaboration among individuals working in health care settings. Definitions will be provided for *collaboration, interprofessional alliances, multidisciplinary, cross-disciplinary,* and *transdisciplinary work.* A theoretical model will be presented to illustrate the process of a successful collaborative alliance. Two case examples will assist the reader to integrate the principles, and concepts, of interprofessional collaborative alliances.

## *DEFINITION OF TERMS*

For the purposes of this chapter, the term *collaborative teamwork* is defined as "an in-depth cooperative effort in which experts from" either the same or "diverse disciplines, clinical experiences, or settings work together to contribute to the study of a problem."[1]

*Interprofessional collaboration* is defined as when two or more experts from different disciplines collaborate in a manner that augments one another's strengths, experiences, and backgrounds.[2] Interprofessional collaboration is one type of work effort that occurs in clinical practice. Increasingly, most workplace and many classroom assignments are being addressed by groups of individuals working as teams.[3] The clinical setting in which most health care professionals currently practice is interdisciplinary, complex, and patient-outcome oriented. An example of interprofessional collaboration in the clinical setting would be when a physician, nurse, physical therapist, respiratory therapist, and a speech therapist participate in a team meeting to arrive at an integrative approach for treating a client hospitalized with a complex condition such as a spinal cord injury (see Figure 14.1). Figure 14.1 illustrates that interprofessional collaboration requires the integration of patient experiences and knowledge with that of the professional clinical team. Although professional contributions such as specialized experiences and knowledge are an important part of collaborative efforts, patient contributions are equally im-

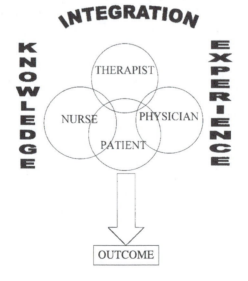

FIGURE 14.1. Interprofessional Collaboration

portant for team approaches. It is believed patients can offer in-depth experiences and knowledge that significantly direct assessment, planning, and treatment outcome.

In the spinal cord injury example, an integrative professional approach is useful because it provides diverse perspectives on a clinical problem. A benefit of the interprofessional approach is that problem definitions and solutions reflect a collective whole versus an individual effort.[4] The solution to a clinical problem generated by an interprofessional team may be more complete or holistic than one devised by a single clinician or even by two clinicians from the same discipline.

However, a goal of collaboration is the creation of value, not merely value as the sum of individual efforts but, more important, value born from the exponential product of the collective interactions among the collaborators. Collaboration describes a process of value creation that our traditional structure of communication and teamwork cannot achieve. The Interprofessional Alliance Model presented later in the chapter illustrates the process of value creation during a successful collaborative effort.

By definition, there are three interpretations of work among and within disciplinary groups.[5] *Multidisciplinary* work is when different disciplines come together based on a commonality. For example, two health care providers who specialize in hematology and oncology respectively may attend a patient care conference based on their common interest in life-threatening illnesses related to blood. The fact that they enter a room together to discuss a patient means just that; they have come together based on a common need to care for a client. *Cross-disciplinary* work is when different disciplines actually work together on a similar question or a similar goal related to a patient. In an acute care center, a physical therapist and a pharmacist may work together to make sure a patient is able to leave the facility with the knowledge and experience he or she needs to take medications and ambulate safely. *Transdisciplinary* work is when disciplines come together but work with a common model. They approach patients together and use their discipline only as a special and specific lens to define an approach that is seen as whole rather than separate and distinct based on individual disciplines. In a true sense, trans-disciplinary work is a formidable example of how to collaborate or build interprofessional alliances (see Figure 14.2).

## *NEED FOR COLLABORATION*

The ability to work collaboratively is quickly becoming one of the top skills desired by employers in health care and business. It is considered not

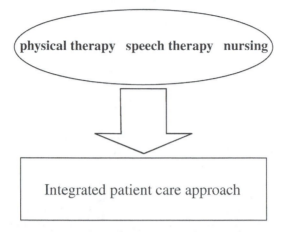

FIGURE 14.2. Transdisciplinary Collaboration. The blending of discipline-specific skills leads to an integrated patient care approach.

only necessary but a mandatory prerequisite by employers in health care systems.[6] Collaboration allows individual power to be joined with the power of others to attain common goals. Future employers desire graduates of health care professional programs to have skills that allow them to collaborate as the highest form of power strategy.[7]

Collaboration is a power-filled strategy because power is considered a mobilization of people's concerted activities, thoughts, and ideas. Working together breaks new ground and brings new knowledge to the workplace. To know something or somebody in a "new way" rather than "no other way" is active rather than passive. Static views of knowledge may occur without collaboration.[8] As such, this type of knowledge discounts and disqualifies various interests and perspectives. This is not what future employers want or need.

A survey conducted with Fortune 500 companies in 1997 indicated the top four desired abilities possessed by new college graduates were teamwork, problem-solving skills, interpersonal skills, and verbal communication skills.[9] Thus, the ability to work collaboratively and effectively is an important skill for students to acquire. Effective collaboration skills can be developed and refined during a student's college years in a safe environment (e.g., a classroom) as preparation for entering the workforce, whether in the capacity of clinical affiliation, internship or practicum or during permanent employment.

For health professionals, collaboration in clinical practice may take place between individuals in the same discipline or in teams composed of providers from different disciplines. Thus, it is imperative allied health students understand the concept of collaboration and be able to develop strategies for creating successful interprofessional alliances. Whether they are formed in clinical practice or academia, interprofessional teams are useful because they provide diverse perspectives on practice, research, educational problems, and/or policy issues.

Health care organizations and businesses are continually requiring that more work be conducted in teams. Although working with others has many benefits, it can also be quite challenging due to the different perspectives, agendas, learning styles, needs, and goals espoused by individual participants.

## CASE EXAMPLE

The following case example illustrates how a university restructured three separate schools (nursing, allied health, and pharmacy) into a single interdisciplinary college of health sciences. The schools were merged to bring the college in line with national agendas that promoted interdisciplinary patient care. The university was also responding to changes imposed by the health care system associated with managed care and the changing demographics of the U.S. population. One such change was the reduction in the number of clinical placement sites for allied health students. The idea behind the schools' merger was to foster a philosophy of interdisciplinary teaching, research, and service agendas among faculty that in turn could be instilled in students.

### Case One

Centered in an urban area, a large university had recently created and supported the integration of three health profession schools—the schools of nursing, pharmacy, and health professions—into a college of health professions. At the same time, a negotiated and grant-supported effort to develop partnerships with eight neighborhood health centers (NHC) and one of the schools received positive reviews in terms of educational, research, and service opportunities for students, faculty, and NHC professional staff. As a result of the merger, all health professions students and faculty were encouraged to creatively integrate education, research, and service as an interdisciplinary initiative.

Faculty began to organize learning and service opportunities for students at the NHCs. This led to a breakthrough of the artificial and real boundaries between the university in a protected separate boundary and the NHCs in the real world of clients. Another reason for expanding the use of the NHCs was the decrease in opportunities for students to gain clinical experience, particularly in an urban setting that experienced strong competition among health care professional schools.

For a long time, faculty and their students were seen as "users" of opportunities at the health centers and received little in terms of research or academic recognition. However, in the process of broadening a beginning partnership with the NHCs, health profession students and their respective clinical faculty worked with health care providers from the NHCs using a common model. In doing this, the collaborative relationship became more than a cognitive exercise—it became a real perspective. Essentially, the plans for student and faculty experiences did not include a conceptual plan for integration of the disciplines nor did they include a plan that operationalized the idea of partnership. Articulation of a collaborative relationship with the NHCs' health providers was little more than an engaging ideal that did not directly address the possibility of sharing a common vision of working together with patients at the NHCs.

At administrative meetings of the college of health sciences there was the perception that the presence of students of different disciplines in collaborative relationships in health care settings was evidence of interdisciplinary collaboration and teamwork.

The reality was that students and faculty had a sense of identity originating from the same university and a special collaborative relationship with the NHCs but little else.

## Discussion About Case One

This first case demonstrates how systematized clinical arrangements can be used to develop a collaborative relationship for partnership's sake but do not contribute to a trajectory of experiences that are based on a sense of mission or intention. If organizations involved in collaborative relationships do not communicate their specific obligations to one another and define what it means to be partners at all levels (within and among one another), there is no relationship. There is also a lack of quality care potential since the system relies on making sure neither organization interferes with the other's established systems of learning and service.

All health care systems are created on the premise that there is a structure and a process that support specific outcomes. Because there is little time to develop systems that we know conceptually are the way things should be, health care systems systemize collaboration from a structural perspective. It is easier to operationalize multidisciplinary and cross-disciplinary work because it means *physically* bringing students, faculty, and other health providers together. However, multidisciplinary and cross-disciplinary work does not address the process of *finding together* a framework or common model in which all feel equal in their contribution as a partnership team.

There are advantages to utilizing a transdisciplinary approach. Some barriers are more pervasive than the need to quickly operationalize partnerships based on an ideal. Contemporary employers are looking for new graduate health care providers that can comfortably forge team relationships or simply become members of a team. When patient care is examined from the perspective of a common team framework, the patient benefits from a whole perspective. This is equally true in health care education. If health care providers and professors created a transdisciplinary approach to education, students would have a wider and broader perspective of care based on ideal and real clinical experiences.

## BARRIERS RELATED TO INTERPROFESSIONAL WORK

Many barriers exist or potentially may be created when individuals from different disciplines work together. These barriers may be related to gender or illusions related to power.[10] Many professionals seem reluctant to admit that the roots of conflict are buried in power plays. Essentially, having control over a situation or others can be a godhead of sorts.[11] Questioning why we hold on to power over one another as professionals or even over patients is often perceived as treason or heresy. Creating boundaries of conversational dissonance between one another will confine and constrict creativity to do something about it. Conversational dissonance is an incongruity or inconsistency in how and why people speak to one another. According to Friedemann, dissonance or lack of congruence refers to the absence of rhythms and patterns that allow energy to flow freely within and between systems and people in those systems.[12]

### Gender Issues

On the other hand, gender differences pertaining to interprofessional work can be particularly difficult barriers in partnerships. Women are acculturated to be collaborators. Women learn to create, maintain, and sustain relationships socially and professionally. Men are acculturated to achieve autonomous success through powerful and competitive relationships. Although this sounds a bit stereotypical, this dynamic has a long history that underlies the potential success of relationships in any health care organization. As a result, when health care disciplines that have a history of being gender seg-regated approach professional relationships, there is a natural progressive dilemma. It is more comfortable for women to gravitate to transdisciplinary work and for men to gravitate to multidisciplinary and cross-disciplinary work by definition.

It has been claimed that women often translate, create group connections, and maintain many interpersonal skills that allow smooth functioning of a team effort.[13,14] They translate and demystify complexity among co-work-ers to keep a project progressing.[15,16] Women create level playing fields of language and experiences by helping members of work groups feel comfort-able with discussions or phases of project experiences. Women often inter-cede to temper interpersonal situations into collaborative interchanges rather than igniting tense, noncommunicative standoffs. Women get people to talk to one another when doing so may be perceived as a concession to inde-pendent ideas or positions.

The majority of employees in academic research settings and in direct provider areas for health care are women.[17] Women often connect individu-als with similar interests to ultimately benefit both the service sector and cli-ents. Women may be the initiators when discussing collaborative options or creating linkages for benefit in grant or award initiatives.[18]

### *Power Illusions*

Another barrier to collaborative relationships is the dissonance that oc-curs between articulating the desire for a partnership and not engaging in a partnership. If individuals who profess to work collaboratively meet infre-quently, do not reflect honestly on their shared vision and the progress made to it, or do not demonstrate care from the perspective of the functional or structural issues in the partnership, the relationship(s) will fail. An illusion of power over others comes from silence. Silence controls the situation and does not allow for change. One feels powerful because the culture of not confronting constructively is reinforced by not causing tension and anxiety in interpersonal interactions. This is illusory because control over a situa-tion does not allow for the possibility of diverse options and diverse solu-tions. Together as professionals, we can examine mistakes and responsibili-ties related to power and redirect how we can work together.

### *Strategies to Reduce Barriers to Interprofessional Work*

Several strategies can be used to decrease the effect of these barriers or prevent them from occuring. These strategies include the following:

1. Legitimizing all work completed in the partnership as a group product
2. Relying on the giftedness of each individual in the collaborative effort and assigning work accordingly
3. Communicating regularly as a group (by telephone, e-mail, meetings, etc.)
4. Meeting at the residences of members to gain an appreciation for their life outside of work
5. Taking time at every other meeting to utilize an evaluative framework that openly allows discussion about the nature of care, reflection, and social support between group members
6. Asking often, "Is this a real partnership or do we just think it is?"

## Educational Strategies for Students to Explore Interprofessional Barriers

By referring back to case one, teachers/leaders can guide students toward an examination of specific barriers by:

- Providing definitions of interdisciplinary and interprofessional collaboration. Discuss the idea of parallel work or synthesis in which a clinician moves from being polite to becoming a partner.
- Examining the benefits of forming interprofessional alliances. Describe how contemporary employers are looking for an expanded repertoire of skills in new allied health graduates that include being team players. Describe other benefits such as becoming a more holistic care provider, especially when patient care is examined from the perspective of an interdisciplinary team.
- Describing examples of barriers to interprofessional alliances, such as those created by professions and those created by individuals.

### Specific Activities to Enhance Collaboration

1. Present the strategy of interprofessional reflection during time-constrained work. Describe the benefits of reflection and the connection between this skill and self-directed professional development in novice and expert clinicians.
2. Share recognition.
3. Acknowledge contributions.
4. Establish group goals and strategies for dealing with conflict.
5. Brainstorm for active group problem solving.

The common theme embedded in these specific activities is the opportunity to refocus group work from the point of view of group goals. A characteristic of a successful group is the generation of group goals. Before beginning any group project it is imperative to establish group goals. The task addressed by collaborators must be a shared and understood goal. A successful group must have a common goal or purpose and group members must be committed to achieving this goal. In addition, the outcome must be significant enough that it demands of individuals more than they can accomplish alone. One strategy for generating group goals and increasing individual commitment to group endeavors is to generate group goals collectively and make them explicit. Making goals explicit means *writing them down* and ensuring that each group member has a copy of the final goals for the project.

### Guidelines for Generating Group Goals

The following is an outline for determining group goals. A suggested number of goals for any group project is three to five. Goals should be written in an objective manner that contains a measurable output. For example, a goal for desired product outcome written as "The group goal is to achieve the best possible outcome for the project" does not contain an objective measurable outcome. The goal would be better stated as "The group goal is to achieve a grade of B+ or better for the final project."

When writing group goals, the following questions may be used as a guide:

1. What is an acceptable result for your efforts?

2. How will decisions be made? Will decisions be made by unanimous agreement of all group members or majority rule? The more shared the group goals are, the more likely a consensus can be developed. This means the process may run smoothly if all group members help define the ground rules for how a group will behave or make decisions. The reason for this is that an individual is more likely to follow rules he or she has developed because the rules reflect how he or she thinks and behaves.

3. What happens in those instances when disagreement occurs (e.g., two or more alternatives are under consideration with no consensus possible)? How can the negative consequences accompanying bad feelings of this unresolved issue be avoided altogether?

There are many different strategies for resolving conflict. A suggested procedure includes identifying areas within the project the group agrees upon. Group members can brainstorm collectively and one person can write down areas of agreement. You may find the group agrees more than it disagrees, and by identifying *agreement* the conflict resolution process begins on a positive note. The following steps may be taken to continue the conflict resolution process: (a) accept an alternative that meets all sides' needs; (b) search for mutual understanding of all points of view involved, of the key issues involved, and of results that would constitute a fully acceptable solution; and (c) commit to creative efforts to build acceptable alternatives based upon understanding of the conflict. However, keep in mind some conflict is good because better ideas often emerge from groups in which there are differing points of view.

4. How are roles going to be identified? What are the group rules for participation, expectations, and consequences associated with the inferior performance of group members?

5. What are the intergroup communication expectations? What approach will be taken to ensure all members are heard and their ideas are considered? What approach is taken to encourage all members to contribute suggestions?

Finally, since they are formed around a shared goal, collaborations tend to dissipate once the goal is either achieved or demonstrated to be unachievable. To address this concern, group goals may need to be rewritten periodically to reflect group progress toward a final product.

*Summary*

Collaborative partnerships require a conscious effort to examine and operationalize how groups can contribute collectively rather than as individuals who are working together out of political correctness. Examining barriers and other professional power issues with students and professional groups that are beginning a project or a practice together is mandatory. It is the explicit group decision making of what group outcomes will be as well as the examination of process and structure that pulls groups together toward a common purpose with great success.

## *INTERPROFESSIONAL ALLIANCE MODEL*

The purpose of this section is to present a theoretical model that demonstrates how successful collaboration is directly correlated with the level of caring, personal knowledge, and degree of social support present in the relationship. A rationale will be provided that supports the use of this model to examine the process by which interprofessional alliances are created, cultivated, and maintained. A case example will illustrate the model, and strategies for working with others will be provided.

There are several models that describe the process of collaboration among health care professionals. Some describe collaboration among those of similar disciplines[19] and others examine interprofessional alliances.[20, 21] The Interprofessional Alliance Model is based on the premise that in a competitive professional atmosphere, collaboration is unlikely to evolve unless clinicians or professionals create an explicit commitment to work together.[22] Within a collaborative team, individuals must feel free to explore, brainstorm, and problem solve, without the limitations imposed by a formal commitment to the positions and ideas held by each respective discipline. It is important to allow a "culture of collaboration"[23] to develop during the establishment of a collaborative team.

## Interprofessional Alliance Model Theory

There are three components to any professional alliance: content, process, and outcome.[24]

### Content

The content of any professional alliance consists of the work or tasks addressed by the collaborative team. Examples of content include issues related to patient treatment approaches, a patient educational module, or an interdisciplinary research endeavor.

### Process

Process refers to a progression of action that leads to a particular result. Describing a process may involve breaking it down into steps to examine what occurs at each stage. The process of any collaborative effort may be examined in relationship to established models. The Interprofessional Alliance Model (IAM) has seven steps or phases that describe how professionals enter and work in collaborative partnerships.

### Outcome

Measurement of the outcome or product of any collaborative effort is one indicator of its success. For example, when examining the impact of the development of a patient education unit, it is important to view the project with regard to learning outcomes. An example of outcome may include a patient being able to independently perform a home exercise program that includes monitoring of pulse rate during ambulation. Evaluating whether students were successful in the completion of the assignment involves assessment of the outcome product. Student assessment can be formative, occurring at several points during the term, and summative when assessment occurs at the program's end point.

### *Necessity of Caring, Social Support, and Personal Knowledge*

The ingredients necessary for a successful collaborative effort include caring, trust, social support, and personal knowledge.[25] Individuals need to be forthcoming about what they hope to accomplish and gain from an interprofessional alliance. This reflects *personal knowledge,* and trust among individual group members is fostered when the personal agendas of group members are openly discussed. With respect to a collaborative effort, each team member must *care* about the success and goals of others. For example, in planning project deadlines or scheduling group meetings, it is important to demonstrate *support* and *caring* related to other academic or job commitments.

The IAM (see Figure 14.3) is circular, contains seven phases, and illustrates that successful collaboration is directly correlated with the level of

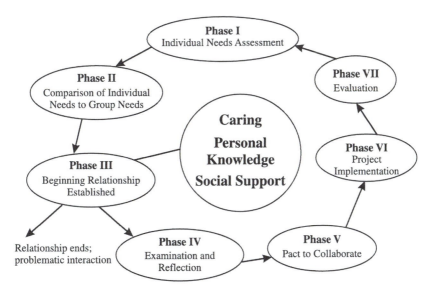

FIGURE 14.3. Interdisciplinary Alliance Model. *Source:* Hayword, DeMarco, and Lynch (2000). Interprofessional collaborative alliances: Health care educators sharing and learning from each other. *Journal of Allied Health* 29: 219-225.

caring, personal knowledge, and degree of social support present within the relationship. Concomitantly, the success and strength of the relationship directly influences individual commitment to the project.

Phase I of the IAM is Individual Needs Assessment. At this point, interdisciplinary team members, in part or as a complete unit, meet and then assess the value represented by a collaborative effort in relation to their own personal agendas and how the collaboration meshes with departmental goals and objectives. Here the individual does a miniature needs assessment of his or her strengths and professional needs. Phase II, Comparison of Individual Needs to Group Needs, describes a meeting of involved parties to evaluate whether a potential fit exists based on individual needs and complementary skill sets. Based on the outcome of Phase II, the individual may choose to proceed to or not to proceed to Phase III, Beginning Relationship Established. During Phase III participants develop a culture of collaboration in which rules and norms for behavior within the group are established. During Phase III and continuing through Phase V, based on the perceived benefit of entering into a collaborative arrangement and the presence of the elements of caring, personal knowledge, and social support, the individual either chooses to end his or her participation in a potentially problematic relationship or continue to Phase IV. Based on how the collaborative process progresses, an individual may decide to exit the relationship at either Stage IV or Stage V of the model.

At this point in the Interprofessional Alliance Model, the decision on behalf of the individual to commit to the collaborative effort has not been solidified. This occurs after the individual has passed through Phase IV, Examination and Reflection. Phase IV represents the individual's continued careful reflection upon the project's feasibility and personal relationships involved, and an evaluation of the relative benefits and likelihood of both a successful relationship and project outcome. It is not until this assessment has been made that the individual is willing to commit to a professional alliance. This commitment is made in Phase V, Pact to Collaborate. Phase VI, Project Implementation, represents the logistical steps required for the eventual implementation of a project. These steps include such factors as necessary funding and Phase VII, Evaluation, whereby individual group members evaluate the relative success of both interpersonal relationships and the outcome. Individual members may decide to either exit the collaborative effort or plan future research or educational efforts with the same or some of the original group members.

## CASE EXAMPLE:
## INTERPROFESSIONAL ALLIANCE MODEL

The following is the case of a patient named Mrs. S. who suffered a cerebral vascular accident in her home.[26] Because Mrs. S. is a patient with a complex diagnosis, she will require the skills of many practitioners, including respiratory therapy, speech therapy, physical therapy, and nursing, as she progresses through many steps within the health care system. Mrs. S.'s initial entry into the health care system would mostly likely be through an emergency room, with progression to an intensive care unit, a neurological inpatient unit, and then to an acute rehabilitation center or skilled nursing facility before discharge.

As a practitioner, one could approach Mrs. S.'s case with respect to evaluation and treatment based solely on discipline-specific knowledge. However, because Mrs. S. is a complex case, she will require the skills of multiple practitioners working together. An *interdisciplinary* approach would involve the collective efforts of practitioners in different disciplines (e.g., physical therapy, respiratory therapy, speech therapy, and nursing) who make an effort to acquire a deeper understanding of the relative contributions of one another. A greater appreciation of practitioner roles would allow an individual in a specific discipline to adapt his or her particular treatment goals and approach to augment the goals and approaches of the other disciplines involved.[27]

### Case 2: Discipline-Specific Approach

The case of Mrs. S. will first be presented from a discipline-specific perspective.[28] Then the case will be revisited using an interdisciplinary approach with the process behind the interdisciplinary collaboration illustrated and explained using the Interprofessional Alliance Model.

### History of Present Illness

Mrs. S. is an eighty-two-year-old female who was found unconscious on the bathroom floor of her home by her daughter. Mrs. S. was transported to a community hospital emergency room where she was unconscious and unresponsive to verbal stimuli. Her right pupil is dilated, and her left pupil is pinpoint. Her right side is flaccid. Her heart rate is 85 beats per minute (BPM), respiration rate is 30, and blood pressure is 186/100.

*Past Medical History*

Mrs. S.'s medical history is positive for more than thirty years of hypertension, peripheral vascular disease, coronary artery disease, a triple coronary bypass graft three years ago, and a mitral valve replacement. She also has osteoarthritis of the cervical spine and hands. Mrs. S. has been taking three medications: Cardizem, Lasix, and Coumadin.

*Psychosocial Issues*

Mrs. S. is a Puerto Rican immigrant who speaks limited English and is a little hard-of-hearing. She lives on the second floor of her daughter's two-family home (her daughter lives downstairs). Her daughter is single and is her primary caregiver. Mrs. S. also has two sons who live in Puerto Rico. Mrs. S.'s family believes she should not be burdened by making medical decisions. Therefore, her family requests they be responsible for all decisions regarding Mrs. S.'s care. In addition, Mrs. S.'s daughter requests that her mother not be told the extent of her current medical condition. Mrs. S. engages regularly in knitting, watching television, and cooking her own meals. However, she has become less active during the past year.

A health care professional of an individual discipline may want to consider these key questions when determining an initial care plan for Mrs. S.:

1. What are Mrs. S.'s risk factors for cardiovascular disease?
2. Based on the cultural beliefs of Mrs. S.'s family, what nonmedical needs should be addressed at this point?
3. What is the overall condition of Mrs. S.? What aspects of care would you stress if you were to write a care plan for her?
4. What would be the immediate goal(s) for Mrs. S.'s care ?
5. What short- and long-term goals would you establish for her?

Five days later, Mrs. S. was discharged from a neurological step-down unit to an acute rehabilitation center. She was intubated for two days and had decreased breath sounds on the right side. She received her medications orally. She was still unable to speak clearly. A computerized tomography (CT) scan of her head confirmed a left hemorrhagic cerebral vascular accident. At this point, her vital signs were stable.

*Physical Therapy Evaluation, Day 5*

Mrs. S.'s muscle tone was checked and it was confirmed that she had increased tone in the right distal lower extremity. She also demonstrated a positive Babinski and slightly increased deep tendon reflexes in her right lower extremity. She had some isolated spontaneous motions in her right hip, knee, and ankle. Her right upper extremity was flaccid. She was able to transfer with moderate assistance from two attendants from bed to chair. She required assistance from one attendant to stand.

### Speech Therapy Evaluation, Day 5

Mrs. S. was choking when taking her medication and had decreased hearing. She seemed to be responsive at the time, moving her head for yes or no and opening her eyes. She was aware of what was going on around her. Spontaneous verbalizations were about 60 percent intelligible.

### Respiratory Therapy Evaluation, Day 5

Mrs. S. had a weak productive cough. Her vital capacity was 60 percent of predicted. Her breath sounds were decreased bilaterally to the bases with scattered crackles throughout the right side noted.

At this point, each discipline could consider the following evaluation questions:

1. What other tests and measures would you need to perform at this time?
2. What does the information provided tell you about Mrs. S.'s condition?
3. What is the primary focus of your intervention?
4. How would you evaluate the effectiveness of your intervention?
5. What would the discharge plan for Mrs. S. include?

## Interdisciplinary Approach to Mrs. S and Application of the Interprofessional Alliance Model

The three disciplines of physical therapy, respiratory therapy, and speech therapy could also approach this case from an interdisciplinary perspective. The following is a reexamination of the case of Mrs. S. using an interdisciplinary approach with the process of collaboration illustrated by the Interprofessional Alliance Model.

### Phase I: Individual Needs Assessment

During phase I, the respective disciplines of physical therapy, speech therapy, and respiratory therapy, in part or as a complete unit, meet and then assess the value represented by a collaborative effort in regards to discipline-specific treatment goals. Each practitioner conducts a miniature needs assessment of his or her discipline-specific treatment goals and plans according to the value presented by a collaborative treatment approach.

Based on her condition, Mrs. S. requires respiratory therapy with a nebulizer and albuterol treatments to decrease the risk of developing pneumonia. Physical therapy treatments could include bed mobility, transfer training, ambulation training, and pulmonary hygiene. Speech therapy could work on swallowing and communication skills. Based on Mrs. S.'s condition and the potential treatments she requires, how might the three practitioners work in a synergistic fashion?

### Phase II: Comparison of Individual Needs to Group Needs

At this point in the model, a formal meeting of the different practitioners occurs. Based on this meeting, the individuals express and compare their discipline-specific treatment goals in relationship to those of the other disciplines involved in Mrs. S.'s care. Discipline-specific goals should also be examined with respect to patient and family goals for the treatment outcome. Evaluation by each discipline occurs to determine if a potential collaborative treatment opportunity exists based on personal and discipline-specific treatment and outcome goals.

### Phase III: Beginning Relationship Established

Based on the perceived benefits of entering into a collaborative relationship and presence of the elements of caring, personal knowledge, and social support, the individual practitioners take a step toward establishing a formal collaborative relationship. For example, if the three disciplines met and brainstormed before treating Mrs. S., they could discuss discipline-specific treatments and then establish the most beneficial priority for treatment administration. However, the respiratory therapist indicated that she was short staffed and had a heavier patient load in the afternoon. The physical therapist articulated that she was flexible and could see other patients before Mrs. S., enabling the respiratory therapist to administer the albuterol treatment first. The respiratory therapist could also perform the pulmonary hygiene portion of the treatment, if needed. The speech therapist indicated that she had a new patient evaluation to complete before Mrs. S. and therefore would not be available in the morning.

Explicitly stating their scheduling needs and staffing concerns reflected personal knowledge because each therapist knew herself well enough to articulate her own strengths and shortcomings. After disclosing these issues, the three practitioners decided to explore the potential for a collaborative team approach to Mrs. S.'s treatment. After a while, their not trusting one another enough to ask for a scheduling accommodation for example was dropped. Each therapist relaxed in knowing that the interchangeable skills (e.g., pulmonary hygiene) could be operationalized by collaborating and drawing upon each discipline's strengths and limitations. Open reflection was possible because each therapist cared about the success of the other's treatment goals and was sensitive to staffing and scheduling needs. As discussion about coordinating Mrs. S.'s care continued, each discipline became more comfortable talking openly with one another. As a result, an atmosphere of trust, caring, and mutual support began to evolve.

## Phase IV: Examination and Reflection

This phase represents individual reflection upon the potential for entering into a collaborative relationship. Each discipline examines the relationship to determine where mutual benefits, such as scheduling flexibility or interchangeable treatment possibilities, exist which also promote discipline-specific goals. Based on the viewpoint of mutual benefit, the successful treatment of Mrs. S. could be viewed as a shared benefit in which each therapist maximizes her treatment goals while taking into account the goals of the other disciplines, the patient, and the family. Mrs. S.'s treatment goals are collectively viewed in the most beneficial manner rather than solely as an individual treatment.

## Phase V: Pact to Collaborate

A decision to commit to a formal collaborative relationship is established by the involved disciplines. At this point, the therapists commit to scheduling and administering treatments in a synergistic fashion in which attention to scheduling and order of treatments occurs in a manner that is most beneficial for Mrs. S.

## Phase VI: Project Implementation

During this phase, the therapists have committed to working together and steps are taken to implement the agreed-upon treatment plan. For example, the order in which each therapist administers treatment now occurs in a complementary fashion. In the case of Mrs. S., for example, complementary treatment would mean that respiratory therapy first administers a nebulizer with albuterol treatment to open her airways and loosen secretions in her lungs. Then, either the respiratory therapist or the physical therapist could perform pulmonary hygiene treatments to increase ventilation and promote the clearance of lung secretions.

Next, physical therapy could work on bed mobility and transfer training to promote increased balance, functional independence, and continued pulmonary hygiene through physical activity. The physical therapist could end Mrs. S.'s treatment by transferring her to a chair in preparation for the speech therapy session. At this point, Mrs. S.'s secretions have been cleared from her lungs and she will demonstrate improved ventilation and oxygenation. As a result of increased oxygenation, she will have an augmented ability to concentrate on a potentially difficult speech therapy treatment. The physical therapist could return at a later time to work on ambulatory training. If the physical therapist had been working in a less complementary manner, she might have had Mrs. S. work on ambulation training before her speech therapy treatment. If this had occurred, Mrs. S. might have been too fatigued to concentrate fully on her speech therapy activities.

Here, three disciplines have worked together in a manner that is complementary. In this instance, the success of Mrs. S.'s treatment was fostered by each therapist's appreciation for one another's roles and for how to maximize versus hinder a treatment.

*Phase VII: Evaluation*

Phase VII refers to a period of retrospective reflection on the collaborative process and outcomes. Also at this time individuals contemplate whether to continue, modify, or terminate further collaboration with team members.

## SUMMARY

This chapter provided students with information regarding the necessity and value of collaboration among practitioners working in health care settings. Definitions were provided for collaboration, interprofessional alliances, and multidisciplinary, cross-disciplinary, and transdisciplinary work. Barriers to effective group work and strategies for dealing with such barriers were also discussed. A theoretical model titled the Interprofessional Alliance Model was provided to illustrate the process behind a successful collaborative alliance. Two case examples assisted students with integrating the principles and concepts of interprofessional collaborative alliances.

## REFERENCE NOTES

1. Gitlin, L.N., Lyons, K.J., and Kolodner, E. (1994). A model to build collaborative research or educational teams of health professionals in gerontology. *Educational Gerontology* 20:15-34; quote from p. 16.

2. Gitlin, L.N., Lyons, K.J., and Kolodner, E. (1994). A model to build.

3. Mello, J.A. (1993). Improving individual member accountability in small work group settings. *Journal of Management Education* 17:253-259.

4. Hayward, L.M., DeMarco, R., and Lynch, M.M. (2000). Interprofessional collaborative alliances: Health care educators sharing and learning from each other. *Journal of Allied Health* 29:219-225.

5. Massey, C.M. (2001). Transdisciplinary model for curricular revision. *Nursing and Health Care Perspectives* 22(2):85-88.

6. Katz, D. and Kahn, R.L. (1978). *The social psychology of organization,* Second edition. New York: Wiley.

7. Huber, D. (2000). *Leadership and nursing care management,* Second edition. Philadelphia: Saunders.

8. Smith, D.E. (1990). *The conceptual practices of power.* Boston: Northeastern University Press.

9. Liebler, J.G. and McConnell, C.R. (1999). *Management principles for health professionals.* Gaitherburg, MD: Aspen.

10. Ginzberg, E., Saltman, R.B., and Brook, R. (1998). Health debate. *Human Resource Executive* 12(6):57-58.

11. Ginzberg, E., Saltman, R.B., and Brook, R. (1998). Health debate.

12. Friedemann, M.L. (1995). *The framework of systemic organization.* Thousand Oaks, CA: Sage Publications.

13. Kritek, P.B. (1994). *Negotiating at an uneven table: Developing moral courage in resolving our conflicts.* San Francisco: Jossey-Bass Publishers.

14. Barnett, R.C. and Rivers, C. (1996). *She works, he works: How two-income families are happier, healthier, and better off.* San Francisco: Harper.

15. Fletcher, J.K. (1995). "Towards a theory of relational practice in organizations: A feminist reconstruction of real work." A paper submitted to the Women in Management Division of the Academy of Management Meeting in Vancouver, British Columbia.

16. Benner, P., Tanner, C.A., and Chesla, C.A. (1996). *Expertise in nursing practice: Caring, clinical judgment, and ethics.* New York: Springer, pp. 280-306.

17. Yoder-Wise, P.S. (1999). *Leading and managing in nursing,* Second edition. St. Louis: Mosby.

18. Sullivan, E.J. and Decker, P.J. (1997). *Effective leadership and management in nursing,* Fourth edition. Menlo Park, CA: Addison-Wesley.

19. DeMarco, R., Horowitz, J.A., and McLeod, D. (2000). A call to intraprofessional alliances. *Nurse Outlook* 48:172-178.

20. Gitlin, L.N., Lyons, K.J., and Kolodner, E. (1994). A model to build.

21. Hayward, L.M., DeMarco, R., and Lynch, M.M. (2000). Interprofessional collaborative alliances.

22. Ibid.

23. Ibid.

24. Donabedian, A. (1985). *The methods and findings of quality assessment and monitoring: An illustrated analysis.* Ann Arbor, MI: Health Administration Press.

25. DeMarco, R., Horowitz, J.A., and McLeod, D. (2000). A call to intra-professional alliances.

26. Belilvoskiy, T., O'Brien, M., Watson, M., Curro, J., Lowe, S., and O'Neil-Pirozzi, T. (2001). Interdisciplinary case studies: Stroke. Retrieved from the World Wide Web, February 1. <http://teaching.bouve.neu.edu/cases/stroke.htm>.

27. Donabedian, A. (1985). *The methods and findings of quality assessment and monitoring.*

28. Belilvoskiy, T., O'Brien, M., Watson, M., Curro, J., Lowe, S., and O'Neil-Pirozzi, T. (2001). Interdisciplinary case studies [paper]. Retrieved from the World Wide Web: <http://www.bouve.neu.edu>.

Chapter 15

# Impact of Technology
# on Allied Health Education

Elzar Camper Jr.
Amani M. Nuru-Jeter
Carole I. Smith

## CASE STUDY

Maria's presentation is due in her anatomy class. She is usually nervous when she gives an oral presentation to her classmates and teacher, but this time she is more confident. She applied the concepts and skills learned from a prior computer course and she is pleased with the results. She used an instructional design model, rehearsed her oral presentation, applied design principles and used graphics software for the handout, and developed a computer slide presentation. She is ready. Her presentation goes well; however, she would prefer not to be the first presenter next time!

Let us take a look at what has occurred as Maria prepared for her presentation. She started her preparations by applying the systematic process of instructional design. Instructional design has many different models, each with its own nuances. However, most models require development of objectives, analysis of audience characteristics, and some form of assessment (evaluation and revision of objectives). Maria modified this process for her presentation. She formulated objectives of what the audience will be able to do after her presentation, analyzed her audience (e.g., she determined their knowledge of the subject matter, age level, number in the audience, and any special characteristics they may have), and applied communication theory to aid with the selection of appropriate media.

Maria's objectives provide the structural framework. Since her topic is an extension of previously covered class materials, she is building upon prior knowledge and adding to the audience's existing information on this topic. Her audience was predetermined (i.e., her classmates), so she is familiar with their general background and knows no one has special needs. She reviewed the list of barriers to effective communication and applied a synthesis of factors from several models of communication theory to determine her choice of media.

The class assignment required that Maria give an oral presentation—it was her choice to add media. She designed and printed a handout to distribute to her classmates. The handout applied graphic design principles she had learned in a technology course. Maria made sure she considered principles such as clarity, simplicity, emphasis, legibility, etc. She applied the elements of font size and color, amount of information, and arrangement of handout and ensured she included and emphasized what was essential to her audience. She collected her information, checked to make sure she was following applicable intellectual property rights and fair use of copyright guidelines, and provided citations for her sources, including those she found on the Internet.

Maria remembered from her studies that intellectual property rights may apply to items that do not have a physical form, e.g., files, documents, images, and other types of items available on the Internet. She also recalled that copyright laws protect the rights of owners of information and their expression of that information from infringement by unauthorized copying and duplicating (Ackerman and Hartman, 2001, p. 262). The issue of copyright infringement was of particular interest because she intends to use this presentation after she graduates. Maria checked her class notes and found the World Wide Web addresses for the government's Digital Millennium Copyright Act of 1998 <http://www.loc.gov/copyright/legislation/dmca.pdf>, and Fair Use guidelines <http://www.loc.gov/copyright>. She selected one of the graphics software programs, used the computer lab at school, printed a copy for herself, and then had electrostatic copies made for each member of the class.

Maria's computer slide project required the use of computer presentation software. Since her presentation included new information on an existing topic, she chose to present review materials in her initial slides. She used progressive disclosure of each text line per slide, to control the display of information and to focus the audience's attention. She liked this process and chose to apply it to the presentation of the new information. Maria really liked the many variations of slide transitions that were available but settled on one method of transition for her entire presentation—remembering the warning of her technology instructor to "keep it simple." Her search of the Internet provided some great graphics and even several audio and video segments. After the initial excitement of having access to these items waned, she decided on one short, fifteen-second movie, which she inserted into her computer slide presentation. However, before including the movie Maria checked with her instructor to make sure the classroom's computer and video projector were compatible. This addressed the interoperability question mentioned in her technology class.

Maria liked the text's legibility and the way the images looked when projected onto the screen in the front of the classroom. All of her information was visible from the rear of the classroom. After her presentation, she and some of her classmates met in the student center and discussed their presentation experiences. Maria felt good about the comments she received from the other students, as well as the feedback she received from her instructor several days later.

Fast-forward several years. Maria is presenting at her alma mater, and she is preparing to give an update of this presentation. She fondly remembers the first time she used this presentation. She has made many revisions over the years, the most recent being the replacement of the floppy disk and Zip disk storage mediums with Internet storage. She is also using video and audio insertions. Although Maria is many miles away from her office, these upgrades will allow her to access her office computer from the site of today's presentation. She will be able to include streaming video from the Internet, MP3 sound bites from several presenters at a recent conference, and case examples from her practice using a cross-platform compact disc she recently produced. Maria reflects on how the technology has continued to evolve from her preservice days, and is glad she has maintained a familiarity with the application of technology as part of her continued professional development.

Maria knows that today's students face many expectations from faculty in content knowledge and presentation skills. She also knows that technological competence is expected by clients.

One of these expectations is that they will be able to communicate effectively by presenting information in a coherent, informative manner with an engaging style. The use of appropriate presentation software and hardware can assist in fulfilling these expectations.

## FAMILIARITY WITH TECHNOLOGY

Access to and application of technology by skilled allied health practitioners who either serve as physician assistants or serve in the areas of physical therapy, occupational therapy, nutrition, clinical laboratory science, and health management will be a major determinant in the quality of health care received by millions of people.

Technology permeates all aspects of the allied health industry. Technology influences the processes of education, research, analysis, diagnosis, and treatment. In turn these processes will impact the practices of information technology, clinics, product development, health care management and administration, biomedical innovations, and the design of instruments and facilities.

Familiarity with a wide range of existing and emerging technological applications is essential for those who are preparing either to enter the allied health field or to engage in continuing education to supplement their skills. Familiarity has many faces, including:

- Delivery of instruction or services via telecommunications as either a supplement to or alternative to face-to-face delivery
- An expanding role for community access television to serve as a resource for delivery of instruction or service to distant clients
- Utilization of distance learning to set the tone for diverse ways to disseminate information and deliver instruction

It is in society's best interest to have well-trained providers. In order to ensure a skilled allied health workforce, it is increasingly important that educational and training programs incorporate the application of technology into traditional educational methods. As the cost of education increases, recent entrants into the allied health fields are finding innovative ways of combining school and work, thus increasing the need for flexible delivery of content within programs for nonhomogeneous student populations.

Access is especially difficult for students that come from backgrounds where discretionary income is not sufficient to match the cost of postsecondary expenses. Income, college readiness, and student and family educational backgrounds are all indicators of whether one enrolls in a postsecondary education program. For health care students in the United States, public policy decisions dealing with technology could help break down lines of demarcation that are being drawn every day. For those who have been traditionally disenfranchised and left behind, there is a clear need to address and remove the access barriers that continue to separate communities.

In a series of reports from both the federal government and private associations, attention is being paid to who has access to technology and the disparity across economic, racial, and ethnic groups both nationally and globally. The phrase *digital divide* is used to describe how not all students seeking entrance to schools or continuing education have equal access to technology. Familiarity with technology promotes acceptance of technology and eases acceptance of innovation and integration of technology into the routine delivery of services by allied health practitioners. The diffusion of innovation model would be a good way to examine the adoption process for cellular telephones, pagers, and personal data assistants by both individuals and groups (Moore, 2003). Additional studies could provide data on accuracy and results of advertising as well as marketing campaigns to promote these devices. No longer novelties, these devices are an indispensable part of our daily existence and their use is stratified by age and impacted by economic levels.

Given the creativity of individuals combined with a capitalistic drive to find new ways to use these and other technological tools, it is apparent wireless transmission of information is not futuristic science fiction but a present reality. Acquiring technology is costly. Students may not be able to secure the technology necessary to participate. These factors may affect who will be prepared for future careers. It is expectations of future rewards that drive current students to engage in the rigors of academic preparation.

## PRESERVICE TECHNOLOGY PREPARATION OF ALLIED HEALTH PRACTITIONERS

In a perfect world, students would look into their collective crystal ball, identify universally acceptable content areas, and secure the necessary resources to benefit from faculty intervention. Since this is not a perfect world, it is critical that those charged with the responsibility of preparing allied health workers decide what skills are needed and then provide the instructional situations for students with diverse levels of preparation to acquire these skills.

It is a simple statement to advocate the integration of technology into the preservice curriculum. The complexity of adding existing technology (that will be used in ways unknown at this time) to the preservice curriculum for allied health students who question its current relevance is a formidable task.

The allied health curriculum is undergoing assessment as part of long-range planning. The assessment is holistic and expands beyond traditional evaluation of student performance. An example is portfolio development. Students are to perform and retain classroom activities and projects as part of an observable display to demonstrate mastery of curriculum objectives and expertise to employers. The portfolio demonstrates proficiencies and is an aid in the evolving roles and shifting performance parameters placed on allied health workers.

## *CORE CURRICULUM AND TECHNOLOGY COURSE*

How students perceive the use of technology in their classrooms is determined by the technology objectives faculty have for students. The requirements for preservice students' application of technology is determined by the objectives of the entire curriculum.

The administrators of post secondary institutions entrust general education computer courses to faculty who by and large are neither trained nor degreed in the allied health fields. Generally, their training is in mathematics, computer science, and/or education. The faculty designs a generic computer course or series of courses with the following goals: (1) to provide students with computer skills that will help them understand the basic concepts of the computers, related accessories, and use of software, and (2) to lay a foundation for the application of these skills in succeeding courses in students' majors.

### *Case Study: Computer Skills in the Core Curriculum of Allied Health Professionals*

I first met Tyrone at a social function. As new acquaintances, our conversation eventually turned toward what we did professionally and we discovered we were both college professors. Tyrone is a computer and technology specialist who is responsible for providing a core curriculum course to allied health students.

Tyrone and I discussed methods of evaluating current course content and what models might be applied to design instruction. As we talked, I was struck by how similar his dilemma might be to a number of professors faced with similar challenges:

- To design a generic course on technology for inclusion in a core curriculum
- To provide a framework for students to apply technology to their major

*Designing for the Use of Technology in a Core Curriculum Course*

Tyrone chose to apply the systematic method of instructional design, which requires the instructor "to plan, develop, evaluate, and manage the instructional process effectively to . . . ensure competent performance by students" (Kemp, Morrison, and Ross, 1994, p. 6). The generic instructional design model is subdivided into objectives, interactive instruction, and assessment. Implementation requires the application of theories of learning and communication and instructional strategies. The instructional design "approach considers instruction from the perspective of the learner" (Kemp, Morrison, and Ross, 1994, p. 6). To achieve this perspective a series of questions must be asked:

- What should the content of the course be?
- How should content be delivered?
- What assessment is best? How should the course be assessed?
- How can we assure that assessment results are systematically integrated into the course?

For Tyrone, it is a daunting task to devise content that will permit both assimilation of the existing technologies and accommodation of undiscovered and undeveloped technologies.

## CONNECTING PRESERVICE THEORY
## AND IN-SERVICE PRACTICE

No matter who you are, sooner or later you will need health care. In the allied health fields public policy decision makers will determine our access to state-of-the-art technology and consequentially the quality of our health care. One of the basic underpinnings of the quality of the nation's health care system is the delivery of reputable service by knowledgeable, well-trained, and adaptable providers. Their collective contributions raise the quality of health care and ultimately the quality of life for all Americans.

The following case study presents factual events. What impact and changes might the application of technology have on this case study? First let's examine the events and then apply the suggestions that follow.

### Case Study: How the Connection Might Be Changed
### by Current and Future Applications of Technology

Carolyn is preparing to go to work. It is a short walk from her front door to her car. As she steps onto the driveway, her foot slips on black ice and she falls. The pain is great, and she is unable to get back up. She shouts several times for her husband, who is inside the house. He hears her and helps her to her feet. They return to the home and eventually her husband transports her to the emergency room. Her injury is diagnosed as ligament damage. The hospital provides her with a shoe and crutches. She is sent home for the day. Six days later she is still wearing the shoe and hobbling.

Carolyn lives in the suburbs where a car is mandatory for travel. She is frustrated because she cannot drive and is dependent upon members of her family for daily transportation to work, to her doctor, and to anywhere else. Wishing to speed the healing process, she chooses to pursue another level of care and selects a sports medicine facility associated with a local university. Over the next several weeks the staff at the sports medicine facility X-ray the injured area and apply a fiberglass cast. Today's visit is to remove the cast. She is told the healing process will involve wearing a boot for another two weeks. She must travel to a medical supply location to obtain the boot. The physical therapist and other staff provide Carolyn and her husband a written list of locations where they can obtain the prescribed boot. Although they called the nearest medical supply house and were assured the item was in to stock, they must visit several different locations to acquire the boot due to miscommunication about the correct size of the boot.

It is now several weeks later and Carolyn's doctor has decided she must continue to wear the boot and begin an exercise routine. Her physical therapist demonstrates several exercises to strengthen and provide flexibility in her foot, and provides a handout of these exercises.

*Technology Assimilation Now and Accommodation in the Future*

How was current technology used/integrated in this case study?

- Automobile for transportation
- Use of telephone to make appointments for visit
- Computer use at hospital and sports medicine facility for entry, storage, and retrieval of medical file, billing, outpatient services, and instructions
- X-ray device and monitoring devices used to obtain blood pressure and heart rate
- Design of the shoe and boot
- Create a list of medical supply house locations using graphic design principles and elements, word processing, and scanning

What might adoption of technological innovation provide in the future?

- Reduction/elimination of duplicate forms at multiple facilities by using computers or personal data assistants (PDA) to record medical information and digitally transmit this and other monitoring, X-ray, and insurance information taken at the hospital to the sports medicine facility

- Language translation devices downloaded from the patient's own personal data assistant (PDA) that provide interpretations from/into Spanish, French, Russian, or another language for an increasingly diversified nation
- Automatic language translation of facility or Web site handouts on where to obtain and purchase and how to use rehabilitation equipment and supplies
- Global positioning system (GPS) to provide location and driving directions
- Transmission systems to electronically contact medical supply houses for availability and price of items, and insurance plan coverage
- Design of Web sites using multimedia, electronic handouts, or digitally mastered compact discs that would permit resizing font to aid readability and fostering of access for those with auditory, visual, and/or physical disabilities
- Animation software for construction of three-dimensional models
- World Wide Web addresses for sites that explain the design, application, advantages, and possible precautions of prescribed devices
- Monitoring equipment to indicate strength and flexibility to reduce or eliminate transportation problems for those whose conditions restrict their access to transportation

The hardware and software technologies just described already exist. Three examples are provided:

- An article in the *Journal of Telemedicine and Telecare* (Maghsudi et al., 1999) reported in Germany that medical communication from emergency scenes using a notepad computer provided reduced time for notification to the admitting hospital. For sixteen patients with life-threatening conditions, time of notification was reduced from 35.5 minutes to 13.6 minutes and more precise information about the patient was transmitted.
- "Given Diagnostic Imaging System is based on the patented M2A Ingestible Imaging Capsule, which records color video images as it glides smoothly through the digestive tract and is naturally excreted" (Given Imaging, 2001). Please note this device is currently undergoing FDA approval and is not commercially available in the United States of America.
- SportBrain First Step. SportBrain's Web site states "this wearable personal fitness assistant will help you set, monitor, and keep track of your fitness goals. Clip this to your waist and it records your physical

activity—how many steps you take each day. At the end of the day, place the SportBrain in the SportPort, and it sends your information through a phone line to your personal SportBrain Web page that keeps track of your activity and progress" (SportBrain, 2001).

The addition of wireless networking provides portable transmission of data from these types of devices, and mass production reduces costs. These two factors, wireless networking and mass production, should assist computer literate generations in using innovative technology for allied health practices.

## DETERMINING AND APPLYING CONTENT

### Student Expectations

For students, within the past several decades the universal application of technology has leaped to the forefront with their expectation of the use of hardware and software in academic and training instruction, presentation, and remediation. Common wisdom urges those charged with preparing allied health workers to provide instruction in the use of technology, e.g., computers. The decision makers (administrators) facilitate the learning process. In varying ways and at different institutions, the confederation between gatekeepers (faculty) and decision makers traditionally entrusts gatekeepers with the design and delivery of content and entrusts decision makers with making it happen by providing the requisite resources.

The gatekeepers' reasons for including topics and decision makers' reasons for supporting these topics within the curriculum may vary from students' reasons for mastering course topics. Students' use of chat rooms, instant messaging, and audio and video transmissions are not always conducted to complete course assignments. For example, it is clear that students attach a social value to e-mail as a way of communicating and exchanging information and there is universal agreement that the Internet is a viable resource.

Issues of privacy, security, First Amendment rights, and censorship arise as students develop classroom presentations and complete assignments on the Internet. At times students' pursuit of Internet research has gone beyond the scope of formal course content and has pushed the parameters of academic justification for providing access to the Web.

Clearly technology has opened a Pandora's box that will test the social and legal interaction of learning and teaching in fascinating and challenging ways for years to come.

## The Challenge to Students

Students entering the same computer class may have diverse skill levels. Some students have access to and experience with computer software and hardware that is better than what they find in class; for others, the term *novice* better reflects their computer skills.

In the past, a number of postsecondary schools required first-year students to partake in a library skills program. If that standard was applied currently, today's students would be asked to partake in an Internet skills program. The content of such a program would cover the organization of and effective strategies for searching and retrieving information from the Internet.

## Do Allied Health Workers Need Only Generic Technology Skills?

The content of most generic computer courses includes word processing; e-mail; basic hardware operation and software organization; presentation software; how to access, search, and evaluate the content of Web pages on the Internet; and to a lesser degree the design and use of databases and spreadsheets. Course content should reflect the divergent needs of students with varying skills and experience.

Word processing is a topic that is often included in entry-level, generic computer courses. Although an argument might be made that some understanding of word processing skills is necessary for e-mail, a stronger argument might be made that proper methods of keyboard typing are a valuable precursor. For example, can a student use e-mail without understanding word processing? Yes, but with today's technology for input can they use e-mail without typing? No. Do most generic computer courses teach proper typing skills e.g., hand placements, which keys to strike with which finger, etc.? Probably not, but I would venture that most teach word processing. Is it not more rational to recognize that a good typist will be able to enter data at a rapid and efficient rate? Strong typing skills would serve well for the entry of data for health management/administration, transcription, or online searching where the speed and accuracy of data entry reduces time and cost needed to complete tasks.

The dilemma that the advocacy of keyboarding instruction presents for the technology provider is symbolic, because it ignores the presence of current and ever-improving voice recognition programs. Why use institutional resources to purchase typing skill programs, and incur the cost to install, uninstall, and discard software, and train personnel when future students and practitioners will use a microphone and voice recognition software for data entry?

## Post Course Application

After completion of a core computer course students generally apply word processing skills to message creation, to e-mail for communication, and to the Internet for researching and searching information. Use of the Internet requires application of communication and information theories. Most Internet users are unaware of the background manipulations of sophisticated computer operations and software instructions that accompany their queries and attempts to communicate.

Information theory components (collection, organization, storage, retrieval, and dissemination) are applied in computer operations involving connection to an Internet Service Provider (ISP), computer/software compatibility, Internet protocol, file transfer protocol (FTP), storage and distribution using a printer, external memory devices (Zip disks), compact disc read (CD-R), and/or compact disc rewrite (CD-RW).

## INTERNET AND SEARCHING

Millions of queries are sent over the Internet every day by people using the World Wide Web (WWW) to find information. The Internet consists of computers with assigned functions, i.e., servers, which are networked to one another. Each server and network computer is assigned an Internet Protocol (IP) address, similar to the system of each residence having a house or apartment address. Servers share stored information using the systematic design of services and resources of the World Wide Web (WWW). Information is shared using the rules of Hypertext Transfer Protocol (HTTP), and is composed in Hypertext Markup Language (HTML). Information is collected and organized at Web sites. Web sites are accessed by their addresses, i.e., their Uniform Resource Locator (URL). URLs are identified by the searchers and entered into their computers. Internet Service Providers allow access to the World Wide Web over telephone and/or cable lines.

### Browsing and Searching

Information on the Web can be found using two fundamental ways—either by subject in directories (browsing) or by keyword using search engines (searching). Search engines provide access to more information, which is stored in databases, than directories. Today's search engines are more sophisticated, and are evolving in structure and techniques designed to ease use and enhance results. Search engines are categorized by their level of sophistication. At the metasearch level, search engines are designed to ask questions and make suggestions for refining queries, and simultaneously use multiple search engine databases. Some are designed to eliminate duplicate findings.

### Search Strategy

Each searcher develops his or her own methods for conducting a search. There are references and books that describe multiple ways for approaching a search. Fundamental is an understanding of how information is collected, organized, stored, retrieved, and disseminated within the databases that one is searching. Such information is provided in the "help" section of search engines, and if applied can greatly improve the effectiveness of a search. For example, most search engines use Boolean search operators such as "or," "and," and "not." The explanation of how best to apply these operators within the context of a search will affect the results or hits of a search:

- To expand a search, use "or"
- To narrow a search, use "and"
- To exclude items from a search, use "not"

### Types of Services

Searches maybe conducted for single-word entry, multiple-word entry, general information, specific subject matter, or combinations. Depending upon the level of sophistication of the results required, whether for a research report or general information, different search terms and engines are employed. For example, a specific search for the effects of prednisone will yield different results than a generic search for steroids. To accommodate diverse purposes, specialized databases for search engines exist, e.g., a same topic search of the "Ask Jeeves" engine <http://www.ask.com> yields different results than a search of the National Library of Medicine's MEDLINE <http://www.nlm.nih.gov/databases/databases_medline.html>.

A good resource for finding other resources on the Web is the Librarians' Index to the Internet, <http//:www. lii.org> (Ackerman and Hartman, 2000, p. 153)

Another set of services are mailing lists and usenet groups. Mailing lists use e-mail. A requestor lists his or her e-mail address with other individuals who share an interest in a common topic. An administrator maintains the list, distributes relevant information, edits, screens, and shares members' comments, but retains control of content and distribution.

Usenet members use e-mail and the Web to exchange collections of articles (i.e., files). Articles are exchanged from one computer system to another. There is no single administrator but rather a community effort on behalf of all participants. Again, membership is topic based.

### How Will Students Acquire These Skills?

Increasingly, computer basics, which earlier may have focused on computer software and hardware configurations, are expanding to address the role of the computer within society. This acceptance of computers is one example of how deeply technology is ingrained in our work and our social and private lives.

The incursion of technology within the social fabric promotes familiarity with new technological terms. The terms *viruses* and *bugs* have led to new definitions of traditional words. Also, we now have discussions on the concepts of copyright and intellectual property. These terms and concepts have gained prominence as society grapples with how to function while ameliorating competing interests within the civil boundaries of our legal and criminal jurisdictions. At stake is how we resolve conflict, maintain civility, and adhere to capitalism, while addressing the technological expansion of the exchange of information and ideas. Information and ideas that are not confined by one nation's legal statutes are now competing with diverse governmental philosophies and accompanying legal statutes in a global marketplace.

Diffusion theory attempts to explain how innovations are adopted by an individual or group. The theory's main elements require an innovation that is communicated through certain channels, over time, and among the members of a social system (Rogers, 1986, p. 117). This theory has particular application in the area of technology since technology by its nature continually requires the adoption of innovations. Rate of adoption is a direct relationship between time of adoption and the number of adopters. This symbiotic relationship of time and adopters is directly correlated to the perceived success of the innovation and can be charted to display an adoption curve.

The rate is graphed as the relationship between the amount of time taken to adopt and the number of adopters. The graph displays an S-shaped adoption curve and reinforces that adoption of an innovation does not occur unilaterally but rather is acceptance at a common time (Rogers, 1986, p. 71).

## POLICY

### Access

The digital divide is a descriptive label used nationally to refer to access to or lack of access to technology. Access is an omnipresent issue, confronting each individual and institution in our national society, and with expansion has increasing global implications. It is an issue with ramifications, as politicians and other policymakers with diverse political viewpoints on regulation/deregulation, marketplace competition, and government involvement advocate positions consistent with their political and social beliefs.

Access to technology reinforces our societal infrastructure. We can demonstrate commitment to reinforcing the societal infrastructure by addressing the access-related areas of universal service and universal access. E-rate services for the elderly and disabled are examples of how to provide universal access by applying universal service models. These services enhance quality of life, which promotes economic development within states, regions, and the nation.

The terms *digital divide, universal access,* and *universal service* are relevant to both current and future populations as indicators of the gap between those who do and will and those who do not and will not have access to existing and cutting edge technologies.

- Transmission lines—modems for telephone and cable, digital subscriber line (DSL), and broadband
- Services—911 emergency/accident for ambulance, monitoring of prescriptions, rehabilitation, wellness, accident notification and treatment, and personal and property protection
- Mastering, copying, editing, distributing video and audio scanners, external storage drives, CD-R, CD-RW creation devices, and affordable software

### Interoperability

Interoperability refers to the ability of different software and hardware to communicate with each other in a fashion that is seamless and reduces technological barriers for the user. Interoperability exists at many levels. Different hardware platforms (Macintosh and IBM clones), network connections such as Asynchronous Transfer Mode (ATM) and ethernet, Universal Serial Bus (USB) and parallel port connectivity of accessories are examples of hardware. Software programs and their compatibility to various computer operating systems are also examples of interoperability. The related issues of hardware performance to software in central processing unit (CPU) speed, random access memory (RAM), formats for CD-R, CD-RW, compact disc read-only memory (CD-ROM), and digital versatile disc (DVD and DVD-R) also impact software selection and operation.

The questions of technology interoperability are not isolated to a single field, e.g., health management or information technology, but transcend all fields, including sonography, radiation therapy, radiography, and nuclear medicine. The potential for networking these disparate fields and coordinating their services was not previously possible.

## *Public Policy, Postsecondary and Adult Education*

Allied health professionals' involvement in the policymaking and regulatory processes of the federal and state agencies that oversee technology, health, and related areas is important, because it can make a difference. For example, the Federal Commerce Department hosts

> the Advanced Technology Program (ATP). The program bridges the gap between the research lab and the market place, stimulating prosperity through innovation. Through partnerships with the private sector, ATP's early stage investment is accelerating the development of innovative technologies that promise significant commercial payoffs and widespread benefits for the nation. As part of the highly regarded National Institute of Standards and Technology, the ATP is changing the way industry approaches R&D, providing a mechanism for industry to extend its technological reach and push out the envelope of what can be attempted. (NIST, 1999)

The Associated Press recently published an article that touched on the future of ATP's federal funding. It noted that "[c]utting ATP has been on the table in Congress for years, with its Republican opponents calling it a form of 'corporate welfare' that should be ended. The former Clinton administration vigorously defended ATP, citing studies that said many companies would not have pursued such research without federal help" (The Associated Press, 2001). The point is that policymakers determine policy, and access to technology is a policy issue.

# TECHNOLOGY AND ONLINE EDUCATION

## Case Study

Cheryl is a twenty-nine-year old single mother of one who is currently working as an assistant at a physical therapy facility. She very much wants to become a physical therapist but cannot afford to leave her job to go back to school full time due to competing financial responsibilities such as child care, mortgage payments, car insurance, and car loan payments, etc. As a young mother with the potential and desire to pursue her career goal but without the resources to realize her dreams, Cheryl settles for a career as a physical therapist assistant. If only there was a way that she could go back to school without having to leave her job and her home!

## Distance Education/Learning

The United States Distance Learning Association defines distance learning as "the delivery of education or training through electronically mediated instruction including satellite, video, audio graphic, computer, multimedia technology, and other forms of learning at a distance" (CDLP, 2003). This is just one definition. There are several, all of which incorporate the same elements. In short, distance education/learning (DE/DL) is a system or process that connects learners with remote resources. It provides students with access to anything any time, anywhere. Students can access courses at any time according to personal needs. They can also access academic resources from anywhere in the world, and can enroll in degree, certificate, and continuing education programs, among others.

As the number of persons seeking and completing postsecondary training increases, current trends in postsecondary education look positive. Distance education has become one of the most innovative ways of meeting the demands of new students who, due to the rising cost of education, must find ways of combining school and work. This is true also for working mothers or fathers who are interested in continuing their education but have competing family demands, and/or scheduling and travel conflicts.

Although distance education is not for everyone, it has brought new hope to growing numbers and has implications for promoting education in all fields including the allied health professions.

## Key Features of Distance Learning Programs

- Separation of teacher and learner in space and/or time
- Use of educational media to unite teacher and learner and carry course content

- Provision of two-way communication between teacher, tutor, or educational agency and learner
- Volitional control of learning by student rather than by distance instructor

*Challenges*

There is growing concern that DE/DL may not provide students with the necessary environment and support available with traditional on-site education. Traditional on-site education includes interactive (synchronous) learning such as classroom lecture and class interaction (class discussion and question/answer) as well as noninteractive (asynchronous) learning using resources such as course syllabi and lecture handouts. Traditional classroom (on-site) education uses tools to assess student progress including quizzes, class exercises, homework, and exams. Finally, on-site education provides students with opportunities outside of the classroom to contact faculty and administrative personnel as well as opportunities to utilize the support available at an institution of higher education, including computer and library facilities.

Distance education/distance learning incorporates most, if not all, of the same aspects as on-site education. DE/DL can involve both asynchronous and synchronous learning. Asynchronous communication includes Web-based materials such as real-time audio lectures (RealAudio), lecture computer slides (PowerPoint, Hyper Studio), video, course materials (syllabi, reading assignments, exercises, and review questions), online exams, peer evaluation, and other Web-based resources. Synchronous communication methods include group discussions, group assignments, and real-time instruction using chat software and other Web implements such as LiveTalk.

*No Significant Difference versus Significant Difference*

Although DE/DL cannot replace the classroom experience, it offers much of the same resources typically available for traditional on-site education. Studies have shown that DE/DL can be as effective a tool as traditional education given the appropriate methods and technology (Wilkes and Burnham, 1991).

There is a growing body of literature assessing the difference between traditional instruction and DE/DL. Much of this literature shows that the type of instructional format (e.g., interactive video, videotape, or live instructor) does not have a significant effect on learning given appropriate technology and content (Wilkes and Burnham, 1991). As with most bodies of literature, there is competing evidence. However, it has not been shown that DE/DL programs are unsuccessful in imparting an adequate amount of knowledge and training in any given field.

The "no significant difference" versus "significant difference" debate will surely continue and will most likely shed light on how DE/DL programs can improve. We already know that any successful DE/DL program includes planning and organization, good teaching, interactive communication and study techniques, and the use of visuals and graphics (Egan et al., 1991; Martin and Rainey, 1993; Schlosser and Anderson, 1994; Coldeway et al., 1980). It has also been shown that interactive communication among students, and between students and teachers enhances the learning experience (Egan, 1991). Therefore, good DE/DL programs incorporate this method of learning using the most up-to-date technology.

## Trends in Distance Learning Programs/Reasons for Distance Learning Programs

From 1995 to 1997/1998, the proportion of public four-year institutions offering DE/DL programs increased from 62 to 79 percent, while the proportion increased from 58 to 72 percent for public two-year institutions (NCES, 2000). In the next three years, 91 percent of both four- and two-year institutions plan to offer DE/DL programs.

There are many reasons for the proliferation of DE/DL programs throughout the country. Distance education/distance learning increases students' access to educational programs, increases enrollment and institutional access to new audiences, and improves the quality of course offerings. For many students, DE/DL programs eliminate travel and scheduling constraints. Furthermore, as the cost of technology decreases, more students from diverse backgrounds will be able to take advantage of such programs and reach their educational goals.

Given current trends in postsecondary education and the proliferation of DE/DL programs, addressing access barriers becomes increasingly important in the digital divide debate. Furthermore, policymakers will have to consider the cost of technology, transmission, improving access, maintenance, infrastructure, production, support, and personnel in their analysis of technical, administrative, political, and economic feasibility.

Over the last several decades we have become familiar with many uses of technology. Many of us have purchased or have access to computers, sophisticated home video game systems, digital still and video cameras, digital audio devices (CD and MP3), wireless and cellular telephones that can connect to the Internet and access e-mail, personal data assistants, and CD recording devices. Our real-world experiences are impacted by the imaginations of computer programmers, graphic designers, and audio and video producers. We must harness and focus these wondrous devices and programs to enhance the ways in which we bring information to the lifelong process of teaching and learning.

Technology for educational use is here and available. A Benton Foundation poll reported in 1994 that most respondents support the aid of technological advancements in the public interest, such as in education and health care, by the government.

## TRENDS IN ADULT LEARNING
## AND POSTSECONDARY EDUCATION

According to the National Center for Education Statistics, adult learning, including postsecondary credentialing programs, has increased from 38 percent in 1991 to 50 percent in 1999 (NCES, 2000). Although adult learning for postsecondary degree training decreases with age, other forms of adult learning, including work-related learning, basic skills training, English as a second language, apprenticeships, and personal development, increase with age. Twenty-one- to twenty-two-year-olds account for 50 percent of the total population in postsecondary credentialing programs and 22 percent of other adult learning programs, while forty-three- to forty-four-year olds account for only 7 percent of those in postsecondary credentialing programs and 48 percent of other adult learning programs. One of the primary contributing factors of this trend is the increasing number of high school graduates who immediately enter postsecondary credentialing programs. Between 1972 and 1998, the number of high school graduates immediately entering college increased from 49 percent to 66 percent, respectively (NCES, 2000).

### Gender, Race, and Age Differences
### in Allied Health Professions

There also appears to be a gender and race difference with respect to trends in postsecondary education (NCES, 2000). The postsecondary enrollment rate is increasing faster for women than for men, particularly at four-year educational institutions. Furthermore, women are more likely to enroll in and earn degrees from allied health professions programs including but not limited to physical therapy, social work, and occupational therapy. Regarding race, although the black-white gap in college enrollment has decreased since 1984, the gap for finishing college has increased. Similarly, the gap in finishing college between Hispanics and whites persists. As with women, racial minorities are more likely to enroll in allied health professions programs than are white males; an aspect of preservice student preparedness, impact on curriculum, and the digital divide discussed earlier.

It is clear the number of Americans who go online is continuing to increase. Yet a large number of Americans do not have access to the basic tools necessary for participation in the information age. Eighty-eight percent of high-income families own a computer, compared to 54 percent of middle-income families and 21 percent of low-income families (NCES, 2000).

## *HEALTH PROMOTION*

One of the basic uses of technology is the facilitation of data collection, storage, transmission, and dissemination. In health promotion various forms of telecommunications technology are utilized in the transmission and dissemination of information. Two of these technologies are cable television and the Internet.

Cable was originally conceived as a method to deliver over-the-air broadcast signals to remote areas. Increasing the availability of the broadcast signal was viewed as an incentive to purchase televisions and to increase the number of viewers. Government regulation of cable as an ancillary service was permitted under the Communications Act of 1934. Over the years there have been congressional modifications to the regulation of cable, stipulation of access channels, and granting of franchises by local municipal authorities.

The Cable Television Consumer Protection and Competition Act of 1992 allowed local and/or state authorities to select a cable franchise and regulate in any areas that the commission did not preempt (FCC, 2000b). Local franchising authorities have adopted laws and/or regulations such as subscriber service requirements, public access requirements, and franchise renewal standards. Under the 1996 Telecommunications Act, Congress noted that it wanted to provide a procompetitive, deregulatory national policy framework designed to rapidly accelerate private sector deployment of advanced telecommunications and information technologies and services to all Americans by opening all telecommunications markets to competition (FCC, 2000b). Although local franchising authorities regulate the rates for the basic service tier, the Telecommunications Act of 1996 terminated the FCC's authority to regulate the rate customers pay for cable programming service provided after March 31, 1999 (FCC, 2000a).

The Internet began as a federally sponsored project to provide data and text communications for Department of Defense interests. During the late 1980s and into the 1990s the Internet was expanded in scope to include the general public, and new protocols (frameworks) permitted graphic, audio, and video transmissions in addition to the text. Federal financial support was withdrawn in the mid 1990s and the Internet took on a commercial appearance.

The transmission of audio and video information across the Internet has also evolved. Today streaming technology allows users to download audio and video files faster than ever. Streaming technology creates a buffer of audio and/or video and begins transmitting as the buffer is replenished. This permits shorter wait times for recipients, and is viewed as preferable to the former method of waiting for the entire audio and/or video to be downloaded before it is heard or viewed. The following are examples of how one urban community is using cable television and the Internet and how they are relating those technologies to the allied health fields.

### Case Study: Cable Television and Community

The cable program *Technology and You: Another Point of View* was created to demystify telecommunications technology for the general public. Produced by Greater Media Cable in Philadelphia, Pennsylvania, and shown citywide on the school district's cable network, the half-hour program was created by Carole I. Smith, founder and executive director of the Workforce 2000 Advisory Council and the Mayor's Telecommunication Policy Advisory Commission as a means to prepare Philadelphia's workforce for the jobs of the future.

Because technology drives the economy, it is important for society to be aware of the various ways technology currently impacts their lives and its future implications. The purpose of *Technology and You: Another Point of View* was to help viewers understand just how pervasive technology is and the many and varied ways it is applied and utilized in all aspects of our lives, including public and private institutions such as colleges and universities, hospitals, nursing homes, rehabilitative centers, health centers, etc., where many allied health professionals train and work.

Three programs that focused on health were "Distance Learning," "Women and Technology," and "Technology and Sports." In each program, the type of technology, the way in which it was used, and the benefit of the application were described and illustrated. "Technology and Sports" focused on a dentist who had developed a joint jaw protector called the Williams Interoral Protective Sports System (WIPSS). Viewers were informed why the protector was needed, how it was used, and the benefit it provided. The program also illustrated the roles of various allied health professionals who were working with the patient and the dentist.

"Women and Technology" focused on an accountant who used technology to automate billings for doctors and other health professionals.

Increasing the availability and variety of learning opportunities was the focus of the "Distance Learning" program. Representatives from a community college, a public television station, and students discussed the pros and cons of distance learning. Since allied health is one of the primary careers chosen by women and minorities who traditionally lack the financial resources to attend college, it is one of the top program areas for distance learning.

## *Internet*

In addition to producing *Technology and You,* Ms. Smith has launched a women's Web site in conjunction with two of her associates, Narissa Wallace and Bernadine Hawes. The site, <DigitalSistas.net>, is designed to link African-American women in technology and new media in an online and offline community. The site was created to respond to the growing needs of African-American women in technology, and provides a portal through which women can identify, link, and collaborate with one another around the world.

DigitalSistas.net has a strategic partnership with The Black World Today, <www.tbwt.com>, and was launched along with their new Women's Portal in March 2001. The Black World Today is one of the oldest and most respected Internet companies in the world. It has a global audience and is visited by more than 2 million persons per month. WebsMostLinked.com currently places the <www.tbwt.com> in the top 1 percent of the Web's most popular sites.

## *Networking*

At the 2001 National Association for Equal Opportunity in Higher Education (NAFEO) conference, Ms. Smith interviewed panelists on the Technology Track, Closing the Achievement and Technology Gaps: Opportunities for Reform and Partnership panel. Regarding career opportunities in the Information Age, one of the workshop participants, a clinical psychologist, discussed the use of technology in her daily activities, continuing education, and community activities. This interview and interviews with other panelists will be uploaded to <www.tbwt.com> and made available on their Internet radio station, Black Talk Radio. Through this mechanism, the community at large can be informed about allied health careers and the uses and applications of technology in the field.

## *Watchdog*

We have advocated the application of technology but we also feel you should be aware that not all claims for using technology are valid or reliable. In November 1998, "over 1200 sites were listed and all received warnings from the Federal Trade Commission that advertisers must have reliable scientific evidence to back up their health claims, and that Web site designers may be liable for making or disseminating deceptive or false claims" (Federal Trade Commission, 1998). An accompanying Web site is Quackwatch <http://www.quackwatch.com>, which bills itself as the guide to "fraud, quackery, and intelligent decisions."

## *SUMMARY*

### *Policy*

Involvement in public policy determines access. A vision of what should be included in models of access to technology and high-quality health care is crucial to the formulation of national, state, and local public policy on health. Access to technology provided at preservice, continuing, and professional development of allied health professionals is required. A society that supports universal service models will continue to produce high quality professionals.

Future policy discussions must include considerations for population changes/shifts. As the face of the nation continues to change, postsecondary training must reflect the diversity of a growing nation and work to create a workforce that can meet a wide variety of health care needs.

## *RECOMMENDATIONS*

### *Preservice*

Future core courses for allied health programs should include worksite and home networking (wired and wireless), Internet search strategies, computer and accessory selection, graphics design, production and use of audio and video, intellectual property rights, copyright and fair use laws and definitions, design and content evaluation of Web sites, and multimedia streaming technology. In providing technology services for students, resources will be needed to construct or enhance current formats for transmission. Public utility commissions of the states and the Federal Communications Commission have been given regulatory control over these transmission formats.

## Access

There is a critical link among access to technology, quality of health care, and lifelong learning opportunities for initial employment and continued professional development.

Allied health professionals should participate in the process of public comment and review. This participation should include but not be limited to the following:

- Planning—to ensure access to technology, high-quality health care, and equity of service
- Transmission—to ensure development linkages are provided for health care facilities, neighborhood communities, schools, and postsecondary institutions
- Regulatory efforts—transmission models for broadcast and ancillary services of telephone, cable, Internet, wireless, and emerging technologies must include a universal service framework to provide universal access that follows guidelines of public interest, convenience, and necessity
- Marketplace—pursuit of open network architecture to provide competition and marketplace forces for technical, software, and hardware development; design; implementation; and evaluation

## BIBLIOGRAPHY

Ackerman, E. and Hartman, K. (2000). *Searching and Researching on the Internet and World Wide Web,* Second Edition. Wilsonville, OR: Franklin, Beedle, and Associates.

Ackerman, E. and Hartman, K. (2001). *Internet and Web Essentials: What You Need to Know.* Wilsonville, OR: Franklin, Beedle, and Associates.

Ask Jeeves (search engine) (n.d.). Available from the World Wide Web: <http://www.ask.com>.

The Associated Press (2001). Bush Budget Cuts Tech Funding Program. *The New York Times,* March 14. Available from the World Wide Web: <http://www.usatoday.com/tech/news/2001-03-14-bush-tech-funding.htm>.

Aufderheide, P. (1999). *Communication Policy and the Public Interest: The Telecommunications Act of 1996.* New York: The Guilford Press.

Benton Foundation (n.d.). Available from the World Wide Web: <http://www.benton.org>.

California Distance Learning Project (CDLP) (2003). *What is Distance Learning?* Available from the World Wide Web: <http://www.cdlponline.org>.

Camper, E., Giles-Gee, H., John, M.E., and Lecca, P.J. (1994). Technology Access and Quality: The Importance of Public Policy. *Educational Record* 75(3):47-52.

Coldeway, D.O., MacRury, K., and Spencer, R. (1980). *Distance Education from the Learner's Perspective: The Results of Individual Learner Tracking at Athabasca University.* Edmonton, Alberta, Canada: Athabasca University.

Cragan, J.F. and Shields, D.C. (1998). *Understanding Communication Theory: The Communicative Forces for Human Action.* Boston: Allyn & Bacon.

DigitalSistas (n.d.). Available from the World Wide Web: <http://www.DigitalSistas.net>.

Egan, M.W., Sebastian, J., and Welch, M. (1991). Effective Television Teaching: Perceptions of Those Who Count Most . . . Distance Learners. Proceedings of the Rural Symposium, Nashville, TN.

Federal Communications Commission (FCC) (2000a). *Cable Television Fact Sheet: The Consumer's Role in Cable Rate Regulation.* Available from the World Wide Web: <http://www.fcc.gov/mb/facts/pubrole.html>.

Federal Communications Commission (FCC) (2000b). *Cable Television Information Bulletin.* Available from the World Wide Web: <http://www.fcc.gov/mb/facts/csgen.html>.

Federal Trade Commission (1998). Remedies Targeted in International Health Claim Surf Day. Available from the World Wide Web: <www.ftc.gov/opa/1998/9811/intlhlth.htm>.

Fijolek, J., Kuska, M., Siriam, M.K., and Davidson, L.S. (Eds.) (1999). *Cable Modems: Current Technologies and Applications.* Chicago, IL: International Engineering Consortium.

Given Imaging (2001). Available from the World Wide Web: <http://www.givenimaging.com/usa/default.asp>.

Grabe, M. and Grabe, C. (2001). *Integrating Technology for Meaningful Learning,* Third Edition. Boston: Houghton Mifflin.

Heinich, R., Molenda, M., Russell, J.D., and Smaldino, S.E. (1996). *Instructional Media and Technologies for Learning,* Fifth Edition. Englewood Cliffs, NJ: Merrill.

Kemp, J.E., Morrison, G.R., and Ross, S.M. (1994). *Designing Effective Instruction.* New York: Merrill.

Librarians' Index to the Internet (n.d.). Available from the World Wide Web: <http://www.lii.org>.

Maghsudi, M., Hente, R., Neumann, C., Schachinger, U., and Nerlich, M. (1999). Medical Communication from Emergency Scenes Using a Notepad Computer. *Journal of Telemedicine and Telecare* 5(4):249-252.

Martin, E.E. and Rainey, L. (1993). Student Achievement and Attitude in a Satellite-Delivered High School Science Course. *The American Journal of Distance Education* 7(1):54-61.

Moore, M. (2003). *Advanced Scientific and Technical Writing, Diffusion of Innovations: Studies.* Available from the World Wide Web: <http://www.u.arizona. edu/ic/moore/414/diffusion_studies.html>.

National Center for Education Statistics (NCES) (2000). *The Condition of Education: 2000.* Available from the World Wide Web: <http://www.nces.ed.gov>.

National Institute of Standards and Technology (NIST) (1999). *Overview of ATP.* Available from the World Wide Web: <http://www.atp.nist.gov/atp/overview. htm>.

National Library of Medicine (2003). *MEDLINE.* Available from the World Wide Web: <http://www.nlm.nih.gov/databases/databases_medline.html>.

National Telecommunications and Information Administration (NTIA) (1999). *Falling Through the Net II: New Data on the Digital Divide.* Washington, DC: NTIA. Available from the World Wide Web: <http://www.ntia.doc.gov/ntiahome/ net2/>.

Overbeck, W. (2001). *Major Principles of Media Law.* Fort Worth, IN: Harcourt College Publishers.

Rogers, E.M. (1986). *Communication Technology: The New Media in Society.* New York: The Free Press. Rogers, E.M. and Shoemaker, F.F. (1971). *Communication of Innovations: A Cross-Cultural Approach,* Second Edition. New York: The Free Press.

Schlosser, C.A. and Anderson, M.L. (1994). *Distance Education: A Review of the Literature.* Ames, IA: Iowa Distance Education Alliance, Iowa State University.

Seels, B. and Richey, R.C. (1994). *Instructional Technology: The Definition and Domains of the Field.* Washington, DC: Association for Educational Technology.

Silbergleid, M. and Pescatore, M.J. (1999). *The Guide to Digital Television,* Second Edition. New York: Miller Freeman.

SportBrain (2001). Available from the World Wide Web: <http://www.sportbrain. com>.

United States Copyright Office (USCO) (1992). *Fair Use.* Available from the World Wide Web: <http://www.copyright.gov/fls/fl102.html>.

United States Copyright Office (USCO) (1998). *The Digital Millennium Copyright Act of 1998: U.S. Copyright Office Summary.* Available from the World Wide Web: <http://www.loc.gov/copyright/legislation/dmca.pdf>.

United States National Library of Medicine (n.d.). Available from the World Wide Web: <http://www.nlm.nih.gov>.

Wilkes, C.W. and Burnham, B.R. (1991). Adult Learner Motivations and Electronics Distance Education. *The American Journal of Distance Education* 5(1):43-50.

Chapter 16

# Allied Health and Public Policy: Making Change Happen

Thomas W. Elwood

The title of this chapter suggests that public policy offers a mechanism for effecting change. Another way of viewing the matter is to consider how public policy can be used to prevent change from happening. For example, as the first session of the 107th Congress drew to a close, HR 2792—the Disabled Veterans Service Dog and Health Care Improvement Act of 2001—was passed by the House of Representatives in late October 2001. If enacted, the legislation would make it possible for chiropractic care to be provided to veterans through all Department of Veterans Affairs medical centers. Physical therapists oppose this expansion on the grounds that proposed new chiropractic services will reduce funding for other needed services such as those furnished by physical therapists. If the latter group is successful in its efforts to block the bill from becoming law, the proposed change will not occur.

The year 2001 affords an excellent illustration of how change can be prevented from occurring when different branches of the federal government work at cross-purposes with one another. This particular situation will be described in much greater detail because of the significant potential impact it would have on the overall economy of the United States.

All three branches of the federal government play a decisive role in the formulation of health policy. Congress produces legislation that is enacted when signed by the president. Typically, statutes lack the fine details that specify how a law should be implemented. That task resides in agencies such as the Center for Medicare and Medicaid Services (which at the time the previously mentioned series of incidents took place was called the Health Care Financing Administration) in the executive branch where rules and regulations for programs such as Medicare and Medicaid are prepared. It is not uncommon, however, for interest groups affected by these rules to challenge them on the basis that they seem to stray far from congressional intent. When divisiveness in interpretation occurs, lawsuits arise and the courts settle these disputes.

A good example of how the three branches of government may clash is illustrated by a final rule on ergonomics (the science of fitting jobs to the individuals who work in them) that was issued on November 14, 2000, by the Occupational Safety and Health Administration (OSHA), a unit within the Department of Labor.[1] The general intent of the rule was to lower the risk of worker exposure to factors that can result in musculoskeletal disorders. A major concern of critics was the enormous financial cost of carrying out the regulation. Almost immediately, fury erupted in Congress because of a belief on the part of many Republican legislators that Democratic President William Clinton had overstepped his bounds by allowing the regulation to be published. In March 2001, the Senate voted 56-44 and the House of Representatives voted 223-206 in favor of a resolution to nullify the rule. Newly elected Republican President George W. Bush signed it into law on March 20, 2001, as PL 107-05.

Many occupations are hazardous, and workers are hurt on the job every day in the United States. Depending on the type of injury, allied health professionals such as physical therapists and occupational therapists play an important role in restoring employees to good health. Although the main intent of promulgating an ergonomics regulation is to enhance worker safety, the ability of health professionals to provide their respective services also would be affected to some extent.

## SEPARATION OF POWERS

As a means of understanding how such political conflicts arise and the impact they often have on the provision of health care services, it is useful to examine the kinds of challenges that had to be faced in the early days of this nation. Even then, the founders of the Republic were greatly concerned with how to structure a government that reflected an appropriate balance of power among its main branches.

During the period 1787-1788, various essays by Alexander Hamilton, John Jay, and James Madison, written under the pseudonym "Publius," were contributed to New York newspapers and collected in a book known as *The Federalist*.[2] The series was undertaken for the specific purpose of convincing the inhabitants of New York State that the federal constitution ought to be ratified.

In No. 37, Madison noted:

> when we pass from the works of nature, in which all the deliberations are perfectly accurate, and appear to be otherwise only from the imperfection of the eye which surveys them, to the institutions of man, in which the obscurity arises as well from the object itself as from the organ by which it is contemplated, we must perceive the necessity of moderating still further our expectations and hopes from the efforts of human sagacity. Experience has instructed us that no skill in the science of government has yet been able to discriminate and define, with sufficient certainty, its three great provinces—the legislative, executive, and judiciary. (p. 269)

In No. 48, he wrote:

> It will not be denied, that power is of an encroaching nature, and that it ought to be effectually restrained from passing the limits assigned to it. After discriminating, therefore, in theory, the several classes of power, as they may in their nature be legislative, executive, or judiciary, the next and most difficult task is to provide some practical security for each, against the invasion of the others. What this security ought to be, is the great problem to be solved. (p. 343)

In No. 51, Madison stated:

> But the great security against a gradual concentration of the several powers in the same department, consists in giving to those who administer each department the necessary constitutional means and personal motives to resist encroachment of the others. The provision for defense must in this, as in all other cases, be made commensurate to the danger of attack. Ambition must be made to counteract ambition. The interest of the man must be connected with the constitutional rights of the place. It may be a reflection on human nature, that such devices should be necessary to control the abuses of government, but what is government itself, but the greatest of all reflections on human nature? If men were angels, no government would be necessary. If angels were to govern men, neither external nor internal controls on government would be necessary. In framing a government which is to be administered by men over men, the great difficulty lies in this: you must first enable the government to control the governed; and in the next place oblige it to control itself. (p. 356)

## *ERGONOMICS*

The Occupational Safety and Health Administration (OSHA) issued its final Ergonomic Program Standard on November 14, 2000, to "address the significant risk of employee exposure to ergonomic risk factors in jobs in general industry workplaces. Exposure to these factors leads to musculoskeletal disorders (MSDs) of the upper extremities, back, and lower extremities" (p. 68262). The rule would not, however, apply to employers whose primary operations are covered by OSHA's construction, maritime, or agricultural standards, or who operate a railroad. This regulation occupied 609 pages of the *Federal Register,* which is published each business day as a means of disseminating proposed and final rules.

The standard included an "action trigger" that identifies jobs with risk factors of sufficient magnitude, duration, or intensity to warrant further examination by the employer. An action trigger would serve as a screen. If an employee reported an MSD, the employer would have to determine whether the MSD was an MSD incident, defined by the standard as an MSD that results in days away from work, restricted work, medical treatment beyond first aid, or symptoms or signs that persist for seven or more days. If it is an MSD incident, the employer would have to check the job using a basic screening tool to determine whether the job exposes the worker to risk factors that could trigger MSD problems.

Risk factors addressed by this standard included repetition, awkward posture, force, vibration, and contact stress. If the risk factors in the employee's job do not exceed the action trigger, the employer would not need to implement an ergonomics program for that job. If an employee reported an MSD incident and the risk factors meet the action trigger, then the employer would have to establish an ergonomics program for that job. The program would have to include the following elements: hazard information and reporting, management leadership and employee participation, job hazard analysis and control, training, MSD management, and program evaluation.

OSHA officials estimated the final standard would affect approximately 6.1 million employers and 102 million employees in general industry workplaces. They also estimated the standard will prevent about 4.6 million work-related MSDs over the next ten years, have annual benefits of approximately $9.1 billion, and impose annual compliance costs of $4.5 billion on employers. On a per-establishment basis, this equals approximately $700. Annual costs per problem job fixed are estimated at $250. The final rule became effective January 16, 2001. Employers would have to provide information to employees by October 15, 2001. After that date, employers would be required to respond to employee reports of MSDs and signs and symptoms of MSDs.

In addition to the activities listed in Table 16.1, OSHA has awarded almost $3 million to twenty-five grant projects that address ergonomics, including lifting hazards in health care facilities. These grant projects have enabled workers and employers to identify ergonomic hazards and implement workplace changes to abate these hazards. For example, the University of California at Los Angeles (UCLA) and the Service Employees International Union (SEIU) both received grants for preventing lifting injuries in nursing homes. Mercy Hospital in Des Moines, Iowa, received a grant to prevent lifting injuries in hospitals.

TABLE 16.1. OSHA's Ergonomics Chronology

| Date | Event |
|------|-------|
| March 1979 | OSHA hired its first ergonomist. |
| Early 1980s | The agency began discussing ergonomic interventions with representatives of labor, trade, and professional associations. |
| August 1983 | The OSHA Training Institute offered its first course in ergonomics. |
| May 1986 | OSHA began a pilot program to reduce back injuries. |
| Fall 1990 | The Office of Ergonomics Support was created and more ergonomists were hired. |
| July 1991 | "Ergonomics: The Study of Work" was published as part of a nationwide education and outreach program. |
| August 1992 | An Advanced Notice of Proposed Rulemaking was published. |
| August 1993 | A survey of general industry and construction employers was conducted. |
| March 1995 | A series of meetings was conducted with various groups to discuss approaches to a draft ergonomics standard. |
| February 1998 | National meetings were held to discuss the standard under development. |
| November 23, 1999 | A proposed ergonomics program standard was published. |
| March-May 2000 | Nine weeks of public hearings were held, generating 18,337 pages of testimony from 714 witnesses. |
| November 23, 1999-August 10, 2000 | OSHA received nearly 11,000 comments and briefs consisting of nearly 50,000 pages collectively into the ergonomics rulemaking docket. |

*Source:* Adapted from *Federal Register* (2000), November 14, *65*(220):68264, table on OSHA's chronology of ergonomics.

### *Elements of the Dispute*

Although the standard was applauded in some quarters, such as the American Occupational Therapy Association, approbation was not universal, for several reasons. The regulatory text required that an employer provide access to a health care professional (HCP) for evaluation, management, and follow-up "when necessary." OSHA's final rule defined health care professionals as "physicians or other licensed health care professionals whose legally permitted scope of practice (e.g. license, registration, or certification) allows them to provide independently or to be delegated the responsibility to carry out some or all of the MSD management requirements of this standard" (p. 68375). When the standard was proposed in 1999, opponents argued that the inclusion of individuals without medical training and experience in the MSD management process was inappropriate. A related issue was whether the employer or the employee would be the one to choose the health care professional who would provide services.

If an employee was allowed to choose the HCP, employers were concerned a doctor might diagnose an MSD without real cause and expose companies to possible fraudulent actions. On the other side of the ledger, employees were worried that a biased opinion might result and the employee's condition might worsen if the employer did the choosing. Another concern was that HCPs chosen by someone other than the employee might be biased in favor of the employer or insurance company in order to obtain future referrals.

Because of this mutual distrust, the final rule included provisions for multiple HCP review. It is OSHA's position that when the employer provides access to an HCP under the final rule, the employer has the right to select the HCP. The employee has a right to a second opinion, however, to review the first HCP's finding at no cost to the employee if he or she disagrees with the employer-selected HCP. If the employee has previously seen an HCP on his or her own, at his or her own expense, and received a different recommendation, the individual may rely upon that assessment as the second opinion.

If the employer's HCP and the employee's HCP disagree, the employer must, within five business days after receipt of the second HCP's opinion, take reasonable steps to arrange for the two HCPs to discuss and resolve their disagreement. If the two HCPs are unable to resolve their disagreement quickly, the employer and the employee, through their respective HCPs, must, within five business days after receipt of the second HCP's opinion, designate a third HCP to review the determinations of the two HCPs, at no cost to the employee. The employer must act consistently with the determination of the third HCP, unless the employer and the employee reach an agreement that is consistent with the determination of at least one of the HCPs. The employer and the employee or the employee's representative may agree on the use of any expeditious alternative dispute-resolution mechanism that is at least as protective of the employee as the review procedures.

## Congressional Reaction to Ergonomics Regulations

By the end of January 2001, Republican leaders in Congress began to consider the possibility of using the 1996 Congressional Review Act (PL 104-121) to nullify the ergonomics standard, along with other rules that were inserted in the *Federal Register* during the closing days of the Clinton administration. This law allows Congress to erase regulations by passing a resolution of disapproval by a simple majority vote of both chambers. A caveat exists, however, insofar as Congress is not able to modify a regulation or disapprove only a portion of it. In addition, once a vote of disapproval occurs, the statute prevents agencies from issuing any new rules in the same area.

At the beginning of the second session of the 106th Congress, Republican leaders hoped all thirteen appropriations bills for fiscal year (FY) 2001 would be completed and signed by President Clinton prior to the end of FY 2000 on September 30, 2000. An added incentive to finish business in a timely fashion was the fact that it was an election year. All House members who wished to be reelected wanted to go on the campaign trail, as did one-third of the members of the Senate, who hoped to remain in office.

Instead, appropriation bills, including the massive one that would provide funding for the Departments of Labor, Health and Human Services, Education, and Related Agencies (commonly referred to as Labor-HHS), languished until after the elections were conducted. Whenever appropriations legislation is not enacted by September 30, Congress must resort to having one or more continuing resolutions (CRs) signed by the president to enable government agencies to continue functioning for short periods of time. A record twenty-one CRs were necessary in 2000 for the aforementioned departments.

One obstacle to completing so-called Labor-HHS appropriations was a provision known as a "rider" that was introduced by Republicans to block OSHA from issuing regulations on ergonomics. On June 8, 2000, the House defeated by a vote of 220-203 an amendment that would have stripped the rider from the Labor-HHS bill. When the legislation was sent to the president in late October, he promptly vetoed it. One reason was because of the rider.

This effort by some legislators to block the issuance of regulations was not the first attempt. A bill titled the Workplace Preservation Act (HR 987) that had 161 cosponsors was introduced in the House on March 4, 1999. It passed by a vote of 217-209 on August 3. A companion bill (SR 1070) was introduced in the Senate on May 18 that same year, but it never went beyond the committee stage. If enacted, the proposed legislation would have directed the completion of a study by the National Academy of Sciences before OSHA could issue a standard or guidelines on ergonomics. (It was anticipated that the study would be completed by the end of 2001.)

Another example of the tension that underlies relations between the legislative and executive branches of government is a law that was enacted on October 17, 2000, known as the Truth in Regulating Act of 2000 (PL 106-312). This act provides that when a federal agency publishes any proposed or final rule, including an interim or direct final rule, which may have an annual effect on the economy of $100 million or more or adversely affects in a material way the economy, a sector of the economy, productivity, competition, jobs, the environment, public health or safety, or state, local, or tribal governments or communities, a chairman or ranking member of a committee of jurisdiction of either house of Congress may request the comptroller general to review such rule.

Carrying out the task will be the General Accounting Office (GAO), the watchdog arm of Congress. After a major rule is proposed, the GAO checks to see how the cost-benefit analysis was done and evaluates the agency's data, methods, and assumptions under the three-year pilot program. The GAO then would have 180 days to complete a report on each rule and send it to Congress. As an example of the magnitude of the challenge, OSHA's ergonomics rule included 1,113 pages of preliminary economic-impact analysis.

### *Litigation Phase Begins*

When the final rule on ergonomics was published in the *Federal Register* on November 14, 2000, opponents responded quickly. The National Coalition on Ergonomics, an alliance representing large and small employers, along with sixty-two associations and companies, filed suits in several different U.S. circuit courts of appeals across the United States on November 20, 2000. Examples of groups belonging to the coalition that sought court action are the Chamber of Commerce of the United States of America and the National Association of Manufacturers.

The nature of the opposition varied. For example, the AFL-CIO filed a motion to intervene on grounds the standard was not sufficiently protective in a number of key respects, although it supported the standard as a whole and had a strong interest in being heard in opposition to the attacks that would be mounted by industry petitioners. Because the standard would not apply to construction employment covered by OSHA, the Associated General Contractors of America filed a motion to have the standard extended to apply to employment regulated by OSHA construction standards and to construction work in general.

A multidistrict litigation office decided by lot on December 1 to transfer these cases to the U.S. Court of Appeals for the District of Columbia. Legal experts predicted that a normal appellate schedule in the U.S. Court of Appeals for the District of Columbia Circuit would result in briefing to be completed by mid-2001, with oral arguments in early fall, and an ultimate decision possible in late 2001 or early 2002.[3] Meanwhile, if Congress wanted to use the 1996 Congressional Review Act to erase the regulations, it would have to do so by mid-spring 2001 because of time limitations imposed by that legislation.

### Why the Standard Generated Criticism

As of November 14, 2000, the only major medical association to previously support the standard and later withdraw its support was the American College of Occupational and Environmental Medicine (ACOEM), an organization of more than 7,000 occupational and environmental medicine physicians. The reason was the standard's lack of a sound medical foundation insofar as the multiple review requirement fails to provide for health care providers who have the ability to make a diagnosis or causal assessment or who have any knowledge of the prevention and treatment of MSDs. In addition, the failure to include a medically accurate definition of an MSD was viewed as confusing and additional cause for litigation. ACOEM President Robert Goldberg stated the standard would be certain to be held up by legal battles for the next several years.[4]

One major complaint was that the final regulation was significantly broader than the rule that was proposed twelve months earlier. Unlike the estimate made by OSHA officials, which predicted the rule would cost $4.5 billion annually, business community estimates of the cost ranged from $18 billion to $125 billion.

Another cause of dissatisfaction was the perceived rush in judgment. The public comment period ended on August 10, 2000, after generating more responses than any prior OSHA rule. Thousands of documents were collected, each ranging in size up to 715 pages. In August, OSHA submitted 2,000 pages of new data at the end of the posthearing submission period, which was before the docket officially closed, but too late for any member of the public to review or comment on them. Requests to reopen the docket to allow additional public comment on this new material were refused.[5]

The entire process from the Notice of Proposed Rulemaking Stage to publication of the final rule took only 358 days. Since 1988, OSHA has published twenty-eight other final rules. The average time for those rules was 1,582 days. Moreover, the ergonomics rule involves broader applicability, a bigger impact on the nation's economy, and a larger record of public comments than any of the other twenty-eight rules. Only one other regulation since 1988 moved at a faster pace, and that occurred in 1999 with the non-controversial rewrite of OSHA's Dip Tank Standard, which specifies safety rules for using dipping processes to paint or coat materials.

Although the ergonomics standard would allow the employer to obtain an opinion from a health care professional (HCP), it would prohibit an HCP from disclosing to the employer information about non-work-related factors that may have caused or contributed to the employee's condition. Employers were concerned this limitation would preclude them from making fully informed decisions regarding the causes of an employee's health problem and the appropriate remedial measures to take. Furthermore, complicating factors such as heredity, fitness, and sports injuries are beyond the control of employers. Another source of apprehension was a concern that disgruntled employees might use the new regulation as a basis for causing trouble for their employers by making accusations to OSHA.

Furthermore, according to the National Coalition on Ergonomics, the proposed rule conflicted with state workers' compensation systems by awarding higher amounts of money. The due-process protections for employers provided under workers' compensation would be denied and there would be no mechanism for determining benefits if the worker had more than one job.[6]

### DISCUSSION

Charles-Louis de Secondat, Baron de Montesquieu, was a member of an influential group of thinkers known as the French Philosophes, aristocratic writers and politicians who greatly spread the ideas of the Enlightenment. His most influential work is *The Spirit of the Laws* (1748).[7]

Viewing the legislature (for the making of law), the executive branch (for the enforcement of those laws), and the judiciary (for the interpretation and scrutiny of the law), de Secondat states:

> ... when the legislative and executive powers are united in the same person, or in the same body of magistrates, there can be no liberty; because apprehensions may arise, lest the same monarch or senate

should enact tyrannical laws, to execute them in a tyrannical manner. Again, there is no liberty, if the judiciary power be not separated from the legislative and executive. Were it joined with the legislative, the life and liberty of the subject would be exposed to arbitrary control; for the judge would be then the legislator. Were it joined to the executive power, the judge might behave with violence and oppression. There would be an end of everything, were the same man or the same body, whether of the nobles or of the people, to exercise those three powers, that of enacting laws, that of executing the public resolutions, and that of trying the causes of individuals. (pp. 151-152)

Were the executive power not to have a right of restraining the encroachments of the legislative body, the latter would become despotic; for as it might arrogate to itself what authority it pleased, it would soon destroy all the other powers. But it is not proper, on the other hand, that the legislative power should have a right to stay the executive. For as the execution has its natural limits, it is useless to confine it; besides, the executive power is generally employed in momentary operations. The power, therefore, of the Roman tribunes was faulty, as it put a stop not only to the legislation, but likewise to the executive part of government; which was attended with infinite mischief. But if the legislative power in a free state has no right to stay the executive, it has a right and ought to have the means of examining in what manner its laws have been executed. (pp. 157-158)

Madison and the other founding fathers had a keen awareness of the problems inherent in designing a government that would function effectively while simultaneously preserving liberty. They knew that not a single one of the colonies had been able to devise a means of effecting a complete separation of powers among the three branches of government.

The system they eventually designed has significant overlapping features. For example, presidents nominate Supreme Court justices, who must then be confirmed by Congress. The same holds true for nominees for posts in the cabinet and other parts of the executive branch. Congress can pass legislation, but the president can veto it. If the president wants to bypass the legislative branch, executive orders and regulations can be issued. If the president's behavior is considered too unacceptable, legislators have the power to impeach that person. In the Senate, the chief justice would preside over the proceedings.

How the three governmental branches operate is a reflection to some extent of the debate over the proper role of government. The contest for the presidency in 2000 pitted candidates representing political parties with different conceptions of where individual and corporate responsibility end and government responsibility begins. Generally speaking, Republicans are more inclined to want to limit the degree of involvement the federal government has in the lives of the populace. Democrats seem more persuaded that the government is a benevolent force for achieving good outcomes that have a positive impact on human existence.

The topic of ergonomics illustrates these dual perspectives. OSHA officials aim to make the workplace safe for employees, yet employers are fearful of any regulation that will have a negative effect on business by imposing added costs. Many legislators worry that such regulations are too overreaching and share the concerns of the business community. The election of George W. Bush led to an end to the controversy for the time being. If Albert Gore had been elected, the regulation more than likely would have remained in place. Congress still might have voted in favor of erasing it, but Gore had indicated during the campaign for the presidency that he would veto any legislation of that nature that crossed his desk. With a Senate evenly divided, at the time, between Republicans and Democrats and with only slightly more Republicans than Democrats in the House, it is most likely that a such a veto would have been sustained. Because of the opposition the rule engendered and the many lawsuits that were filed, the next step would have been for the courts to wade into the controversy, with the final outcome perhaps not being decided for many years.

The term *ergonomics* was unknown to the framers of the U.S. constitution. Yet based on a close reading of history and remarkable intuition, they had a clear sense of the immensity of the task of creating a suitable balance of power among the three branches of government. Were they able to survey the scene today, it can be imagined they would recognize the recent debate over ergonomics as being equivalent to adding just another pinch of spice to the constitutional broth that has been simmering for more than 200 years.

## OTHER DETERMINANTS IN MAKING PUBLIC POLICY

The federal government is not the only level at which public policy is formulated and implemented. The United States is a large, multifaceted society that lacks a single, unified health care system. Instead, many different kinds of components of a system characterize how health care is financed and delivered in this country. Major elements of the system include the following:

- Constructing and operating health care facilities such as hospitals, nursing homes, and ambulatory care sites
- Financing biomedical research
- Educating personnel such as allied health professionals

- Manufacturing health commodities such as pharmaceutical products and a wide assortment of medical devices
- Operating academic institutions such as schools of allied health that are involved in research, service, and the educational preparation of health professionals
- Developing financial mechanisms such as the aforementioned Medicare and Medicaid programs[8]

The federal government plays a substantial role in providing many of these components. It is involved in collecting and disseminating information; educating and training personnel directly, and providing financial support to them; operating health care institutions; furnishing other direct health services; and participating in financing, supporting, and carrying out research, planning, evaluation, and regulatory functions. The same may be said of the fifty states and other jurisdictions such as the District of Columbia and the Commonwealth of Puerto Rico, although there are variations in the degree to which such activities are performed at different locales. The states become a major focal point when health professions groups compete with one another over scope of practice issues.

Although state health departments tend to be highly visible, city health departments also are engaged in providing many essential services in areas such as maternal and child health. Other activities include tuberculosis control, immunization programs, and control of sexually transmitted diseases. Although the situation differs from one state to another, certain jurisdictions have large, dynamic county health departments. California provides a good example of a state that is organized to provide an extensive array of health care services at the county level.

In addition, nongovernmental agencies have an important role to play. Professional organizations, such as the Association of Schools of Allied Health Professions (ASAHP), have members who serve on government advisory committees, who evaluate funding proposals through peer review activities, and whose staff carry out federally funded projects to advance the objectives of the U.S. Public Health Service and other government agencies. Consumer organizations such as AARP and Families USA sponsor national research projects that have an impact on how public policy is formulated and they often also administer a wide range of programs that are funded by the federal government.

Washington, DC, exists in large measure as a place where laws are enacted, regulations are produced to explain how these laws will be implemented, and items such as transmittal letters are prepared to clarify regulations. More than 100,000 pages of information have been written by officials at the Center for Medicare and Medicaid Services (CMS) to explain how the

Medicare program should be operated. Depending on which aspect of public policy is being addressed, an army of federal and nonfederal employees derives its livelihood from the whole process. This army, in turn, is comprised of legions, each of which specializes in developing proposed legislation, responding to legislative initiatives, reporting on what is happening in Congress, and then repeating all these same kinds of activities for regulations that follow the enactment of legislation.

The legionnaires include employees of individual members of Congress; committees and subcommittees on Capitol Hill; the Congressional Research Service; the General Accounting Office; agencies of the executive branch such as the Department of Health and Human Services; consulting firms; think tanks; publishing firms specializing in journals, newsletters, magazines, and newspapers; radio and television talk shows; public relations firms; and trade, consumer, and professional associations. No state can match this vast array of activity, but on a lesser scale, much of it transpires in state capitals such as Albany, New York; Boston, Massachusetts; and Sacramento, California.

## INTEREST GROUPS

The sixteenth edition of *Health Groups in Washington* lists more than 900 groups that either have headquarters in metropolitan Washington, DC, or have some type of government relations activities being carried out there on their behalf.[9] They tend to belong to the following categories:

- Professional organizations (e.g., Association of Schools of Allied Health Professions)
- Consumer organizations (e.g., AARP)
- Pharmaceutical manufacturers and medical supply companies (e.g., Amgen)
- Voluntary organizations (e.g., American Cancer Society)
- Provider organizations (e.g., American Hospital Association)
- Health insurers (e.g., Kaiser Permanente)
- Accrediting bodies (Joint Commission on Accreditation of Health Care Organizations)
- Educational institutions (University of California)

Several of these entities also have chapters and state affiliates that are active in state and local affairs involving public policy. Each group has good reasons for wanting to be in a position to influence events both in Washington, DC, and in state capitals. Examples follow:

- Having a law enacted that will have a positive impact on the interest group it represents
- Seeking to amend an existing law for the same reason
- Influencing the writing of a regulation that will be to the advantage of the constituency represented
- Preventing issues from ever becoming part of the legislative agenda
- Opposing a law or a regulation that imposes hardships
- Attempting to influence how an agency carries out its mandate
- Influencing the appropriations process successfully so that more funds are directed toward the interest in question

The term *interest group* is often used disparagingly to describe the activities of those who engage in these activities. Candidates for office are fond of railing against them, pledging during election campaigns that they will not be the tools of so-called special interest groups. Although it is true that handgun manufacturers and tobacco companies are examples of such entities that attract a lot of public attention, the field is rather crowded indeed. It includes AARP acting on behalf of improved health benefits for the aged, the Association of Schools of Allied Health Professions providing information about the extent to which minority students are underrepresented in health professions' academic institutions, and the American Cancer Society pointing out the advantages of adequately funding biomedical research.

Since the keen French observer Alexis de Tocqueville visited the United States in the nineteenth century to study the American penal system and subsequently wrote his landmark book *Democracy in America,*[10] other writers also have argued that interest groups have improved the performance of the political system and the quality of American society in several ways. First, interest groups increase opportunities for participation. Second, they are a training ground for an active citizenry, providing experience in the practice of democracy. Third, they provide decision makers with information, drawing on a knowledge of technical problems often beyond the capacity of government itself to provide. Fourth, interest groups not only identify problems or potential solutions but solve them either by working in partnership with government agencies or running their own programs as an alternative to governmental activity.[11] For example, shortly after George W. Bush became president in 2001, he proposed that more resources be directed to faith-based groups so that they could be more involved in the operation of various social programs.

## Political Action Committees

Some interest groups form political action committees (PACs), which can raise funds from members to be spent in various ways, such as giving money to candidates directly. PAC activities must be disclosed to the Federal Election Commission and the funds involved must fit within certain contribution limits. Although many PACs are active in American elections, a majority of corporations, trade associations, and membership organizations do not have PACs. They are more common among labor unions, but some unions have not formed PACs or have terminated PACs that were once active.[12] Just as individuals become more effective political actors by forming groups, individual groups increase their effectiveness and maximize their resources by forming coalitions. A coalition may be either termporary or semipermanent in nature. Examples in order of size from small to large include the

- Allied Health Round Table Group
- Health Professions and Nursing Education Coalition (HPNEC)
- Friends of HRSA (Health Resources and Services Administration)

The HPNEC group focuses on health professions education programs under Titles VII and VIII of the Public Health Service Act, including Section 755, Allied Health and Other Disciplines Program. The Friends of HRSA group embraces both HPNEC and the round table group while directing its attention to a much broader array of programs.

Coalitions provide good venues in which information can be exchanged and the validity of rumors confirmed or denied. Oftentimes, one member of a coalition will take responsibility for calling meetings and arranging for the distribution of information and materials to its members. Another common activity is for coalition members to split the division of duties and visit congressional committee members in small groups to ensure that all committee members are contacted.

How influential are interest groups? Influence is affected by several factors, including the type of issue, nature of the demand, availability of resources, and structure of the political conflict. In direct efforts to influence legislation, influence will be weaker on highly salient, visible issues that also are ideological or partisan in nature. This point of view suggests the better informed the voters are on an issue, the less important interest groups are. Interest groups have more success on nonsalient, expert issues in which there is little media coverage or public interest. If interest groups can tie their desired policies to strong public support, their chances of success are enhanced. Many powerful interest groups fought against the passage of

Medicare, but the strong preference for health care coverage for the aged led to its enactment.[13]

## *CONCLUSION*

Russian literary theorist Mikhail Mikhailovich Bakhtin (1895-1975) alerted scholars to the multivoiced nature of language by his use of the key term *heteroglossia*. In "Discourse in the Novel," Bakhtin describes heteroglossia as a complex mixture of languages and worldviews.[14] Voices arise from many different sources, including legislators, staff on legislative committees and subcommittees on Capitol Hill, executive agency personnel, and persons representing consulting firms, think tanks, publishing firms specializing in material that covers governmental activities, radio and television talk shows, and public relations firms, as well as trade, consumer, and professional associations.

Wendy B. Young, who served on the staff of Senator Tom Daschle (D-SD) when he was Senate minority leader, noted that the restructuring of congressional committees and increasing ease of travel between home districts and the Capitol have erased any clear distinction between campaigning and policymaking activities. Members of Congress are readily accessible to constituents and can engage in the policymaking agenda of most committees. Hence, they must have information that is current and framed to be consistent with their platform. An industry has emerged to supply such tailored information on a just-in-time basis similar to the management strategies used by Japanese manufacturers to shorten production time and enhance market competition.[15]

Opening committee appointments dispersed power and expanded the agenda as the policymaking process engaged more participants and a wider range of perspectives. All committees and subcommittees acquired staff and the latter expanded the agenda to provide a showcase for members and the special issues they espouse. The market for policy information grew from the relatively permanent and exclusive group of staff that serves a few senior members of Congress, to a large and diverse range of staff serving each member of Congress who expressed interest in a particular policy issue. Washington, DC, thus began to see a proliferation of advocacy, lobbying, consulting, and think-tank organizations seeking to supply information to those involved in an expanded and more diverse policymaking process. On a different scale, similar developments have also taken place at the state level.

Outsourcing information requests to these various groups have the advantage of shortening the time required to produce policy and political materials to advance the message of the moment when legislation begins to move at a quicker pace. Both the purveyors and the consumers stand to benefit from the relationship. A legislator can obtain condensed information from research reports, government reports, the media, and polls that is tailored to fit into his or her political message, while advocacy groups gain advance notice of intended tactical and legislative changes.

Clearly, allied health professionals have an important role to play by dispensing information to policymakers. In order to be effective, they need a keen understanding of how policy decisions are made. Moreover, they must learn not only how to identify key points in the process where it becomes advisable to intervene, but also to be cognizant of when it is propitious to do so.

## REFERENCE NOTES

1. Elwood, T.W. Ergonomics: Situated at the Crossroads of Conflict Among the Three Branches of Government. *Journal of Allied Health.* 2001, 30:55-60.

2. Hamilton, A., Madison, J., and Jay, J. ([1788] 1966). *The Federalist.* Edited by Wright, B.F. Cambridge, MA: The Belkings Press of Harvard Universtiy Press.

3. National Coalition on Ergonomics. Litigation Status Report. December 4, 2000.

4. American College of Occupational and Environmental Medicine. "Occupational Physicians Withdraw Support for OSHA Final Ergonomics Standard." Chicago, IL, November 14, 2000.

5. Employer Policy Foundation. Policy Backgrounder. Washington, DC: November 6, 2000.

6. National Coalition on Ergonomics. "Proposed Workplace Safety Rule Will Cost State Billions, Study Shows," Washington, DC: November 1, 2000.

7. Montesquieu, Charles de Secondat, baron de ([1748] 1949). *The Spirit of Laws.* Translated by Nugent, T. New York: Hafner Press.

8. Jonas, S. *An Introduction to the U.S. Health Care System,* Third Edition. New York: Springer Publishing Company. 1992. pp. 1, 4-8, 10-12, 34-35.

9. National Health Council. *Health Groups in Washington.* Sixteenth Edition. Washington, DC: National Health Council, 2001.

10. deTocqueville, A. *Democracy in America.* Translated by Mansfield, H.C. and Winthrop, D. Chicago, IL: University of Chicago Press, 2000. p. 832.

11. Wilson, G.K. Interest Groups in the Health Care Debate. In Aaron, H.J. (Ed.), *The Problem That Won't Go Away: Reforming U.S. Health Care Financing,* (pp. 110-143). Washington, DC: The Brookings Institution, 1996.

12. Rozell, M.J. and Wilcox, C. *Interest Groups in American Campaigns: The New Face of Electioneering.* Washington, DC: CQ Press, 1999.

13. Weissert, C.S. and Weissert, W.G. *Governing Health: The Politics of Health Policy.* Baltimore, MD: The Johns Hopkins University Press, 1996.

14. Bakhtin, M.M. "Discourse in the Novel." In M. Holquist (Ed.), *The Dialogic Imagination: Four Essays*. Translated by Caryl Emerson and Michael Holquist. Austin, TX: University of Texas Press, 1981. pp. 259-422.

15. Young, W.B. "The Market for Information in Health Policy: Using the 'Just-In-Time' Strategy." In Lewin, M.E. and Lipoff, E. (Eds.), *Information Trading: How Information Influences the Health Policy Process*. Washington, DC: Institute of Medicine, 1997. pp. 11-26.

Chapter 17

# Gaps in Knowledge and Research Needs

Kevin J. Lyons

## *INTRODUCTION*

As a group, the allied health professions are relatively young but growing fields. Each is on an evolutionary path moving from clinical specialties that are concerned solely with providing specialized services to physicians or dentists, to more autonomous providers of health care. The typical pattern of this evolution includes a number of intermediate stages, each requiring increased education and a focus on developing a body of knowledge specific to each discipline, eventually leading to professional status. Prior to 1960, the primary method of preparing allied health professionals was on-the-job training. There were fewer than fifteen colleges of allied health in the country.[1] With increased federal money in the late 1960s and 1970s, a sharp increase in the number of programs occurred. Some of these programs were located at community colleges, but many others were housed in university settings, either as departments in medical schools, or as freestanding schools of allied health. Those located in large universities were faced with certain changes in expectations for the programs and the faculty teaching in them. As members of the university community, faculty were required to adapt the culture of academe, which is steeped in requirements for scholarship and research. This transition has been a difficult one.

True professions have a number of accepted characteristics, two of which are particularly important. The first is a long, extended period of education. In the pursuit of this goal, there seems to be some progress. Although many allied health programs are still at the associate degree level, most have moved to the baccalaureate level and beyond. For example, physical therapy and occupational therapy now require education beyond the baccalaureate level, and speech pathology requires a master's degree for entry into the profession. A few others, most notably audiology, require a doctorate as the entry-level degree. The second characteristic of true professions is the possession of a specific body of knowledge that sets it apart from other professions.

This poses a dilemma for allied health professionals. The key to the development of a body of knowledge is sound, scientific research. However, the evolution of the allied health professions has been rooted in clinical practice and remains tied to those conventions, which lack a tradition of research or a culture that values the pursuit of knowledge. This clinical culture often views knowledge as experience which is passed down from those skilled as clinicians to those who are novices. Because of the ambivalent way in which the allied health professions approach education and the transmission of knowledge, there exist gaps in their knowledge base. There is also a lack of a systematic research approach to fill these gaps.

Consider an example of what might happen in a clinical setting.

## CASE STUDY

Professor Harrington is a clinical coordinator in occupational therapy. She is working with one of her students, Gina, in a large rehabilitation hospital. Gina has just learned a new therapeutic technique in her class at the university that is supposed to help patients recovering from strokes improve their functional ability. Professor Harrington is not familiar with the technique and is very comfortable with the procedure she has been using over the past ten years. Obviously, Gina is anxious to use what she has learned in class, although it conflicts with the way Professor Harrington prefers to see things done. When Gina asks about trying the new technique, Professor Harrington refuses, saying, "The technique we've been using has always worked well; there isn't any reason to change the way we do things now." Gina persists, however, and asks, "Isn't there a way to find out if the new procedure works as well or better than the traditional procedure?" Professor Harrington responds, "There might be, but I don't know how it could be done." Gina spends the remainder of her clinical rotation learning and using a therapeutic technique that many would consider outmoded.

In this scenario the inability to assess whether a new treatment is effective could potentially compromise the quality of patient care and delay the advancement of professional knowledge. The problem, in part, is the lack of research knowledge and skill on the part of Professor Harrington.

Was there a way to find out if the new technique was superior to the old in its ability to improve patient function? In this particular case, a small research study would have been able to provide some evidence for the effectiveness of one technique over the other. Since this is a very large rehabilitation hospital, there are many stroke patients admitted each month. Since Professor Harrington's method has worked well in the past and the new technique has been successful in other settings, it would not be unethical to implement a two-group comparison study. In the study, one group of patients would receive Professor Harrington's treatment and another group would receive therapy using the new technique. At the end of a certain period the groups could be compared on a measure of functional ability.

Why does Professor Harrington not have the knowledge or skills to conduct this relatively simple study to compare the effectiveness of the two techniques? There are at least three reasons for this.

The first is the historical roots of the professions that were discussed earlier. Providing specialized services to patients, based on authoritative judgments of others, results in a certain outlook on life. For example, one difference between researchers and clinicians is what has been called time orientation.[2] An individual's time orientation tends to be situationally based and is dependent upon the amount of time required to obtain feedback regarding one's actions on the job. For example, clinicians usually receive relatively quick feedback regarding their decisions, and their responsibilities tend to be organized into short periods of activity during the workday. Researchers, on the other hand, often have a different time orientations with longer periods of time transpiring between action and feedback. This orientation translates into behavior. It influences the expectations regarding the speed at which a project should move and how tasks are delineated and described. This difference may seem minor, but it is very important and a potential source of conflict and misunderstanding in the relationship between researchers and clinicians.

The second reason is the lack of a research culture or tradition in allied health. One feature of a research culture is the desire to think critically and to continually question what exists. A major goal of researchers is the building of a knowledge base. In the allied health professions, the goal is to apply what is known in a profession, with little thought given to increasing the amount known. Professor Harrington would not even consider research because of the nature of the clinical culture (i.e., giving treatments to patients that she knows works), and because of the historical tradition of passing down knowledge to novices.

A result of these two conditions, the third reason is the lack of educational experiences to prepare new professionals to do research. Since allied health professionals do not have a history of conducting research, their educational experiences tend to be very clinically oriented. Even with the increased educational requirements of some of the professions, programs tend to emphasize the development of clinical skills rather than research skills. There are very few doctoral programs which traditionally serve as the training ground for researchers. Most allied health professionals, whether they are clinicians or faculty members at universities, receive a master's degree in their field. If they earn a doctorate, it is usually in a discipline other than their allied health field (e.g., education, which is also an applied discipline).

The other, more research-oriented, professions have developed a different educational approach. For example, someone in the basic sciences will take a very specific career path to reach his or her goal. They will enter a doctoral program in their discipline that is mainly research based. They will have a substantial amount of course work, but they will also spend significant time in a laboratory conducting research under the tutelage of a mentor. Once they graduate they will then spend a minimum of two to three years doing postdoctoral research, again, in the laboratory of an established investigator. Some will take more than one postdoctoral experience. So, by the time they complete their training, they will have had considerable research experience under other knowledgeable researchers. Consider the difference between these individuals and an allied health professional. Not only has Professor Harrington not been exposed to a research culture, she also has not been provided the opportunities in her educational programs to learn the skills necessary to conduct research. In a sense, she does not value the process, nor does she have the skills to deal with it.

## IMPORTANCE OF RESEARCH
## TO THE ALLIED HEALTH PROFESSIONS

Research and scholarship is critical to the further evolution of the allied health disciplines to become true profession. Research will also take on an increasingly important role as our nation's health care system changes in response to the environment of the twenty-first century. As health care units are forced to continually assess the way they operate, more and more emphasis will be placed on providing cost-effective care. Allied health professionals will be challenged to show that the outcomes of any treatment are effective. They will also need to engage in what has been called "evidence-based practice." Evidence-based practice simply requires you to base interventions on the best available evidence. To do this, health care professionals will need to be aware of the literature in their field and to select treatments for each condition based on research that has assessed its effectiveness. Where there is no data, evidence will have to be generated through research.

Contrary to prevailing belief, however, research skills are very similar to the skills that are needed for effective clinical practice. Research is not a set of discrete skills separate from those that are needed to practice in the clinic. Rather, it is a way of thinking. To be a good clinician, you need to be able to think critically about a problem that presents itself, i.e., you need to assess the problem, collect as much information as you can about it, consider alternative approaches, decide and carry out the best approach and, finally, evaluate the results. It is a systematic process by which you ask questions and logically think through possible answers. Research requires the same kind of thinking process. In its simplest form, research is a way of finding answers to questions or, in some cases, identifying important questions in an area. Although research and clinical practice require different skills, the most important quality that should be brought to both processes is the way you think about what you are observing.

As a researcher, you would observe some phenomenon in your practice and then ask the question, "Why is this happening?" Once you've asked the question, you then set out to find the answer to it. For example, in the case study just discussed, the question would be, "Is one of the treatments better than the other for improving a patient's functional ability?" One way to find the answer to the question would be to compare both treatments. To do this, a group of stroke patients assigned to rehabilitation would identified and asked if they would like to participate in a study. The group would be divided in half. Both groups would then be assessed for their functional abilities. One group would receive Professor Harrington's standard treatment and the other would receive Gina's new treatment. At the end of the rehabilitation period, both groups would be tested again for their functional abilities. If one of the groups made more improvement than the other, or if they both showed similar improvement, you would have an answer to your question. The correct answer to the question provides you with more knowledge to provide better care to your patients, while at the same time advances the knowledge base of your profession. This, obviously, is an oversimplified example. There are a number of details you would have to attend to, such as making sure qualified therapists gave both treatments, ensuring the groups were as similar as possible at the beginning, and using correct measuring and analytical tools. However, it does show that the process of research is very similar to the process followed in clinical treatments.

To summarize the previous section:

- Research is necessary for the development of a profession.
- Most allied health professionals have not developed a culture of research, nor have they been trained in conducting research.
- Research is necessary to advance the knowledge base of each of the allied health professions and improve patient care.
- Research is a way of thinking and this way of thinking is similar to the thinking that occurs in effective practice.
- Critical thinking is a research skill as well as an important clinical skill.
- The move toward evidence-based practice will require an understanding of research.

## TYPES OF RESEARCH BEING CONDUCTED
## BY ALLIED HEALTH PROFESSIONALS

As each of the allied health professions evolve, there has been a growing awareness of the importance of research and scholarship in many of the professions. Although still not comparable to many of the more mature professions, strides are being made. Allied health researchers are becoming engaged in both basic and applied research. Basic research is research that strives to develop and expand our theoretical understanding of an issue. This type of research may include studies such as those that lead to a better understanding of the workings of a cell or the development of a theory of occupation. It is research that is not concerned with any practical application; it is concerned with a better understanding of a phenomenon. Applied research, on the other hand, is exactly what its name implies. It is research that takes what is learned from basic research and applies it to practical situations. Because the allied health fields are predominately applied fields, most of the research conducted is of an applied nature. However, researchers in some fields are also conducting basic research.

The types of research being conducted by allied health researchers are diverse and cut across many fields and areas of interest. An occupational therapist or physical therapist might be involved in research on rehabilitation issues. For example, there are research studies aimed at enhancing the functional ability of frail elderly people through home environment modification. Some studies are designed to promote optimal aging in the home, and others are designed to help those recovering from stroke regain some of their physical abilities. Clinical research studies have also focused on such things as osteological analyses of bone spurs in the heel, analyses of the walking styles of frail elderly people with the goal of preventing falls, and studies to predict the effectiveness of muscle endurance exercise for people with multiple sclerosis. There is a large amount of educational research being conducted in a variety of settings. Occupational therapists and speech-language pathologists often work in public and private school settings. Therefore, they might study innovative occupational therapy or speech services in the schools, or conduct other studies that investigate optimal therapeutic practices in early intervention with children at risk, or compare different methods to prevent stuttering.

Allied health researchers also conduct basic science research. Those in the laboratory science areas such as medical technology or cytotechnology have conducted studies on the molecular analysis of genetic mutations in visual diseases. Other studies investigated the molecular basis of inherited macular degeneration. These are just a few of the examples of research that can and has been done by allied health professionals who opt for a research career.

## *STRATEGIES FOR BECOMING PROFESSIONAL*

Although many allied health professions have made considerable progress in advancing research, more needs to be done. There are at least two approaches to this problem. The first applies to the disciplines themselves. Each of the allied health fields will have to consider its priorities and preparation programs. Changes will need to be made in the expectations for students and the roles graduates will play. The second approach applies to individuals. As in the biomedical sciences, future allied health professionals will be responsible for developing the skills they need to become more proficient in research if they expect to advance the knowledge base of their professions and contribute to the health care system.

The following sections will provide practical suggestions for the allied health professions and for students who desire to become professionals. There are at least six strategies the professions can use.

### *Professionwide Strategies*

1. Develop a research infrastructure.
2. Provide research opportunities in educational programs for both future clinicians and scholars in two different curriculum tracks: one for clinicians to learn to read research and another for scholars to learn to do research.
3. Develop a cadre of researchers by creating more doctoral programs in each discipline.
4. Stress the importance of interdisciplinary approaches to research.
5. Encourage more collaboration between clinicians and researchers at universities.
6. Encourage more faculty research development programs.

The professions need to go beyond addressing specific research areas in isolation and work on the development of a national research infrastructure. A major step toward creating a research infrastructure would be to develop more research-oriented doctoral programs from which a cadre of allied health researchers will emerge. These programs need to be rigorous PhD programs, not professional doctorates. If there is not a sufficient body of knowledge in an allied health discipline to warrant a PhD program, then efforts should be expended to develop this body of knowledge, not to implement professional degrees.

As the allied health professions build a cadre of researchers, the content of research training programs must be taken into consideration, particularly in light of a new health care system that is more responsive to individual, community, and population-based needs. Currently, most professions put little emphasis on teaching research to students. If there is an emphasis, it tends to focus on traditional research designs that inevitably lead students to conduct narrow, clinical trial type studies. Although classical research designs are important, they are generally taught to the exclusion of other, equally appropriate approaches. A more responsive strategy would be to include epidemiological approaches, decision analysis, cost-effectiveness analysis, health services research, single-subject designs, case study methodology, participant-action research, participant observation, and cross-cultural studies in research preparation programs, in addition to basic statistics.

Doctoral training need not, and should not, be the only avenue for advancing research in the allied health professions. Training at the master's level should also be explored as a vehicle for advancing knowledge. However, this training needs to be based on a different premise than that which exists in current practice, which is to teach soon-to-be-clinicians the same material as beginning PhD students. The practice is justified by claims that the objective is to make clinicians educated consumers of the research literature. Research training at the master's level might be more effective if it had two separate tracks: the first track designed to provide preliminary training for future PhD students, the second to provide "terminal" research training for those whose interests do not lie in a research career. At the very least, content in this track would focus on the skills needed to identify researchable problems, read and understand the literature, and work on a research team. In effect, this track would train clinicians to be reflective research practitioners.

### Individual Strategies

In addition to changes in each of the health professions, individuals can help establish their own approach to developing a research career. Planning a research career is a systematic process. One example of a systematic plan is presented here:

Step I: Build a set of research credentials at state and local levels.
Make presentations at local professional meetings.
Write an article about a research topic for state or local publications.

Offer to write a book review for your professional journal.
Work on a research team with more experienced investigators.
Network with more experienced researchers in your profession.
Apply for faculty-development seed money at your university.
Step II: Build on previous experience.
Submit abstracts to national conferences based on your research.
Write your presentation for submission to your professional journal.
Continue to network with more experienced researchers.
Apply for researcher-development money from agencies in the federal government.
Seek foundation money for your research projects.
Step III: Continue to build on previous experience.
Apply for federal funding as an independent investigator.
Seek opportunities to present at national and international conferences.
Continue to network with other researchers.
Participate in multisite studies.

As you can see, this outline presents a series of steps that an allied health professional can take to launch a research career. Doing so requires that you develop a plan for long-range professional development. Ask the question, "Where do I want to be three to five years in the future?" This may seem a long time, but becoming an accomplished researcher takes time and patience. The first step is to build a set of individual credentials. As you build these credentials, you are expanding your own knowledge base about certain aspects of your profession. You are also providing evidence to others that you are becoming a more accomplished researcher. Such a reputation will help you obtain more opportunities to expand your career.

There are three general components that help build your career: presentations, publications, and the actual conduct of research. There are numerous ways to become involved in each of these components as a beginner. The first is to identify one or two areas of research interest. These should be broad areas that have potential for long-term investigation, and should be of sufficient interest to keep your attention. They should also be areas of interest to your profession. Begin by making presentations on your chosen topic at meetings of your local professional society. These presentations can then be turned into articles for local newsletters or journals. Your professional journal is always looking for members to write book reviews on new texts or abstracts of pertinent articles. These are all relatively easy ways to break into print the first time. You also might offer to serve as a reviewer for abstracts submitted at meetings of your professional society.

In addition to gaining local recognition for writing and presenting, you should start to develop your skills at conducting research. The first place to start would be your university. If you become a faculty member, you could volunteer to work on a research project of a funded investigator in exchange for gaining experience. If you are working in a clinic or laboratory, you could also offer your services as a researcher.

Many universities have small amounts of seed money for novice researchers to conduct pilot studies. Ask your department chair if this money is available and how you apply for it. In addition, many professional associations have money for small research studies. Announcements about these funds are usually found in professional journals or newsletters. Each of these strategies will help start your career as a researcher. They will give you experience making presentations and writing for publication. They will also help refine and advance knowledge in your area of interest and help you learn some of the skills needed to conduct research. From this beginning you can then expand your horizons.

Once you have gained experience at local levels, consider gaining regional or national exposure. If you have received seed money to conduct a small research study, the results of this study can be used to justify a larger study. Many government agencies and foundations have money available for those who are beginning a research career. Having data from a pilot study will help in the competition for this money. Submitting abstracts for a presentation at a national conference will give you additional exposure and experience. As you did with local presentations, write your presentation for submission to your national professional journal. These strategies should be continued at more advanced levels. Each presentation, publication, and research study should build on the previous one, so that in a few years you will have a consistent track record of work in a specific area. You will also have advanced the knowledge base of your profession.

Another strategy is to collaborate with more experienced researchers. If you have offered to work on a research study at your university, continue to collaborate on other studies in more responsible roles. If the primary researcher is planning to write a grant proposal for another project, ask if you can work with him or her on the proposal. This person might also agree to mentor you in your career. If his or her area of research is not consistent with your career plans, then you should find someone experienced who has more similar interests. If no one at your university is working in your area of interest, look outside the institution. From the literature, you will know who is doing work similar to yours. Contact these people, ask for their help, and ask if you can contribute to their work. Many researchers are flattered when a novice investigator asks for their help.

Systematic planning to develop a research career is just one step in the process. There are certain skills, attitudes, and abilities common among researchers. Most of these can be learned.

The first learned skill is an understanding of the research process. These are the technical skills or the "nuts and bolts" of doing research. They include knowledge of research designs, knowing how to develop research questions, knowing the parts of research proposals, understanding funding sources and how to access them, and knowing how to conduct an efficient literature review.

Once you have mastered the essentials, it is very important to develop what is called *domain expertise.* This is simply an in-depth understanding of the knowledge base of your profession: What are the major theoretical models upon which practice is based? What are the major studies in the field? What is the philosophy of your profession? Who are the influential writers and researchers?

Clearly related to research skills are abilities. These are certain personal characteristics that can be developed. Successful researchers tend to be very organized. The caricature of the researcher as an absent-minded professor is a myth. Research is as complicated as any clinical intervention. Most researchers are systematic in their approach to problems and disciplined in following research protocols. It is also important to think critically as well as creatively about a problem. Questions to continually ask are: What is going on here? What could have caused this particular situation?

Along with being systematic and organized, a good deal of flexibility is also required. What would happen if a study you were conducting did not turn out the way you had hoped? The flexibility to think about why it did not work would be very helpful. Researchers are enthusiastic about their work, but always remain a little skeptical if things go too easily. Because of the nature of research and the fact that not everyone will agree with you, it is also necessary to be able to accept criticism. Finally, because things often go wrong, a good sense of humor is always helpful.

In addition to research skills, all allied health professionals, whether they are clinicians or faculty members, will face certain barriers to conducting research. Once these barriers are known and expected, it is possible to devise strategies to overcome them. Some of the major barriers include lack of time, mentoring, financing and resources, institutional support, and a research culture. Each of these will be discussed along with possible ways to overcome such barriers.

Lack of time is one of the greatest problems faced by allied health professionals, both in clinical settings and at universities. In clinical settings, the efficient handling of patients or clients is a priority, particularly in this new cost-conscious marketplace. Most laboratories are shorthanded and there is a high priority placed on the fast, accurate handling of specimens. At universities, faculty often have a larger teaching load than do their counterparts in the more research-oriented disciplines. There is also a heavy committee load and myriad administrative tasks that must be performed. Research takes time—time for reflection, time for writing, and a need for a certain amount of solitude. It is extremely difficult to overcome this number-one barrier to research. In some cases, the solution to this obstacle is an individual one. To do research individuals need to organize and manage their time efficiently. Choices have to be made and priorities set. Where possible, faculty members must say no to committee work or to other responsibilities. Deadlines need to be set and kept. It also may be possible to lobby to receive research credit for part of the regular heavy workload. In many universities, faculty members are given one day per week to conduct research. When this happens, it must be taken advantage of and not wasted. At clinical or laboratory sites, it may not be possible to make this arrangement, and research may have to be conducted after hours. Research is not a nine-to-five job and everything cannot be accomplished in an eight-hour day.

To summarize the previous section:

- There is a growing awareness of the importance of research among the allied health professions.
- Strides are being made to advance the research missions of the allied health professions.
- Allied health researchers engage in a wide variety of research approaches, both basic and applied.
- In order to continue to advance the research missions of the allied health professions, a national infrastructure must be developed to develop and support allied health investigators.
- Allied health professionals should plan their research careers through a series of systematic steps.
- There are certain skills, abilities, and attitudes that can be developed to improve the ability to conduct research.

## CONCLUSION

Research is the hallmark of a profession. The allied health disciplines are evolving from clinically oriented occupations to professional careers. In order to continue along this evolutionary pathway, an increased emphasis must be placed on research. Although there are a number of impediments to this advancement, they can be overcome. Surmounting these barriers requires that a concerted effort be made by professional associations, by university faculty, and, most of all, by individual allied health professionals. Professional associations must move to support a national research infrastructure and provide research support to its members. University faculty need to consider and develop more research-based doctoral programs for their professions. Individuals who desire a research career should develop a systematic long-range plan to guide their movement from novice to expert investigator. They should also work to develop the research skills, abilities, and attitudes necessary for a successful research career. A concentrated effort on the part of all three groups will allow the allied health professions to realize true professional status.

## NOTES

1. Lyons, K.J. and Abrams, L. (1995). Role of allied health in health care. *Medicine and Health Care into the 21st Century.* In Majumdar, S.K., Rosenfeld, L.M., Nas, D.B., Audent, A.M. (Eds.) Easton, PA: The Pennsylvania Academy of Science. pp. 289-300.

2. Lawrence, P.R. and Lorsch, J.W. (1969). *Organization and environment.* Homewood, IL: Richard D. Irwin Inc.

Chapter 18

# Preparing Future Allied Health Leaders

Gail A. Nielsen

### CASE STUDY: WHAT WOULD THE LEADER DO?

Manager Michael Reed shook his head in disbelief as he held the worn rubber tip from the examining room footstool. How could such a little thing cause so much trouble? Reed had been summoned from the cafeteria an hour earlier by the vice president of patient services, who reported a patient had just fallen in Reed's department. A subsequent review of the patient's condition in the hospital's emergency department and discussion with the employee who had been with the patient when he fell had shaken Reed's usual calm composure. The discussion with the vice president had raised his blood pressure, but news that the CEO wanted to see him at 3 p.m. had rattled him. Reed seldom saw his CEO, except in large group meetings, and he had never been summoned for problems in his own department.

Preparing for his meeting with the CEO, Reed reviewed his discussions with his employee and his vice president. The employee reported that the patient, while stepping down from the examination table, had apparently pushed too hard on the handle of the step stool, which skidded across the floor as he was stepping down and caused him to lose his balance and fall to the floor. The employee had caught the patient partway down, but could not break the fall enough to keep the patient's chest from striking a footstool and fracturing a rib.

Following his discussion with the employee, Reed found the worn rubber tip which may have contributed to the skidding of the footstool. Normal wear and tear caused these rubber tips to wear through and they needed to be replaced from time to time. Who had neglected to replace this one? Should the employee be disciplined for using defective equipment? Should the vice president of patient services be disciplined for failing to keep track of the

---

This chapter is dedicated to the future health and success of the graduates of the Coalition for Allied Health Leadership.

condition of the rubber tips? How many more worn rubber tips were currently in the department? Could Reed find less expensive rubber tips and keep more of them on hand? Were his staff members knowledgeable about the policies for keeping equipment in good condition? Whose responsibility would ultimately be questioned?

The vice president had different questions: Was the employee properly trained to keep watch on the rubber tips? Could this fall have been prevented? Was the employee properly trained to assist unstable patients? What were the related department policies and procedures? Would Reed have an incident report filed by morning? Would someone's job be threatened? What plans did Reed have for correcting the problem and preventing future accidents?

No review could have prepared Reed for the ensuing discussion with his CEO, Hal Baker. A large, imposing man, Baker was known for his strict, no-nonsense leadership style. Baker began the meeting with a question: "Do you remember the infamous incident at the Dana-Farber Cancer Institute in 1994 in which a *Boston Globe* health columnist died after receiving a massive overdose of chemotherapy? Since that time," he went on to explain, "we, and other leaders across the country have felt similar tragedies could happen at our own institutions. How can we keep it from happening here?" Baker then described the patient safety program he had presented to the hospital's board of directors the previous evening. It was soundly approved and the program would be introduced in the coming month. Although the board acknowledged that improving patient safety could add significant cost to operations and the return on investment would be difficult to prove, the cost of errors would add thousands of dollars to a patient's care, not to mention possible disability or loss of life.

Could today's accident be the facility's first opportunity to act under the new patient safety program's guidelines? It could be a concrete example of a situation that would resonate with employees. Baker would be participating firsthand in this and future reviews of risks to patient safety, and planned to review this particular incident himself. He wanted to know what happened, not who did it. "Have we told the family the whole thing and not held back about the worn rubber tip on the foot stool?" Baker asked. He was passionate about the importance of patient safety and the culture needed to improve and protect it. Baker intended to create a system for identifying potential problems before things happened, one that enabled employees to report errors, unsafe conditions, and potential problems freely without fear of reprisals or punishment. Ultimately, he wanted to engender the trust needed for a safe environment across his entire health system.

## Case Study Questions

On his train ride home that evening, Reed thought long and hard about the three different reactions exhibited that day by his CEO, his vice president, and himself. What were the qualities demonstrated by these three individuals? Whose conversation and thought processes showed more leadership qualities? Who demonstrated more managerial qualities?

Tables 18.1 and 18.2 relate excerpts of leadership and management qualities from two well-known, contemporary authors on the topic of leadership: Warren Bennis (1994) and John P. Kotter (1990). The reader is encouraged to review the conversations and thought processes of the case study characters and outline the leader versus manager qualities each displayed. The reader is also encouraged to become aware of the growing body of evidence of the impact of medical error in the United States and the many opportunities for clinical improvement being studied and implemented today.

TABLE 18.1. Leader versus Manager Description

"I tend to like to think of the differences between leaders and managers as the differences between those who master the context and those who surrender to it. There are other differences, as well, and they are enormous and crucial" (pp. 44-45).

| Leader | Manager |
| --- | --- |
| Innovates | Administers |
| Develops | Maintains |
| Focuses on people | Focuses on systems, structures |
| Inspires trust | Relies on control |
| Has a long-range perspective | Has a short-range view |
| Asks what and why | Asks how and when |
| Has an eye on the horizon | Has an eye always on the bottom line |
| Originates | Imitates |
| Challenges status quo | Accepts status quo |
| Is his or her own person | The classic good soldier |
| Does the right thing | Does things right |

*Source:* From ON BECOMING A LEADER by WARREN BENNIS. Copyright © 1989, 1994 by Warren Bennis, Inc. Reprinted by permission of Basic Books, a member of Perseus Books, LLC.

TABLE 18.2. Leadership versus Management

| Leadership | Management |
|---|---|
| To provide direction through a vision and specific strategies | To use planning and budgeting strategies for achieving results |
| To align people needed to accomplish the vision and strategies | To use organizing and staffing approaches in carrying out a plan |
| To motivate and inspire people to produce | To monitor results by controlling and problem solving |
| To bring about change or new products | |

*Source:* Adapted from Kotter, J.P. (1990). *A Force for Change: How Leadership Differs from Management.* New York: The Free Press.

## WHY ALLIED HEALTH PROFESSIONALS SHOULD PREPARE FOR THE FUTURE

Why should busy students of allied health, working professionals, or educators concern themselves with the concepts of leadership? After all, mastering the necessary clinical and technical skills is an overwhelming and honorable task. Aren't educators already leaders?

The complexities of the current health care system have grown to a level that eliminates our ability to function in a business-as-usual atmosphere. Shortages of trained professionals, pressures of reduced resources and funding, and the need to reduce error in medical care now combine with the burgeoning growth of required mastery of new knowledge. Additional stresses come from consolidation resulting from managed care or the impact from other reimbursement strategies, an aging and diversifying society, and technological advancements requiring training or retraining. Awareness of the need to reduce the volume of errors in health care and significant harm resulting from medical error, adds new stresses to reduced resources.

Resulting frustrations create an atmosphere that is driving young and experienced professionals away from health care. These frustrations also undermine our ability to understand the root causes of problems and develop good solutions. The ultimate result is increased potential for harm to patients receiving health care and preventive services. In the words of Peter Drucker (1997): "Management's biggest problem is that the work in which they learned to manage no longer exists" (statement made at the second annual Worldwide Lessons in Leadership Conference, October 1997).

Solutions and changes to the delivery of health care that begin to attract the brightest and best to the health professions will come from leadership. Leadership skills can be learned and developed by everyone. Regardless of our role or station, the ability to hold a long-range perspective, to ask why, to master problems rather than surrender to them, and to do the right thing, are possibilities that open a new realm of solutions for a better tomorrow (Bennis, 1994; Headrick, 2000; Kotter, 1990; Leape et al., 2000).

The need for leadership in health care has been recognized and discussed in many venues for a number of years. It is time to move the mountain out of our way or drill through it by encouraging allied health students and professionals to understand and learn leadership skills and apply them in everyday settings. The following are more specific references or evidence that more leadership is needed. Observational comments are also included "from the field" by allied health professionals, managers, and educators.

### *Commission on Allied Health Findings and Recommendations*

In response to growing pressure to examine issues related to the allied health workforce, the 102nd Congress authorized Section 302 of the Health Professions Education Extensions Amendments of 1992 to establish the National Commission on Allied Health (NCAH). The commission conducted a comprehensive review of the issues, problems, and potential solutions pertaining to the education, supply, and distribution of allied health professionals throughout the United States. NCAH identified, in its report, that "with the right support, allied health educational and professional leadership could effectively surmount barriers that impede prompt and appropriate responses to the unmet needs of a rapidly changing health care system." Recommendation 10 of the commission's report states, "Allied health professions must undertake concerted proactive efforts to create formal programs for educational and professional leadership and mentoring" (Department of Health and Human Services [USDHHS], 1995, pp. 13-14).

On the subject of leadership in education, the commission recommended:

> Exceptional allied health leadership supported by appropriate incentives is needed to encourage the development of alternative approaches to more traditional educational practices in order to meet the needs of the marketplace for reducing cost while improving access and quality of health care. (USDHHS, 1995, p. 64)

> What is needed most in bringing about allied health workforce reform, the Commission identified, is leadership in the professions, education system, and health care system. Appropriate leadership is essential to begin to move allied health education programs toward a

more fundamental reorientation and restructuring of their curricula
and educational experiences. (p. 72)

## *Pew Health Professions Commission Findings and Recommendations*

According to the Pew Health Professions Commission report of 1993,
the need for leadership is coupled with the need for individual allied health
professionals to reevaluate their own skills portfolios to ensure their educational choices and work experiences advance versatility as well as expertise
(Pew Health Professions Commission, 1993).

## *Implementation Task Force of the NCAH Report: Building the Future of Allied Health*

The Implementation Task Force of the NCAH was formed to ensure that
the recommendations of the Commission were not forgotten, but were acted
upon and embraced by the allied health community and its many stakeholders. Key areas recommended for immediate focus were: education reform, outcomes research and collaboration. The recommendations of the
Implementation Task Force included the reminder that in its report, the National Commission on Allied Health made several references to the need to
develop leaders within the allied health community. According to NCAH,
the task force pointed out, individuals must be prepared by experience and
training to participate in meaningful collaboration with all other health care
stakeholders. Such collaboration could then lead to a more thoughtful use of
allied health professionals. Preparation to participate in meaningful collaboration should include leadership development.

## *Center for the Health Professions Findings and Recommendations*

In "The Hidden Health Care Workforce," the Center for the Health Professions, UCSF, reported the following:

> At all levels of workers, employers have difficulty attracting workers
> with critical thinking, communication and computer skills as well as
> strong work ethic. While turnover rates were often qualitatively de-
> scribed as problematic and many current and future labor shortages
> were identified, few leaders in human resources departments are ad-
> dressing these challenges with long-term solutions. Many were simply
> mired in the day-to-day work of staying afloat in a highly competitive

marketplace. As a result, few could articulate the repercussions of changes impacting the workforce such as new technology, the transfer of care to long term and outpatient settings, or a rapidly diversifying patient base. If the health care delivery system does not address these and other work force issues, it will be at risk of facing greater recruitment and retention challenges and an even smaller pool of qualified practitioners willing to work in the health care system. Ultimately, these issues will determine an organization's viability in the evolving health care environment. (Ruzek et al., 1999, pp. 6-7)

### The Health Professions Network Vision

The Health Professions Network (HPN) is a gathering of health care provider organizations, educators, accreditors, and administrators who are concerned with exploring current issues and advancing the allied health professions. The organization was established as an interactive, cooperative group in which the needs of allied health in general are put before the needs of an individual organization. HPN's vision is to be the premier network of health professions working to positively influence the delivery of quality health care. Knowing that leaders are needed to continue to develop the vision and mission of the allied health network and to engage in collaborative work, HPN sought to create a leadership "boot camp" to foster development of emerging leaders of allied health professional associations. The expectation was that bringing future leaders of diverse disciplines together to learn advocacy and leadership skills would foster a deeper understanding of many disciplines among the participants. These future leaders would then be equipped to collaborate, share resources, solve problems together, and ultimately improve the quality of health care.

### Collaborative Education to Ensure Patient Safety, a Joint Report to the Secretary, HHS

In September 2000, the Council on Graduate Medical Education (COGME) and National Advisory Council on Nurse Education and Practice (NACNEP) met in a joint venture to collaborate on patient safety. Following are five findings for which they suggest major change will be required to achieve needed improvements in patient safety:

1. Patient safety cannot be accomplished without interdisciplinary practice approaches.
2. Patient safety gains are unlikely to be achieved at a satisfactory pace in the absence of revolutionary changes.

3. Current systems discontinuities need to be confronted with a goal of building a true safety-oriented system of care.
4. A significant cultural change in medicine and nursing is required to achieve the needed gains in patient safety.
5. Patient safety requires that patients become acculturated to the need to participate actively in their own health care. (COGME-NACNEP, 2000)

The COGME-NACNEP report aligned with the Institute of Medicine's report, theme 1: "Establishing a national focus to create leadership through research, tools, and protocols to enhance the knowledge base about safety" (Institute of Medicine, 1999, p. 6). Throughout the COGME-NACNEP deliberations on patient safety, the need for national leadership was stressed. Leadership is needed at all levels to provide the resources and solutions that will be required to sustain a major systems development that affects the entire health care field (COGME-NACNEP, 2000).

Findings from the Breakthrough Collaboratives at the Institute for Healthcare Improvement report indicate that successful efforts to change systems and prevent error tended to have strong leadership, clearly defined aims, careful use of an improvement model, measures of progress, interdisciplinary teams, early involvement of stakeholders, and practical changes in work processes are key components of successful efforts to improve patient safety (Leape et al., 2000; Headrick, 2000).

## OBSERVATIONS FROM THE FRONT LINE

The following are observations from health care administrators on the front line:

- "Staff show minimal evidence of foresight or vision."
- "There is a general lack of advanced education."
- "Staff show little desire to achieve a greater knowledge base; any outside professional or self-development readings are minimal."
- "Technologists must increase scholarship pursuits and increase research."
- "One of my own long-term goals is to get my doctorate. However, the cost ($8,000 to $10,000 per year) plus job, family (my youngest is ten), and professional commitments make this difficult."
- "Staff members show a lack of interest to volunteer in professional organizations on a local, state, or national level."
- "Minimal efforts are seen where employers support participation in advance pursuits or professional volunteerism at the front-line level."

- "More opportunities are needed for professional development."
- "It is difficult to find mentor role models (nearby or easily accessible) even though many leadership guides recommend using mentors."
- "Based on my own and my colleagues' observations, there seems to be a drought in the quality of administrators entering higher education. While we have plenty of PhDs, we are lacking individuals with excellent communication and problem-solving skills that are needed to lead education out of its doldrums. We essentially are lacking people with *vision*."
- "I look at recent hirings in my district and see individuals being promoted into positions that they are not suited for. And I'm speaking about presidents, deans, and executive directors. I'm bothered by this turn of events based partially on my Coalition for Allied Health Leadership (CAHL) experience. I now know the difference between a leader and manager. And I don't see a lot of true leaders entering higher education."
- "Although I took the personal initiative to seek leadership courses, my hospital made some attempts at 'management' courses in house; opportunities for leadership development were lacking."
- "I do not see leadership and/or allied health issues in my professional journals. I am now on the editorial board of our journal and may be able to influence inclusion of articles on leadership."
- "I am exploring taking some credit courses in leadership for nonprofit organizations."

Comments regarding the hopefulness for the future:

- "I am an optimist and know we can improve the situation."
- "I believe there is certainly synergy gained by having a unified Allied Health Professionals' (AHPs) voice. Many AHPs can learn from one another."
- "CAHL is one excellent forum to network, gain leadership skills, and further develop one's potential; funding is needed to continue the efforts."

Comments from the front lines from allied health associations:

- "Our association is very concerned about leadership in our profession. The key thing that concerns us is the difficulty and sometimes inability to fill candidate slots on ballots at both the state and national level."

- "This year's association president has established a special committee on leadership development. As a member of that committee I can tell you that we find it an overwhelming task."
- "We have begun to tackle leadership development through several venues. We have asked our education committee to develop an Individual Independent Study Packet on Leadership to be used by school programs. Second, we are publishing articles in our association newsletter."
- "Declining [numbers of] leadership volunteers underscore the need for programs such as CAHL."
- "I do *not* see a real emphasis on addressing leadership skills in allied health personnel, and I worry about this."

## Other Leaders Speak Out

V. Clayton Sherman, chairman of Management House, a health care consulting firm, and author of *Raising Standards in American Healthcare: Best Practices, Best People, Best Results,* pointed out that "The larger management community outside of health care judges managers within the industry to be insular, outmoded and guilty of creating their own problems. Because much of what is done in management does not represent current best practice, the industry suffers from nothing less than management malpractice" (quoted by Lovern, 2001, p. 38).

In "Wanted: A Few Good Leaders," author Mary Chris Jaklevic examines the serious shortage of qualified top executives able to direct health care organizations through today's troubled waters. Jaklevic discusses a twelve-month collaborative effort, funded by a grant from the Robert Wood Johnson Foundation to address the training of future health care leaders. The 2001 effort was a first-ever industry summit (Jaklevic, 2000).

Jeptha Dalston, president and CEO of the Association of University Programs in Health Administration, has acknowledged that graduate education in health care today is "simply out of sync with the demands of the 21st century" (Jaklevic, 2000, p. 38).

Thomas Dolan, president and CEO of the American College of Healthcare Executives, has said he is disturbed that "health care systems are dropping the ball when it comes to mentoring and continuing education for midcareerists" (Jaklevic, 2000, p. 38). Dolan says there is too little leadership development in health care when compared with the business world.

## COALITION FOR ALLIED HEALTH LEADERSHIP (CAHL)

In 1998 the Health Professions Network (HPN), the Association of Schools of Allied Health Professions (ASAHP), and the National Network of Health Career Programs in Two-Year Colleges (NN2), collaborated to conduct a leadership development program supported by a cooperative grant from the Bureau of Health Professions, U.S. Department of Health and Human Services. The allied health community provided the remaining funding through its professional associations, their members, and their employers. Believing success in today's health care environment requires the allied health professions to identify, develop, and mentor new leaders, the Bureau of Health Professions, ASAHP, HPN, and NN2 have continued to support the Coalition for Allied Health Leadership. The fourth-annual class of thirty participants was enrolled in January of 2001.

### The CAHL Experiential Model

Heavy emphasis on experience-based strategies and mentoring are hallmarks of the Coalition for Allied Health Leadership. Changing an individual participant's paradigm from unidisciplinary to interdisciplinary in a short time appears to require multiple exposures to the value of collaboration across disciplines. Peer counseling, team projects, sharing of mutual issues and concerns, and multiple small-group exercises have been successful in catalyzing long-term networking and collaboration among CAHL graduates.

### Role-Playing and Capitol Hill Visits

The spring session program content for the Coalition on Allied Health Leadership is designed to develop participants' confidence to interact with governmental agencies and elected representatives. Participants receive instruction on the basics of meeting and influencing their elected representatives as well as staff and assistants. Through role-playing with their classmates, confidence is built in preparation for meetings "on the Hill" with their own senators and representatives. Each class has the opportunity to visit congressional offices and meet with White House advisors, federal budget experts, and agency representatives. Issues of concern to the professions and professional associations are reviewed. Emerging issues and talking points are developed which enable CAHL participants to lead discussions and prepare informational documents for Senate and other congressional offices. Participants are encouraged to develop relationships with their senators and representatives, to offer ongoing resources for information, and to continue the dialogue in the coming months.

In addition to the experience participants gain by advocating their interests on the federal scene, participants also learn about existing models of grassroots networks, state organizations of allied health professionals, and consumer advocacy associations. Participants learn how to influence their professional associations and employers' health care facilities by promoting National Allied Health Week through the use of packaged materials. Participants are prepared to use their newly acquired advocacy skills to continue building ongoing relationships with their own state and federal legislators.

## Leaders Learn Best from Experience:
## The Learning Model

The diversity of disciplines, educational preparation, ethnicity, gender, and age, plus a wide variation in skill mix, lends experience to CAHL participants. In addition, class members share mutual issues and concerns plus a range of experience in leadership within their own state and national professional associations. Faculty members and mentors challenge the participants with experience-based learning opportunities, work projects, and small group exercises.

Each year CAHL participants engage in long-distance teamwork on projects focused on allied health issues. Project concepts are recommended by the allied health community and federal agencies, and are consistent with the recommendations of the Implementation Task Force of the National Commission on Allied Health's 1999 report. These projects also support the expectations of the Bureau of Health Professions' strategic plan with regards to quality improvement in health professions practice.

Required work projects force learning through individual experience in long-distance communication and relationship building with a purpose. Each participant is required to engage in a team project of his or her choice to research an area of interest related to the needs of the collective allied health community. Project teams range in size from two to five members who work together for six months, from April to September, to research their issues and create a product. A deliverable product, such as an article for publication, research paper, or monograph, is presented as evidence of leadership development upon returning to the fall education session. Examples of completed work projects include white papers for professional associations, published articles, and an allied health Web site. Other tools include a how-to manual for understanding the process of influencing and collaborating with federal and state agencies and elected officials, and an allied health week celebration package. Publications include articles on clinical outcomes assessments, outcomes research using a collaborative distance approach, a call to action for allied health professional representation, a proposed model for a middle school mentoring program, cost-benefit analysis of clinical education in two-year college allied health programs, and scholarship resources documentation for minority allied health students.

The process of working together for six months to produce a product for the allied health community is an overwhelming task for most teams. However, the overwhelming size of the task is exactly what students of leadership need to challenge their skill building, to help them personally experience the value of interdisciplinary team participation, and to gain a higher-level perspective. Through this sometimes painful process, participants discover the leadership dynamics of group process: forming, storming, norming, and performing. And perform they do. Outcomes from completed projects have provided useful information and assistance to the allied health community.

## *Developing Leadership Skills*

The fall session of the CAHL program includes leadership content intended to increase awareness and build personal as well as team skills. Interactive learning techniques are introduced to engage participants in leadership experiences. A consultant experienced in conducting 360-degree personal assessments walks participants through an intense process of receiving and processing feedback on their leadership skills, as seen from the perspective of their bosses, peers, and employees. The personal insight and assistance with interpreting feedback are crucial instruments of the growth process. To further support participants during this tense and reflective time, the skill of peer counseling is introduced. Participants work in teams to listen and advise one another in a safe environment that allows reality checks and mutual support too often unavailable in the workplace.

Through their presentations of the summer research projects, students experience the joys and challenges of speaking and presenting material. Each team presents the outcomes and products they produced during their summer research and collaboration. Further learning for all participants comes through the discussion of each team's findings following team presentations.

Additional topics explored in the fall session on leadership include:

- Leadership in times of change
- Leadership and stress management
- Decision making and prioritizing
- Team building and problem solving
- Personal conflict management
- Association leadership

## CAHL Outcomes

Reports of personal growth of CAHL graduates show evidence that the first three years of the program have had strong positive impact on the futures of individual participants. Job promotions, new job opportunities, elected offices, and professional appointments are just a few of the accomplishments graduates have attributed to the growth they achieved through participation in CAHL. Graduates also report they have experienced changes in personal perspectives and an enhanced self-awareness.

One of the outcomes, anticipated to be of long-term significance, is also the most difficult to demonstrate in the short term: a growing awareness and deepened understanding of the value of collaboration among health professionals from diverse clinical backgrounds. A specific example was seen when one of the project teams presented the results of their efforts. Diverse in age, sex, professional training, and cultural and ethnic backgrounds, this team got off to a stormy start. In fact, one team member asked to be reassigned. In their final report, the team included a testimonial tribute to the project process, which succeeded in bringing the team members together. By September, all members were not only working as a team, they had become fast friends. Professional by professional, team by team, class by class, planners and faculty have observed leadership growth and a renewed enthusiasm for the future of health care in the United States. Continued networking across the country and across disciplines promises to bring a new perspective to future problem solving.

Graduates report their progress attributable to the CAHL experience:

- "CAHL has provided me with a wealth of tools and insights to allow me to grow professionally and personally."
- "I have been appointed by the governor to the Radiologic Technology Licensing Board."
- "I am the lead instructional designer, working with a cross-functional group of allied health and nursing faculty in addressing on-going curriculum issues; we are revamping the core curriculum."
- "I have more confidence in my abilities to lead people."
- "My dissertation topic is an outgrowth of the summer project I worked on for CAHL."
- "The increased confidence in myself that I gained as a result of CAHL has just opened many doors for me. I am now a partner in business in a medical clinic in Michigan."
- "I was elected to the board of directors of the National Network of Health Career Programs in Two-Year Colleges."

- "I have joined the chamber of commerce."
- "I am no longer intimidated to speak to legislators and insurance companies to fight for what is right!"
- "I am enrolling in credit courses in leadership in nonprofit organizations."
- "I have joined the American Society of Association Executives."
- "Now that I am on the editorial board of our journal, I may be able to influence the journal to begin to include articles on leadership."
- "I am applying the skills I gained from CAHL in my current position."
- "I have found CAHL to be a wonderful experience and sing its praises wherever I go."
- "I have been appointed to the Nuclear Medicine Technology Certification Board."
- "I have established professional links with other health educators that I might not have without the CAHL experience."
- "I am running for a position as a member of the Society of Nuclear Medicine Executive Board."
- "I have become a formal member of our grassroots network for the American Society of Radiologic Technologists. Our combined efforts have resulted in the successful introduction of the Consumer Assurance of Radiologic Excellence (CARE) Act by Congressman Rick Lazio."
- "I am planning a trip to Capitol Hill to support the CARE Act."
- "I am now serving on my association's Government Relations Committee."
- "I was elected secretary of the American Art Therapy Association."
- "I successfully completed my PhD."
- "I was hired for a full-time faculty position."
- "I entered a PhD program in education and just completed twenty-one credits."
- "I was elected vice president of internal affairs for the American Association for Respiratory Care."
- "I was voted in as vice president for external affairs and appointed representative for the Health Professions Network for the American Association for Respiratory Care."
- "I have been asked to mentor a new author on adapting her 200-page college thesis to a format for journal submission."
- "I was appointed to the editorial board of the *Journal of Diagnostic Medical Sonography.*"
- "I believe I have a responsibility to accept the reins of leadership as an ongoing commitment to CAHL."

## Collaboration of the Associations (HPN, NN2, ASAHP)

Leadership growth has also been displayed by the three organizations that have partnered to plan and facilitate the CAHL. Although each organization desired a leadership program for its respective membership, the vision for each program varied considerably from that of other organizations. Through collaboration to manage the grant from the Bureau of Health Professions, and collaboration to design and conduct the CAHL program, new relationships among the three organizations have developed. Shared resources and meeting planning are evidence that collaboration has been a powerful return on investment.

# RECOMMENDATIONS FOR STUDENTS OF ALLIED HEALTH

### Value of Collaboration Across Disciplines: The Need for Awareness

When collaboration on issues of common interest brings health professionals from different disciplines together, the resulting common knowledge of their mutual needs, concerns, and fears builds confidence and interest in working together. Even when the short-term outcomes are small, the long-term benefits of realizing opportunities to share resources becomes a powerful force. Changes in health care have begun to take a toll on professional associations, from membership declines to diminishing volunteerism and declining financial reserves. How will these professional associations continue to serve their constituents and communities?

Associations are beginning to see they can share annual meeting venues, exhibition space, and costs. Some allied health educational programs are exploring ways to combine educational resources in new ways. When professionals, educators, and administrators have a mutual understanding of one another's needs and strengths, further collaboration becomes a reality. The CAHL seeks to ensure that future leaders of allied health professional associations enter their leadership roles equipped with the perspective that collaboration with other associations and disciplines opens new avenues of success for the future of their professions and for the improvement of quality in U.S. health care.

- Students of allied health education programs should take the initiative to seek out other disciplines and collaborate in education, practice, community outreach, improving patient care, health care advocacy, patient safety, and leadership development.

### Value of Association Outreach

In times of greatest challenge from diminishing resources, allied health professional associations often become introspective and cut off their outreach activities. Future association leaders should be prepared with a more global knowledge of potential opportunities and resources that enable them to make tough leadership decisions and balance the internal and external needs of their membership. Outreach can enable allied health associations to become part of collective efforts to improve the health of the nation.

- Students of allied health education programs should participate in their own professional associations. Students should influence their associations to develop leadership among members and reach out to other disciplines to improve the health of the nation.

### Value of Expansion of Knowledge in Leadership Development

The need for leadership development is everywhere in health care. Each professional in the workforce and in education programs is a leader of something. Enhanced leadership skills benefit our relationships with others, enhance our value to our professions and to our employers, and enable our contributions to improve the health of the nation.

- Students of allied health education programs should develop their own leadership skills. Students should develop a vision of the future and strategies to get there, energize people to overcome barriers, challenge the status quo, and inspire innovation.

### SUMMARY

Leadership skills are needed everywhere in health care today. The challenges we face in the delivery of affordable health care for the entire nation will touch every health profession, health system, and U.S. citizen. If we are to increase access to affordable, safe health care for all citizens, health professionals with leadership skills are needed. The capacity for substantive change and the energy and enthusiasm to create change must come from leadership.

Leadership development is needed for individual allied health professionals, for leaders of allied health professional associations, and for educators in allied health. Opportunities for development are being successfully provided by the Coalition for Allied Health Leadership. Allied Health professionals who have engaged in leadership development through CAHL have reported job advancements, greater job satisfaction, and greater interest in active participation in advanced education and professional associations. Students of allied health education programs should be aware that leadership is a learned skill and that leadership in health care will be in demand in coming years.

## REFERENCES

Bennis, W. (1994). *On Becoming a Leader*. Reading, MA: Addison-Wesley Publishing Company.

Council on Graduate Medical Education and National Advisory Council on Nurse Education and Practice (2000). *Collaborative Education to Ensure Patient Safety*. Rockville, MD: U.S. Department of Health and Human Services, Health Resources and Services Administration, Bureau of Health Professions, Division of Nursing, Division of Medicine and Dentistry.

Drucker, P. (1997). "Shared Leadership in the New Workplace: Thriving on True Teamwork." Presented at the second annual conference on Worldwide Lessons in Leadership Series, October 23-24.

Headrick, L.A. (2000). "Learning to Improve Complex Systems of Care." *Collaborative Education to Ensure Patient Safety*. Rockville, MD: U.S. Department of Health and Human Services, Health Resources and Services Administration, Bureau of Health Professions, Division of Nursing, Division of Medicine and Dentistry.

Institute of Medicine, Committee on Quality (1999). *To Err Is Human: Building a Safer Health System*. Washington, DC: National Academy Press.

Jaklevic, M.C. (2000). "Wanted: A Few Good Leaders." *Modern Healthcare*, October 2, 38-40.

Kotter, J.P. (1990). *A Force for Change: How Leadership Differs from Management*. New York: The Free Press.

Leape, L., Kabcenell, A.I., Gandhi, T.K., Carver, P., Nolan, T.W., Berwick, D.M. (2000). Reducing Adverse Drug Events: Lessons from a Breakthrough Collaborative. *The Joint Commission Journal on Quality Improvement*, 26:321-331.

Lovern, E. (2001). "Tough Love for Healthcare Executives." *Modern Healthcare*, February 26, p. 38.

Pew Health Professions Commission (1991). *Healthy America: Practitioners for 2005: An Agenda for Action for United States Health Professional Schools*. Durham, NC: HRSA.

Pew Health Professions Commission (1993). *Schools in Service to the Nation*. San Francisco, CA: HRSA.

Ruzek, J.Y., Bloor, L.E., Andersonm J.L., Ngom M., and the University of California at San Francisco Center for the Health Professions (1999). *The Hidden Health Care Workforce: Recognizing, Understanding and Improving the Allied and Auxiliary Workforce.* San Francisco, CA: UCSF Center for the Health Professions.

Sherman, V.C. (1999). *Raising Standards in American Healthcare: Best Practices, Best People, Best Results.* San Francisco: Jossey-Bass.

U.S. Department of Health and Human Services (USDHHS) (1995). *Report of the National Commission on Allied Health.* Rockville, MD: U.S. Department of Health and Human Services, Public Health Service, Health Resources and Services Administration, Bureau of Health Professions, Division of Associated, Dental, and Public Health Professions.

U.S. Department of Health and Human Services (USDHHS) (1999). *Building the Future of Allied Health: Report of the Implementation Task Force of the National Commission on Allied Health.* Rockville, MD: U.S. Department of Health and Human Services, Public Health Service, Health Resources and Services Administration, Bureau of Health Professions, Division of Associated, Dental, and Public Health Professions.

Chapter 19

# Employment Opportunities in Allied Health

Peggy Valentine
Pedro J. Lecca

## *INTRODUCTION*

Health services is one of the largest industries in the United States, and the future outlook is very promising. There are an estimated 11 million jobs in the health field, with a projected 26 percent increase through 2008. This industry is expected to grow due to an aging population and new technologies that are widely available. More allied health professionals will be needed to fill employment positions.

A recent dilemma in allied health is the decline in enrollment for many programs, despite robust job openings. For example, clinical laboratory science projects a need for 9,000 technologists each year through 2008, yet there are only 5,000 of these professionals produced annually. This creates a shortfall of 4,000 professionals. Another dilemma is the aging of allied health professionals. Many are approaching retirement age, which will create further shortages in the allied health professions.

It is estimated that 40 million Americans will be over the age of sixty-five in 2010. By 2030, this number of elders is expected to grow to 66 million as baby boomers born between 1946 and 1964 reach retirement age. There will be a greater need for more home health care, nursing, and personal care. By 2008, the need for medical assistants is projected to increase by 58 percent and the need for physician assistants by 48 percent. The demand for dental care will increase as more middle-aged and older persons retain their natural teeth.

## *PREPARING FOR CAREERS IN A HIGH-TECH AGE*

More allied health professionals will be needed in high tech positions. We are living in a time of major advances in medical technology. Many of these technologies are being used in hospitals, physicians' offices, and ambulatory care centers. The demand for all types of diagnostic imaging is now at the forefront of medicine, and cross-trained imaging technologists are in great demand. Diseases are being diagnosed and treated earlier and more people are using technologies such as total body scanning as prevention tools. There is also a high demand for information technology to improve care and efficiency. Telemedicine, picture archiving, and communications systems demands will increase. Palm Pilots or handheld computers, for example, are an efficient way of reducing record-keeping errors and reducing paper waste. Using these devices, notes and vital signs are recorded and later transferred to a main database. This is important because health information is increasingly processed by computers and transmitted by communications technology.

In addition to having good computer skills, allied health professionals need to know about health informatics, which is the application of computer and information sciences. Health informatics encompasses mathematics, statistics, and computing, and applies engineering, management, and information sciences to problems arising in biology, medicine, and the delivery of health care. This technology is useful to health care professionals, hospital administrators, and government planners, and the collected data is used to make effective health care decisions.

Smart cards, which resemble credit cards, are also being used to store large amounts of patient information. This technology allows patients to keep their medical records with them, thereby promoting efficiency and reducing errors by health workers.

Continued advances in medical technology will also improve the quality of life for persons with chronic disabilities and improve the survival rate of severely ill and injured patients. Advances in gene therapy are improving cancer treatment, and less-invasive surgical techniques are speeding recovery time.

### Staying Abreast of Changes in Health Care

Allied health professionals will need to remain current in their discipline and stay abreast of changes in the health care field that may affect future employment. Health services, for example, will continue to emphasize a shift from inpatient to less expensive outpatient care. Since the early 1990s, numerous hospitals have merged or been reduced (Ruzek et al., 1999). Health networks will continue to become larger as a result of mergers, adding to the complexity of these organizations. More health managers and support personnel will be needed to manage these organizations, and specialized clinical training in health services will serve as an asset for these administrative jobs.

## WHERE ARE THE JOBS?

More than 469,000 organizations make up the health services industry. The majority of jobs are in the private sector (92 percent). Most of these are in offices of physicians, dentists, and other health practitioners. Although hospitals make up only 2 percent of health services organizations, they employ approximately 40 percent of all health workers (Bureau of Labor Statistics, 2002).

Eight segments of the health services industry hire health workers:

*Hospitals* provide complete health care, including diagnostic services, surgery, inpatient and outpatient care, emergency care, and continuous nursing care. They employ workers at all levels of education and training. An estimated 25 percent of hospital employees are registered nurses, and about 20 percent are service occupations. Hospitals also employ physicians, physician assistants, therapists, social workers, a large number of technicians, and administrative support workers.

*Nursing and personal care facilities* provide inpatient nursing, rehabilitation, and health-related personal care to individuals who need continuous health care but do not require hospitalization. These facilities include nursing homes, assisted living facilities, and convalescent homes. Most employees are nursing aides and other service occupations. Allied health professionals are often hired through contractual arrangements to provide rehabilitation and other services.

*Offices and clinics of physicians and osteopaths* include freestanding clinics, emergency care centers, ambulatory surgical centers, group practices, and more. These practice settings utilize many health professionals, including medical technologists, therapists, physician assistants, nutritionists, nurses, health managers, and others. Physicians are more likely to work as salaried employees of these facilities now than in the past.

*Home health care services* involve skilled nursing or medical care often provided in the home under physician supervision. This is one of the fastest-growing health care industries in the United States. Recipients of this care include the elderly, chronically ill, terminally ill, and others. The home health setting employs a host of health professionals to deliver respiratory care for persons with chronic lung disease, intravenous transfusions for cancer treatment, rehabilitation services for stroke patients, and more. Physicians, physician assistants, or nurse practitioners make house calls for follow-up care.

*Offices and clinics of dentists* provide general or specialized dental care and dental surgery. These practices often employ dentists, dental hygienists, dental assistants, and support staff. It is estimated that one out of every four health facilities is a dentist's office. Major advancements in the dental field over the past twenty years have led to improved retention of natural teeth and improved oral health well into old age.

*Offices and clinics of other health practitioners* include a variety of professionals who deliver specialized services, including rehabilitation, complementary health care, nutritional counseling, etc. Types of providers include chiropractors, optometrists, podiatrists, occupational and physical therapists, psychologists, audiologists, dietitians, acupuncturists, hypnotists, and naturopaths. The demand for these services has increased through public awareness of these professionals. Hospitals and other health facilities may contract these services.

*Other health and allied services* include establishments that provide a variety of outpatient and community-focused services. These include kidney dialysis centers, drug treatment facilities, childbirth preparation classes, and blood banks.

*Medical and dental laboratories* provide services to the medical community or follow a physician's order. Health workers in these settings analyze blood, complete diagnostic imaging studies, and perform electrocardiograms and other clinical tests. Dental workers make dentures, artificial teeth, and other orthodontic appliances.

## *Types of Jobs*

Health services employs workers in professional specialty, service, managerial, administrative support, and technician occupations. Most allied health professionals fall within the professional specialty, technologist/technician, and managerial occupations, and a college degree is usually required.

*Professional specialty* occupations include physicians, registered nurses, social workers, therapists, etc. Examples of allied health professionals are shown in Figure 19.1. These individuals often supervise other workers, provide services, and conduct research. Degree requirements vary, and may range from an associate's to a master's; however, given the high level of responsibility and complex duties of these disciplines, they are considered professional. It should be noted that some of the professional organizations of these disciplines do not consider themselves allied health.

*Service occupations* often require little or no specialized education or training and include nursing and psychiatric aides, dental and medical assistants, and personal care and home health aides. Service workers may advance to higher-level positions with experience, further training, and education.

## Health Diagnosis and Treatment Professionals

Audiologists
Dietitians and Nutritionists
*Occupational Therapists
Optometrists
*Physical Therapists

*Physician Assistants
Radiation Therapists
Recreational Therapists
Speech-Language Pathologists
Other Therapists, Naturopaths

## Other Professionals and Technicians

Anesthesiology Assistants
Art Therapists
Audiometrists
Athletic Trainers
Cardivascular Technologists
  and Technicians
Clinical Laboratory Scientists
Cytogenetic Technologists
Dental Hygenists
Dental Laboratory Technicians
Diagnositc Medical Sonographers
Electroneurodiagnostic Technicians
EMTs and Paramedics
Genetic Counselors
Health Information Technicians
Kinesiotherapists
Low Vision Therapists

Medical and Clinical Laboratory
  Technologists
Medical Transcriptionists
Medical Records and Health
  Information Technologists
Music Therapists
Nuclear Medicine Technologists
Orthopists
Orthotists/Prosthetists
Perfusionists
Pharmacy Technicians
Psychiatric Technicians
Radiologic Technologists
  and Technicians
Respiratory Therapy Technicians
Sonographers
Surgical Technologists/Technicians

## Mental and Behavioral Professionals

Community Counselor
Family Counselor
Mental Health Counselors

Social Workers
Substance Abuse Counselors

*These professions may not self-identify as allied health.

FIGURE 19.1. Examples of Allied Health Professions. *Source:* Adapted from Bureau of Labor Statistics (2001).

*Technicians* and related support occupations are among the fastest-growing health occupations and include health information technicians and dental hygienists. These individuals operate technical equipment and assist health practitioners. Formal training is required and may range from one to three years after high school but less than four years of college.

*Health managers* often have a clinical specialty or training in health services administration, or they may have a general business education. Formal education often requires a minimum of a baccalaureate degree, although a master's degree is usually preferred. These individuals keep organizations running smoothly.

## Other Opportunities

Most allied health careers provide opportunities for clinical practice, research, leadership, and education. In clinical practice, the allied health professional applies knowledge and skills gained for health care delivery.

The allied health field is advanced through research. New knowledge that is acquired through research may improve health care outcomes for clinical practice. Research opportunities are available with pharmaceutical companies, governmental agencies such as the National Institutes of Health, and other agencies.

Allied health leaders work in a variety of positions including educational program directors, department heads, deans, presidents of national organizations, and administrators of clinical units. Leadership development often begins through professional affiliation at the local chapter level. Opportunities exist for health professionals to serve as elected officers or committee chairpersons. Through continued professional development and experience, one may prepare for higher leadership positions in education, work settings, or professional organizations.

In educational settings, allied health professionals may serve as faculty members and educate new generations of students. In these positions as faculty, expected duties include teaching, research, and service. Teaching may be provided to discipline specific allied health students and students enrolled in other programs. To be promoted as an educator, faculty members must also conduct research, publish papers, and present their work at professional meetings. Service to the college and profession is another expectation for advancement.

## Working Conditions

Many health service facilities, such as hospitals and nursing personal care facilities, operate around the clock. Health workers in these settings often work in shifts when they are needed at all hours. Shift workers commonly include nursing personnel, physician assistants, medical technologists, and diagnostic imaging technologists.

It is estimated that a large portion of the health workforce averages thirty-three hours worked per week. More than 15 to 20 percent of the health care workforce is employed on a part-time basis. Many of these part-time workers include students, parents with young children, older employees, and individuals holding dual jobs.

Health workers involved in direct patient care must take precautions to prevent back injuries from lifting patients and equipment, exposure to radiation and chemicals, and infectious diseases such as HIV, tuberculosis, and hepatitis.

## *MAXIMIZING THE UNDERGRADUATE EDUCATIONAL EXPERIENCES FOR FUTURE EMPLOYMENT*

Most allied health programs are undergraduate in nature and offer baccalaureate degrees. The educational program often provides two years of prerequisite courses in English, mathematics, science, humanities, and an additional two years of discipline-related course content. At the community college level, allied health programs are usually two years in length, with fewer prerequisite courses and greater concentration in the specific discipline.

In preparing for an allied health career, students can enhance their educational experiences by acquiring additional skills that would give them the edge over others with similar training.

### *Shadow a Professional*

Most allied health careers provide employment opportunities in a variety of settings. These include hospitals, clinics, physician offices, and community-based organizations. Students can use their educational experience to meet as many types of providers in their discipline as possible. Students can learn about providers' backgrounds, job duties and functions, emerging roles, and any need for cross-training in a specific area. Weekends, evenings, and holiday breaks are good opportunities to gain these experiences. It is often wise to communicate and acquire clearance from school personnel before shadowing a professional in a work setting for insurance liability purposes.

### *Gain As Many Experiences As Possible*

Acquire as many different learning experiences as possible. Clinical rotations or internships are a great way to gain a variety of learning experiences in rural, urban, or inner-city settings. Learn as much as you can about different cultures and ethnic groups. Volunteering at a homeless shelter, soup kitchen, Native American reservation, and other settings provide life-long memories and sensitivities for working with underserved populations. Some schools offer study-abroad opportunities through which students can complete a semester or academic year in another country. These experiences make for an impressive résumé.

### *Acquire Leadership Skills*

Numerous leadership opportunities exist for students. On most college campuses, there are student governments and organizations. Most educational programs provide opportunities for students to elect class officers. There are also opportunities for students to gain leadership skills by organizing events such as clothing drives for the homeless, tutoring at the local boys and girls club, or hosting a fund-raising event for students to attend a professional organization's conference.

## MAXIMIZING THE GRADUATE EDUCATIONAL EXPERIENCES FOR FUTURE EMPLOYMENT

The standard for a number of allied health programs is increasing. Physical therapy, occupational therapy, speech and audiology, for example, now require graduate degrees. More than 40 percent of physician assistant programs now offer master's degrees. Other allied health professionals may return to college for graduate degrees to enhance employment opportunities and skills. For example, to become a faculty member at a college or university, a graduate degree is often required. Numerous opportunities exist for graduate students to contribute to their profession through research and publications. The educational experience affords the opportunity for students to work alongside faculty experts in the field and to receive guidance for future career endeavors.

### *Acquire Skills in Research and Writing for Publication*

Most graduate programs require students to complete a research project. This may range from an empirical research project to a clinical literature review article. Students can use this opportunity to develop a special research interest and contribute to allied health literature for years to come. As a student, there is access to professors with expertise in a given area who are usually pleased to provide guidance to young researchers and budding authors.

## *Research/Teaching Assistant Opportunities to Work with Faculty Experts*

As a graduate student, there are often opportunities to apply for research and teaching assistantships. These student jobs provide needed funds for living, and they also provide unique opportunities to work with a professor. As a research assistant, students may gain experience in conducting literature reviews, writing first drafts of papers, preparing presentation materials for a professional meeting, and editing articles. On some occasions, graduate assistants may be listed as secondary authors on a publication. As a teaching assistant, students may also gain experience in course management. This may include updating lecture materials, preparing educational materials for lecture, maintaining a student database of attendance and performance, and participating in learning exercises. These experiences constitute work experience and may be viewed favorably by potential employers.

## *SUMMARY*

Allied health professionals are in great demand, with shortages projected to the year 2008. Shortages have resulted primarily from an increasing elderly population, declining enrollment for some allied health programs, and advances in health care technology. Allied health professionals will need to be technologically savvy during this high-tech age.

Most allied health professionals fall within professional specialty, technologist/technician, and managerial categories, and college degrees are usually required. These professionals work in all eight sectors of the health care industry, with the largest concentration in hospitals, offices, and clinics of physicians and other health professionals.

Most allied health careers provide opportunities for clinical practice in which professional knowledge and skills are applied to safe and effective patient care, research to advance professional knowledge, leadership to effect health care policy, and education to promote development of the next generation of allied health professionals. The undergraduate and graduate educational experiences of allied health students provide ample opportunities for future professionals to prepare for unique career opportunities.

## REFERENCES

Bureau of Labor Statistics (2001). Occupational Employment Projections to 2010. *Monthly Labor Review 124*(11):57-84.

Bureau of Labor Statistics (2002). *Occupational Outlook Handbook, 2002-03 Edition.* Available from the World Wide Web: <http://www.bls.gov>.

Ruzek, J.Y., Bloor, L.E., Anderson, J.L., Ngo, M., and the University of California at San Francisco Center for the Health Professions (UCSFCHP) (1999). *The Hidden Health Care Workforce: Recognizing, Understanding, and Improving the Allied and Auxiliary Workforce.* San Francisco, CA: UCSFCHP.

# Conclusion and Recommendations

In reflecting on the content in this book, it is obvious that allied health has become a major contributor to health care in America. The field is continuing to advance as new technologies and a changing health care environment are creating new and emerging roles for these professionals. Although these accomplishments can be celebrated, a number of issues presented in this book should be addressed concerning allied health education and practice.

The first issue is the need to develop a common understanding of allied health. As indicated in Chapter 1, allied health is not well defined. Many definitions have been given and each has its limitation. Some agencies have linked allied health as one profession when in fact it constitutes a number of professions. As each discipline has its own regulatory agency, there are different rules concerning accreditation, practice, and education requirements. It is clear that allied health professions have evolved into a major provider of health services in the United States. As Harry E. Douglas III points out in Chapter 1, "the collective voice of allied health has not maximized its influence in the health policy and educational arenas." Allied health professions need to come together to define themselves. This is an important agenda for the twenty-first century, and the definition should be communicated to all health care professions, providers, and clients.

Another issue for allied health professionals is access to health care services. Americans are living longer, and the aging baby boomer population presents significant challenges for the health care system. As Richard E. Oliver and Stephen L. Wilson point out in Chapter 10, "A greater incidence of health problems and greater need for assistance are an inherent part of the aging process." Allied health professionals will have to be more than technically prepared to serve an older population. They will have to be particularly sensitive to the aging process and demonstrate a professional attitude in delivering care.

Health care access is a continuing issue for ethnically diverse populations. The United States has become more ethnically diverse than ever before. By 2030, ethnic minorities, when combined, are expected to constitute the majority. All health care systems will be responsible for providing accessible, sensitive care. As Cheryl T. Samuels indicates in Chapter 12, allied health educational programs will need to include cultural sensitivity in clinical practice in the curriculum so that quality health care is enhanced for those with individual and cultural differences. These changes in diversity will also affect the allied health provider population, and more attention should be given to recruiting and retaining an ethnically diverse student body for future professional roles. Currently, people of color constitute nearly 30 percent of the U.S. population, yet they represent less than 10 percent of the allied health population.

Another access to health care issue is lack of insurance. About 44 million Americans are currently uninsured, and approximately 60 percent of those individuals live in families with incomes below the federal poverty level. Given immigration and an increasing trend of part-time employment without health benefits, it is expected that the number of uninsured will continue to rise over the next decade.

A great challenge in allied health education is ensuring the curriculum addresses core knowledge of specific disciplines while staying abreast of new and emerging issues. By their very nature, allied health professionals play critical roles in primary health care, rehabilitation, and diagnostic services. As John Echternach points out in Chapter 4, allied health professionals are part of the health care team, regardless of work environment. Rarely does an individual with a serious disease or injury receive care from only one individual.

As educational institutions address core knowledge issues in the curriculum and build on the team approach to learning, there are additional challenges of meeting learner needs for flexible program schedules. Distance learning is becoming more popular in allied health education and some programs are completely online. To remain competitive, educational programs are challenged to provide a variety of teaching and learning methods to meet the demands of its technologically savvy constituents.

It is also clear the federal government has played a major role in supporting allied health education and curricular innovation, as stated by Norman L. Clark in Chapter 2. The federal government has supported distance-based learning programs in academic health centers and community colleges where new technologies are being used to deliver education material to learners at distance sites. These programs are addressing the isolation barriers of many underserved and rural areas, as well as the lack of human resources and the inability of practitioners to work face to face in many instances.

This book also highlighted new content that should be included in the curriculum. Such information as complementary health care is of great interest to the general public. As Barbara F. Harland points out in Chapter 6, many people are seeking complementary medicines for contributions to youthfulness, body building, and sexual enhancement. These products (both efficacious and harmful) are strongly advertised and readily available via the media and Internet. Some of these products are considered risky because of possible unintended drug interactions and contamination. Allied health professionals need to stay abreast of these products in order to provide sound advice to the general public.

Other hot topics for the allied health curriculum include the human genome and bioterrorism. As highlighted by Thomas W. Elwood in Chapter 13, information on the human genome sequence and proteomics is likely to change medicine in the area of reproductive health and permit health professionals to make diagnoses in earlier stages. The allied health professions have already seen the value of adding this information to the curricula for a number of health disciplines.

After the events of September 11, 2001, bioterrorism has become a topic for inclusion in many allied health curricula, specifically for clinical laboratory science, respiratory therapy, and physician assistant programs. Equally important, all students in the health sciences can benefit by training to assist others during disasters. As K. Habib Khan indicates in Chapter 8, active listening skills, and empathy are crucial as well as other communication skills. Patients expect a lot from health care professionals and to be effective in their work health care professionals need to understand their strengths and weaknesses. Allied health professionals are not super humans and at times they might need therapy.

As educational programs work to maintain a vibrant curriculum they are further challenged by the accreditation process. As John E. Trufant points out in Chapter 11, there is a lack of agreement on the purpose(s) of accreditation and a lack of coordination across and within agencies. Most schools of allied health are accredited by multiple agencies; a few may have as many as fifteen to twenty allied health programs that are accredited by separate agencies. This is a very expensive and time-consuming process. Some allied health deans are in favor of school accreditation rather than program accreditation.

A unique challenge for educational programs has been maintaining a steady enrollment during changes in the health care environment. In the early 1990s, allied health enrollment peaked across the nation. With changes in health care, specifically managed care, allied health enrollment began to drop in the late 1990s and some programs have since closed. Physical therapy, occupational therapy, and other occupations experienced major job cuts in the health sector, and enrollment sharply declined in a number of allied health schools. Now, there are job shortages for these and other allied health professionals. It is estimated by the year 2008, job shortages will be experienced in all allied health professions.

A number of other reasons have been cited for the decline in allied health enrollment, including challenging curricula with high science requirements, lack of recognition by some professions, and misinformation about employment opportunities. As fewer students enter allied health programs and current professionals reach retirement age, job shortages will become more severe. In clinical laboratory science, for example, there will be 9,000 job openings per year with only 5,000 new graduates per year. This will create a national problem for many hospitals. In addressing this crisis, professional organizations have begun to work with schools of allied health on student recruitment issues and marketing of these exciting yet not-well-known educational programs.

We must work to replenish the workforce by informing young people about the range of opportunities within allied health professions. We must work to renew the workplace by developing new prototypes and collaborative models that encourage teamwork, and by providing support for new and experienced providers. Educational institutions must work with the health care industry to retain health care staff. We must work with one another to improve our image and practice of health care in this complex era of change.

The retention of allied health professionals for clinical practice is crucial. As health practice moves away from hospitals and toward community-based organizations, which focus on primary, secondary, and tertiary care, more allied health professionals will be needed as acknowledged by Ivan Quervalu in Chapter 9.

The increased use of technology is another practice issue of importance. As Elzar Camper Jr., Amani M. Nuru-Jeter, and Carole I. Smith point out in Chapter 15, technology permeates all aspects of the allied health industry. Technology influences education, research, analysis, diagnosis, and treatment. In turn these processes will impact information technology, clinic, product development, health care management and administration, biomedical innovations, and the design of instruments and facilities. Familiarity with a wide range of existing and emerging technological applications is essential for those who are preparing to either enter the allied health field or are continuing their education to supplement their skills.

As each of the allied health professions evolve, there has been a growing awareness of the importance of research and scholarship. As Kevin J. Lyons states in Chapter 17, "the types of research being conducted by allied health researchers is diverse and cuts across many fields and areas of interest." In order to advance allied health research, each of the disciplines will need to consider their priorities and their preparation of students and graduates as future contributors to the literature. Allied health professionals in the future will be responsible for developing skills needed to become proficient in research in order to advance the knowledge base of their profession and contribute to the health care system.

Another important role for allied health professionals to play in advancing their professions is dispensing information to policymakers. According to Elwood in Chapter 16, in order to be effective, allied health professionals need a keen understanding of how policy decisions are made. The federal government plays a substantial role in providing many of these components. It is involved in collecting and disseminating information, educating and training personnel directly and providing financial support to them, operating health care institutions, furnishing other direct health services, and participating in financing, supporting, and carrying out research, planning, evaluation, and regulatory functions. Nongovernmental agencies have an important role to play as well. Professional organizations such as the Association of Schools of Allied Health Professions (ASAHP) have members who serve on government advisory committees and evaluate funding proposals through peer-review activities, and have staff who carry out federally funded projects to advance the objectives of the U.S. Public Health Service and other government agencies. The National Society of Allied Health also has members who serve on national task forces to effect policy development for the improvement of access to health care in communities of color.

Another issue of importance is the need for leadership development in allied health education and clinical practice. As Gail A. Nielsen points out in Chapter 18, "students of allied health education programs should be aware that leadership is a learned skill and that leadership in health care will be in demand in coming years." The Coalition for Allied Health Leadership has prepared a number of educators and practicing allied health professionals for leadership roles. Participants in this program have reported job advancements, improved job satisfaction, and greater participation in professional associations.

To advance the allied health agenda, there must be greater collaboration among the professional associations, schools, the health care industry, and policymakers to address the issues we have presented in this book. Concerted efforts must be directed to forge greater recognition of allied health among the general public. Allied health professionals have been major contributors to quality health care in this nation, and they will continue to play a key role in health care throughout the twenty-first century.

# Appendix

# Allied Health Organizations and Affiliates

**Accreditation Review Committee for the Education of Anesthesiologist Assistants**
2941 Country Club Drive
Pueblo, CO 81008
Phone: 719/545-4668
Fax: 719/545-4668

**Accrediting Commission for Education in Health Services Administration (ACEHSA)**
Accreditation Operations
730 11th Street, NW, Suite 400
Washington, DC 20001
Phone: 202/638-5131
Fax: 202/638-3429

**Alliance for Cardiovascular Professionals**
Member Services Director
910 Charles Street
Fredericksburg, VA 22401
Phone: 540/370-0102
Fax: 540/370-0015
<http://www.acp-online.org>

**Alliance for Cardiovascular Professionals**
4456 Corporation Lane, #120
Virginia Beach, VA 23462
Phone: 757/497-1225
Fax: 757/497-0010

**American Academy of Anesthesiologist Assistants (AAAA)**
University Hospitals of Cleveland
Department of Anesthesiology

11100 Euclid Avenue
Cleveland, OH 44106
Phone: 216/844-7318
Fax: 216/844-3781
<http://www.anesthetist.org>

### American Academy of Anesthesiologist Assistants (AAAA)
P.O. Box 13978
Tallahassee, FL 32317
Phone: 850/656-8848
Fax: 850/656-3038
<http://www.anesthetist.org>

### American Academy of Anesthesiologist Assistants (AAAA) (Organization Address)
P.O. Box 81362
Wellesley, MA 02181-0004
Phone: 800/757-5858
Fax: 617/239-3259

### American Academy of Physician Assistants
Executive Vice President
950 North Washington Street
Alexandria, VA 22314
Phone: 703/836-2272
Fax: 703/684-1924
<http://www.aapa.org>

### American Art Therapy Association (National Office)
1202 Allanson Road
Mundelein, IL 60060-3808
Phone: 888/290-0878
Fax: 847/566-4580
<http://www.arttherapy.org>

### American Art Therapy Association
8020 Briar Summit Drive
Los Angeles, CA 90046
Phone: 323/650-5934

### American Art Therapy Association/National Coalition of Arts Therapies Association
Mount Mary College
2900 N. Menomonee River Parkway

Milwaukee, WI 53222
Phone: 414/258-4810

**American Association of Bioanalysts (AAB)**
918 Locust, Suite 1100
St. Louis, MO 63101
Phone: 314/241-1445
Fax: 314/241-1449
<http://www.aab.org>

**American Association of Bioanalysts (AAB)**
   **Associate Member Section (AMS)**
1501 East 10th Street
Atlantic, IA 50022
Phone: 712/243-5402
Fax: 712/243-7553

**American Association of Bioanalysts (AAB)**
10820 Fairview Boulevard, SW
Port Orchard, WA 98376
Phone: 630/874-2677
Fax: 360/895-5540

**American Association of Blood Banks**
CEO
8201 Glenbrook Road
Bethesda, MD 20814-2749
Phone: 301/907-6977
Fax: 301/907-6895
<http://www.aabb.org>

**American Association for Clinical Chemistry**
2101 L Street, NW, Suite 202
Washington, DC 20037
Phone: 202/857-0717 x715
<http://www.aacc.org>

**American Association of Community Colleges (AACC)**
Development
One Dupont Circle, NW, Suite 410
Washington, DC 20036
Phone: 202/728-0200 x228
Fax: 202/833-2467
<http://www.aacc.nche.edu>

**American Association of Electrodiagnostic Technologists**
P.O. Box 79489
North Dartmouth, MA 02747
Phone: 401/846-5446
Fax: 401/846-5826

**American Association of Electrodiagnostic Technologists**
11012 Corundite, NW
Massillion, OH 44647
Phone: 330/543-8397

**American Association of Medical Assistants**
20 North Wacker Drive, Suite 1575
Chicago, IL 60606-2903
Phone: 312/899-1500
Fax: 312/899-1259
<http://www.aama-ntl.org>

**American Association of Medical Dosimetrists**
P.O. Box 1928
Deer Park, WA 99006
Phone: 509/464-5131
Fax: 509/468-2942
<http://www.medicaldosimetry.org>

**American Association of Physicists in Medicine,
   Southwest Chapter (SWAAPM)**
c/o Baylor College of Medicine
Department of Radiology
One Baylor Plaza
Houston, TX 77030
Phone: 713/794-7190
Fax: 713/794-7825

**American Association for Respiratory Care**
11030 Ables Lane
Dallas, TX 75229
Phone: 972/243-2272
Fax: 972/484-2720
<http://www.aarc.org>

**American Association of State Colleges and Universities**
1307 New York Avenue, NW
Fifth Floor
Washington, DC 20005-47041

Phone: 202/293-7070
Fax: 202/296-5819

**American Board of Registration of EEG and EP Technologists**
P.O. Box 916633
Longwood, FL 32791-6633
Phone: 407/678-6308

**American College of Cardiology**
616 Quick Silver Drive
De Soto, TX 75115
Phone/Fax: 972/223-7619

**American College of Healthcare Executives (ACHE)**
One North Franklin, Suite 1700
Chicago, IL 60606-3491
Phone: 312/424-9493
Fax: 312/424-0023

**American Dental Assistants Association**
203 N. La Salle Street, Suite 1320
Chicago, IL 60611
Phone: 312/541-1550
Fax: 312/541-1496
<http://members.aol.com/adaai/index.html>

**American Dental Hygienists Association**
444 North Michigan Avenue, Suite 3400
Chicago, IL 60611
Phone: 312/440-8932
<http://www.adha.org>

**American Dietetic Association**
216 West Jackson Boulevard
Chicago, IL 60606-6995
Phone: 312/899-0040 x4872
Fax: 312/899-4817
<http://www.eatright.org>

**American Health Information Management Association**
919 North Michigan Avenue, Suite 1400
Chicago, IL 60611-1683
Phone: 312/787-2672
Fax: 312/787-5926
<http://www.ahima.org>

**American Healthcare Radiology Administrators (AHRA)**
111 Boston Post Road, Suite 100
Sudbury, MA 01776
Phone: 978/443-7591
Fax: 978/443-8046
<http://www.ahraonline.org>

**American Healthcare Radiology Administrators**
Iowa Health Systems
1200 Pleasant Street
Des Moines, IA 50309-1406
Phone: 515/241-8626
Fax: 515/241-5059

**American Healthcare Radiology Administrators**
Fayetteville Medical Clinic PC
101 Yorktown Drive
Newnan, GA 30214

**American Medical Technologists**
Frances Simpson, President
710 Higgins Road
Park Ridge, IL 60068
Phone: 256/386-1621
Fax: 256/386-1716
E-mail: fkain1@aol.com

**American Music Therapy Association**
8455 Colesville Road, Suite 1000
Silver Spring, MD 20910
Phone: 301/589-3300
Fax: 301/589-5175
<http://www.musictherapy.org>

**American Occupational Therapy Association**
4720 Montgomery Lane
P.O. Box 31220
Bethesda, MD 20824-1220
Phone: 301/652-2682
Fax: 301/652-7711
<http://www.aota.org>

**American Optometric Association**
243 N. Lindburgh Boulevard
St. Louis, MO 65141

Phone: 314/991-4100
Fax: 314/991-4101
<http://www.aoanet.org>

**American Physical Therapy Association**
1111 North Fairfax Street
Alexandria, VA 22314
Phone: 703/684-2782
Fax: 703/706-8519
<http://www.apta.org>

**American Public Health Association**
1015 Fifteenth Street, NW, Suite 300
Washington, DC 20009
Phone: 202/789-5600
<http://www.apha.org>

**American Registry of Radiologic Technologists**
1255 Northland Drive
St. Paul, MN 55120
Phone: 651/687-0048
Fax: 651/687-0349
<http://www.arrt.org>

**American Society for Clinical Laboratory Science**
7910 Woodmont Avenue, Suite 530
Bethesda, MD 20814
Phone: 301/657-2768
Fax: 301/657-2909
<http://www.ascls.org>

**American Society for Clinical Pathology**
2100 West Harrison Street
Chicago, IL 60612-3798
Phone: 312/738-4893
Fax: 312/738-0101

**American Society for Cytotechnology**
1500 Sunday Drive, Suite 102
Raleigh, NC 27607
Phone: 919/787-5181
Fax: 919/787-4916

**American Society of Echocardiography**
1500 Sunday Drive, Suite 102
Raleigh, NC 27607

Phone: 919/787-5181
Fax: 919/787-4916
<http://www.asecho.org>

**American Society of Electroneurodiagnostic Technologists (ASET)**
428 West 42nd Street, Suite B
Kansas City, MO 64111
Phone: 816/931-1120
Fax: 816/931-1145
<http://www.aset.org>

**American Society of Extra-Corporeal Technology National Office**
11480 Sunset Hills Road, Suite 100E
Reston, VA 22090-9955
Phone: 703/435-8556
Fax: 703/435-0056
<http://www.amsect.org>

**American Society for Healthcare Human Resources Administration (ASHHRA)**
One North Franklin
Chicago, IL 60606
Phone: 312/422-3721
Fax: 312/422-4577

**American Society of Radiologic Technolgists (ASRT)**
15000 Central Avenue, SE
Albuquerque, NM 87123-3917
Phone: 505/298-4500 x1258
Fax: 505/298-5063
<http://www.asrt.org>

**American Speech-Language-Hearing Association**
10801 Rockville Pike
Rockville, MD 20852
Phone: 301/897-5700
Fax: 301/571-0469
<http://www.asha.org>

**Association of Academic Health Centers**
1400 16th Street, NW, Suite 720
Washington, DC 20036
Phone: 202/265-9600
Fax: 202/298-5063
<http://www.ahcnet.org>

**Association for Applied Psychophysiology and Biofeedback**
10200 W. 44th Avenue, Suite 304
Wheat Ridge, CO 80033-2840
Phone: 303/422-8436
Fax: 303/422-8894
<http://www.aapb.org>

**Association of Educators in Radiologic Sciences**
P.O. Box 90204
Albuquerque, NM 87199-0204
Phone/Fax: 505/823-4740
<http://www.aers.org>

**Association Management Group**
8201 Greensboro Drive, Suite 300
McLean, VA 22102
Phone: 703/610-9000
Fax: 703/610-9005

**Association of Polysomnographic Technologists**
Sleep Disorders Institute
St. Jude Medical Center
1915 Sunny Crest Drive
Fullerton, CA 92835
Phone: 714/446-7240
Fax: 714/446-7245

**Association of Surgical Technologists**
7108-C South Alton Way
Centenial, CO 80112
Phone: 303/694-9130 x234
Fax: 303/694-9169
<http://www.ast.org>

**Association of University Programs in Health Administration (AUPHA)**
730 11th Street, NW
4th Floor
Washington, DC 20001
Phone: 202/638-1448 x131
Fax: 202/638-3429

**Association of Vascular and Interventional Radiographers**
2021 Spring Road, Suite 600
Oak Brook, IL 60521

Phone: 630/571-2266
Fax: 630/571-7837

**Board of Registered Polysomnographic Technologists**
924 33rd Street, NW
Rochester, MN 55901
Phone: 507/284-6308
Fax: 507/284-7772

**Cerner Corporation**
2800 Rockcreek Parkway
Kansas City, MO 64117-2551
Phone: 816/201-2845
Fax: 816/201-8845

**Citizens Advocacy Center**
1424 16th Street NW, Suite 105
Washington, DC 20036
Phone: 202/462-1174
Fax: 202/265-6564

**Clinical Laboratory Management Association (CLMA)**
989 Old Eagle School Road, Suite 815
Wayne, PA 19087
Phone: 610/995-9580
Fax: 610/995-9568

**Commission on Accreditation of Allied Health Education Programs (CAAHEP)**
35 East Wacker Drive, Suite 1970
Chicago, IL 60601-2208
Phone: 312/553-9355 x24
Fax: 312/553-9616
<http://www.caahep.org>

**Commission on Graduates of Foreign Nursing Schools (CGFNS)**
3600 Market Street, Suite 400
Philadelphia, PA 19104
Phone: 215/222-8454 x226
Fax: 215/662-0425

**Health Resources and Services Administration (HRSA)**
Bureau of Health Professions
Division of State, Community, and Public Health

Allied, Geriatrics, and Rural Health Branch
5600 Fishers Lane
Parklawn Building, Room 8C-09
Rockville, MD 20857
Phone: 301/443-0062
Fax: 301/443-0650

**International Hearing Society**
Washington Council
600 13th Street, NW
Washington, DC 20005
Phone: 202/756-2005
Fax: 202/756-8087
<http://www.ihsinfo.org>

**Joint Commission on the Accreditation of Healthcare Organizations (JCAHO)**
601 13th Street, NW, Suite 1150N
Washington, DC 20005
Phone: 202/783-6655
Fax: 202/783-6888
<http://www.jcaho.org>

**Joint Commission of Allied Health Personnel in Opthalmology, Inc. (JCAHPO)**
2025 Woodlane Drive
Woodbury, MN 55125-2995
Phone: 651/731-2944
Fax: 612/731-0410
<http://www.jcahpo.org>

**Joint Review Committee on Education in Electroneurodiagnostic Technology (JRC/END)**
3350 South 198th Road
Goodson, MO 65659
Phone: 417/253-5810
Fax: 417/253-3059
<http://www.aset.org>

**Joint Review Committee on Education in Nuclear Medicine Technology (JRCNMT)**
PMB #418
2nd Avenue East, Suite C
Polson, MT 59860-2107

Phone: 406/883-0003
Fax: 406/883-0022

**Joint Review Committee on Education in Radiologic Technolgy (JCERT)**
20 North Wacker Drive, Suite 900
Chicago, IL 60606
Phone: 312/704-5300
Fax: 312/704-5304

**Mind Media Institute**
3166 E. Palmdale Boulevard, Suite 214
Palmdale, CA 93550
Phone: 805/947-2534
Fax: 805/947-4127

**National Association of County and City Health Officials**
1100 17th Street, NW, 2nd Floor
Washington, DC 20036-4631
Phone: 202/783-5550 x247
Fax: 202/783-1583
<http://www.naccho.org>

**National Association of Emergency Medical Technicians**
102 W. Leake Street
Clinton, MS 39056
Phone: 601/924-7744
Fax: 601/924-7325
<http://www.naemt.org>

**National Association of Home Care**
228 Seventh Street, SE
Washington, DC 20003-4306
Phone: 202/547-7424
Fax: 202/547-3540
<http://www.nahc.org>

**National Association of Social Workers**
750 First Street, NE, Suite 700
Washington, DC 20002-4241
Phone: 202/408-8600
<http://www.socialworkers.org>

**National Athletic Trainers Association, Inc.**
2952 Stemmons Freeway, Suite 200

Dallas, TX 75247
Phone: 214/637-6282
Fax: 214/637-2206
<http://www.nata.org>

**National Certification Board for Therapeutic Massage and Bodywork**
8201 Greensboro Drive, Suite 300
McLean, VA 22102
Phone: 703/610-9000
Fax: 703/610-9005
<http://www.ncbtmb.org>

**National Coalition of Art Therapy Associations, Inc.**
Route One, Lake of Woods
Bruceton Mills, WV 26525
Phone/Fax (call first): 304/379-3301
<http://www.ncata.com>

**National Consortium on Health Science and Technology Education (NCHSTE)**
2410 Woodlake Drive, Suite 440
Okemas, MI 48864
Phone: 517/347-3332
Fax: 517/347-4096
<http://www.nchste.org>

**National Council of Community Hospitals**
1700 K Street, NW, Suite 906
Washington, DC 20006
Phone: 202/728-0830
Fax: 202/296-7689

**National Health Council, Inc.**
1730 M Street, NW, Suite 500
Washington, DC 20036
Phone: 202/785-3910
Fax: 202/785-5923
<http://www.nhcouncil.org>

**National Network of Health Career Programs in Two-Year Colleges (NN2)**
Greenville Technical College
P.O. Box 5616
Greenville, SC 29606-5616

Phone: 864/250-8263
Fax: 864/250-8462
<http://www.nn2.org>

**National Skills Standards Board**
Healthcare Industry Consultant
1441 L Street, NW, Suite 9000
Washington, DC 20005

**National Society of Allied Health**
13603 Waterfowl Way
Upper Marlboro, MD 20774
Phone: 301/390-5652
<http://www.nsah.org>

**National Society for Histotechnology**
4201 North View Drive, Suite 502
Bowie, MD 20716-2604
Phone: 301/262-9188
Fax: 301/262-6221
<http://www.nsh.org>

**North American Society of Pacing and Electrophysiology Council of Allied Health Professionals (NASPE/CAHP)**
Sherman Hospital
Cardiac Arrhythmia Center
935 Center Street
Elgin, IL 60120
Phone: 847/429-8988
Fax: 847/429-8929
<http://www.naspe.org>

**Northeast Association of Allied Health Educators (NAAHE)**
207 Riverview Road
Rexford, NY 12148
Phone: 518/262-3938
Fax: 518/262-5927

**Plexus Consulting Group**
National Skills Standard Board
1620 Eye Street, NW, Suite 900
Washington, DC 20006
Phone: 202/785-8940
Fax: 202/785-8949

## Section for Magnetic Resonance Technologists
2118 Milvia Street, #201
Berkeley, CA 94704
Phone: 510/841-1899
Fax: 510/841-2340
<http://www.ismrm.org>

## Society of Diagnostic Medical Sonography
278 Amfield Court
Gahanna, OH 43230
Phone: 614/475-6511
Fax: 614/471-6905
<http://www.sdms.org>

## Society of Nuclear Medicine
1850 Samuel Morse Drive
Reston, VA 22090-5316
Phone: 703/708-9000 x1241
Fax: 703/708-9015
<http://www.snm.org>

## Society of Vascular Ultrasound
4601 President Drive, Suite 260
Lanham, MD 20706
Phone: 301/459-7550
<http://www.svnet.org>

## SSG Wellness Center
HQ SSG/MSOW (US Air Force)
200 East Moore Drive
MAFB-Gunter Annex, AL 36114
Phone: 334/416-5656
Fax: 334/416-6620

# Index

AARC (American Association for
    Respiratory Care), 11
AARP, 311, 312, 313
AAS (associate in applied science),
    physical therapy, 66
Academic health centers, 180
Acceptance of patient by
    psychotherapists, 143, 152
Access to technology, 273-275, 285,
    286, 291, 295
Accreditation, 187-188, 211-212
    ACOTE, 68
    agencies, 193-195
    allied health education issues,
        197-200
    AMA involvement in, 9
    CAAHEP. *See* Commission on
        Accreditation of Allied Health
        Education Programs
    competition, 205-206
    continuous reporting, 199, 202-203
    costs, 196-197, 208-209
    documentation, 204-205
    Flexner Report, 8
    historical overview, 191-192
    increased value of, 208-209
    innovation, 200, 210-211
    institutional, 15-16, 190-191,
        192-193
    interest groups, 312
    organization of, 192-193
    outcomes standards, 198, 201-202
    predictability, 209-210
    processes, 195-196
    program autonomy versus
        intrusiveness, 199
    public information, 206-207
    purposes of, 15-16, 188-190, 197,
        211
    rating scales, 207-208
    SASHEP, 20-21
    site visits, 195, 198-199, 203-204,
        210

Accreditation *(continued)*
    specialized (programmatic), 15-16,
        190-191, 192-193
    standards, 196, 210
Accreditation Council for Occupational
    Therapy Education (ACOTE),
    68
ACOEM (American College of
    Occupational and
    Environmental Medicine),
    307
ACOTE (Accreditation Council for
    Occupational Therapy
    Education), 68
Action trigger, 302
Active listening skills, 141-142
Acupressure, 166-167
Acupuncture
    Chinese therapy, 3
    medical philosophy, 227, 229
    traditional Oriental medicine, 165,
        166-167
Acute care
    defined, 63
    emergency medicine, 54
    example, 63-64
    integration of services and care, 50
Administrators
    cost-effective measures, 59
    observations on future leaders,
        340-342
    secondary care provider, 48
    technology instruction decisions,
        280
Adolescents as vulnerable populations,
    163
ADRs (adverse drug reactions), 244
Advanced Technology Program (ATP),
    286
Adverse drug reactions (ADRs), 244
Advisory Committee of Education, 21
Affiliations, 76
AFL-CIO, 306

Africa, 2-3
African-American complementary and alternative medicine, 168
Aging. *See* Elderly
Aging population trend, 173-177, 220
AHP (Allied Health Professionals), 341
Alcohol
    CASAC (counselor), 160
    hospital detoxification units, 157
    screening for abuse, 161
    stress and, 150, 153
    wines, 114-116
Alexander technique, 227-228
Allicin, 108
Allied health, defined, 193
Allied Health and Other Disciplines Program, 314
Allied Health Grant Program
    authorization, 39
    funding, 38
    role of government, 33
Allied Health Personnel Training Act of 1966, 19-20, 22
Allied Health Professionals (AHP), 341
Allied Health Round Table Group, 314
*Allied Health Services: Avoiding Crises* (1989), 22-23
*Allium sativum*, 108
Allopathic medicine, 225
Allopathic school graduates (MD), 56
Alternative medicine. *See* Chemical and dietary therapies; Complementary and alternative approaches
AMA. *See* American Medical Association
American Academy of Speech Correction, 70
American Association for Respiratory Care (AARC), 11
American Association of Schools of Allied Health and the National Society of Allied Health, 5
American Board of Ophthalmology, 16
American Cancer Society, 312, 313
American College of Occupational and Environmental Medicine (ACOEM), 307
American College of Physicians Executives, 78

American Hospital Association, 312
American Medical Association (AMA)
    accreditation, 192, 194
    accrediting allied health professions, 9-10
    allied health, defined, 4-5
    certification system, 16
    Committee on Medical Education, 14
    echinacea herbal remedy, 109
    history, 6, 26
    medical education reform, 8
    SASHEP, 21
American Occupational Therapy Association (AOTA)
    ergonomics dispute, 304
    history, 67
    purpose, 68
    specialty certifications, 69
American Physical Therapy Association (APTA), 64-65
American Registry of X-ray Technicians, 14
American Speech Language/Hearing Association (ASHA), 70, 71
American versus Japanese decision making, 95-96
Americans with Disabilities Act, 243
Amgen, 312
Anacin caffeine content, 113
Analytic factors for laboratory tests, 121, 124
Ancient medicine, 1-3
Anesthesiologist assistant, 194
Angelou, Maya, 168
Antioxidants, 105-106
Anxiety screening, 161
AOTA. *See* American Occupational Therapy Association
Aphasics, treatment of, 70
Appel, M., 230
Application process, 40-41
Apprenticeship, 13-14, 359, 361
APTA (American Physical Therapy Association), 64-65
Aqua-Ban caffeine content, 113
Arkman, Dan, 75, 98
Armstrong, W., 220
Art therapy, 194, 228
Arterial blood gases laboratory test, 133

Artificial sweeteners, 111-112
ASAHP. *See* Association of Schools of Allied Health Professions
ASHA (American Speech Language/Hearing Association), 70, 71
"Ask Jeeves" search engine, 283
Assisted living residences, 176
Associate in applied science (AAS), physical therapy, 66
Associated General Contractors of America, 307
Associated Press, 286
Association of Schools of Allied Health Professions (ASAHP)
   administration of Allied Health Personnel Training Act, 19-20
   CAHL development, 343
   collaboration of associations, 348
   interest groups, 312, 313
   members on government advisory committees, 367
   public policy roles, 311
Association of University Programs in Health Administration (AUPHA), 78
Aston-Patterning, 227-228
Asynchronous Transfer Mode (ATM), 286
ATG marker, 239
Athletes, caffeine intake, 113
Athletic trainers, 77, 194
ATM (Asynchronous Transfer Mode), 286
ATP (Advanced Technology Program), 286
AuD (doctor of audiology), 71
Audiology
   CAAHEP accreditation, 195
   education, 71
   educational requirements, 319
   employment statistics, 18
   history, 71
   language pathology and, 69-70
   occupational statistics, 77
AUPHA (Association of University Programs in Health Administration), 78
Authorizing language, 39
Ayurveda, 221, 222, 226

β-sitosterol (SIT), 110
Baby boomers. *See* Elderly
Bacteria, prebiotics and probiotics, 104-105
Bakhtin, Mikhail Mikhailovich, 315
Banda, Chira, 215
Barnard, Marvin, 45, 119
Barr, J. T., 121
Beck's Anxiety Scale, 161
Behavioral services, 156-157, 357
Benchmarking, 91, 97
Bennis, Warren, 138, 335
Benson, Herbert, 228
Benton Foundation poll, 290
Bilingual personnel
   communication skills, 158
   cultural sensitivity, 178-179, 219
   students' backgrounds, 222
Billings, J., 220
Bioenergetics, 228
Biomarkers, 103
Biomolecular medicine, 225
Biotechnomagnetic applications, 165
Bioterrorism, 365
Black Women's Health Study (BWHS), 169
Black World Today, 293
Blood bank tests, 129, 194
Blood pressure control, 105, 106
Board of trustee management responsibilities, 77-79
Bodywork, 227-228, 229
Boston University's Black Women's Health Study (BWHS), 169
Botanical medicine, 225
Brainstorming sessions, 97
Brand, R., 220
Breakeven analysis, 93-94
Breakthrough Collaboratives, 340
Brown, S., 220
Buckingham, R. W., 140
*Building the Future of Allied Health,* 224
Bureau of Health Manpower Education, 19-20
Bureau of Health Professions
   application process, 41
   CAHL grant, 343
   genetics and health professions, 245
   history, 34

Bureau of Health Professions
  *(continued)*
  leadership training, 344
  publishing grant information, 37
  training administration, 35
Bureau of Labor Statistics, 17, 18
Bureaucracy, 81-82
Burlington Northern Santa Fe Railway,
  243
Bush, President George W.
  embryonic stem cell research, 244
  ergonomics law, 300, 310
  interest group influence on policy,
    313
Business plan, strategic planning, 84,
  88-89
Buyouts, 76
BWHS (Black Women's Health Study),
  169


CAA. *See* Complementary and
  alternative approaches; Council
  on Academic Accreditation
CAAHEP. *See* Commission on
  Accreditation of Allied Health
  Education Programs
Cable television, 291, 292-293
Cable Television Consumer Protection
  and Competition Act of 1992,
  291
Caffeine, 112-114, 150, 153
CAGE (alcoholism screening), 161
CAHEA (Committee on Allied Health
  Education and Accreditation),
  192, 194
CAHL. *See* Coalition for Allied Health
  Leadership
CAM (complementary and alternative
  medicine), 221
Camper, Elzar, Jr., 271, 366
Cancer
  breast cancer and nutrition, 106
  case study, 101
Capitol Hill visits, training for, 343-344
CAPTE (Commission on Accreditation
  of Physical Therapy
  Education), 66

Carcinogens
  alcohol, 115
  smoked and blackened foods,
    110-111
Cardiology, 55
Cardiovascular technology, 194
Carotenoids, 105-106
Cartesian dualism, 3
Cartwright, D., 230
CASAC (certified alcohol and
  substance abuse services
  counselor), 160
Case studies
  chemical and dietary therapies, 101
  diagnostic services, 120-121
  distance education, 287, 292-294
  impact of technology on education,
    271-273, 276-279, 292-294
  interdisciplinary behavioral
    approach, 157-160
  Interprofessional Alliance Model,
    263-268
  interprofessional collaborative
    alliance, 253-255
  knowledge and research gaps,
    320-322, 323
  leadership, 333-336
  primary health care, 45-46
  rehabilitative therapy, 61-63
CBC (complete blood count), 125-126,
  133
CCC (certificate of clinical
  competence), 71
CD-R (compact disc read), 282, 285,
  286
CD-ROM (compact disc read-only
  memory), 286
CD-RW (company disc rewrite), 282,
  285, 286
Census (2000)
  population shifts, 172
  racial and ethnic diversity, 216-217
Center for Complementary and
  Alternative Medicine, 221
Center for Creative Instruction, 41
Center for Medicare and Medicaid
  Services (CMS), 311-312
Center for the Health Professions
  (UCSF), 338-339
Central point of reference, 59

Central processing unit (CPU), 286
Centralization structure, 89, 90-91
Certificate of clinical competence
    (CCC), 71
Certification, 16
Certified alcohol and substance abuse
    services counselor (CASAC),
    160
Certified Occupational Therapy
    Assistant (COTA), 68, 69
CES-D (depression screening), 161
CFR (Code of Federal Regulations),
    36-37
Chamber of Commerce of the United
    States of America, 306
Chamomile (tea), 108
Chaparral, 108
CHEA (Council for Higher Education
    Accreditation), 193
Chemical abuse. *See* Substance abuse
Chemical and dietary therapies, 116
    case study, 101
    complementary and alternative
        medicine, 102-104
    dietary supplements. *See* Dietary
        supplements
    food facts, 110-116
Chemistry studies, 126-129, 133
Chemoprotection, 103
Child abuse, reporting of, 165
Children's Health Insurance Program
    (CHIP), 182
Chimpanzee genome, 238
Chinese traditional medicine, 3, 221,
    226
CHIP (Children's Health Insurance
    Program), 182
Chiropractic
    growth of profession, 221
    medical philosophy, 228
    treatment methods, 166
    veterans' benefits, 299
Cholesterol control
    flavonoids, 105, 106
    garlic, 108
    phytosterols, 110
    wine consumption and, 115
Chondroitin sulfate research, 169
Chopra, Deepak, 226
Chronic care, 48, 50

Church pastoral counselors, 165
Clarification by health worker, 143-144
Clark, Norman L., 31, 364
Clarke-Tasker, Veronica A., 119
Client-centered service philosophy, 141
Clinical chemists, 48
Clinical ecology, 225
Clinical laboratory science, 245
Clinical Laboratory Sciences
    Occupational Therapy, 194
Clinical laboratory technologists and
    technicians
    CAAHEP accreditation, 195
    employment statistics, 18
Clinical pathways, defined, 81
Clinton, President William
    ATP funding, 286
    ergonomics law, 300, 305
    genetics issues, 238, 243
    health system overhaul, 139, 176
Cloning, human, 243-244
CMS (Center for Medicare and
    Medicaid Services), 311-312
Coagulation studies, 130, 133
Coalition for Allied Health Leadership
    (CAHL), 341
    collaboration of associations, 348
    experiential model, 343
    goals, 348, 349, 367
    learning model, 344-345
    outcomes, 346-347
    participant experience, 342
    program development, 343
    role-playing and Capitol Hill visits,
        343-344
    skill development, 345
Coalitions, 314
Cocoa, 112
Code of Federal Regulations (CFR),
    36-37
Coffee, 112
COGME (Council on Graduate
    Medical Education), 339-340
COHEHRE (Consortium of Institutes
    of Higher Education in Health
    and Rehabilitation in Europe),
    230
Collaboration, association, 348
Collaborative teamwork, defined, 250
College model of education, 13-15

Collier, Stephen H., 11
Collins, F., 236, 240
Comfrey, 108
Commission on Accreditation of Allied
    Health Education Programs
    (CAAHEP), 9, 27
  accreditation standards, 196
  history, 192
  members, 194
  program accreditation, 77-78
Commission on Accreditation of
    Physical Therapy Education
    (CAPTE), 66
Committee on Allied Health Education
    and Accreditation (CAHEA),
    192, 194
Committee on Medical Education, 14
Committee on the Future of Primary
    Care, 46-47
Committee to Study the Relationships
    of Medicine with Allied
    Health Professions and
    Services, House of Delegates,
    9-10
Communication
  bilingual personnel, 219
  future demand, 354
Communications Act of 1934, 291
Community-based folk care practices,
    167
Community-based health care
  behavioral approaches, 156
  case study, 157-160
  complementary and alternative
    medicine, 165-169
  depression in primary care, 160-161
  focus, 155-156
  health services, 162-165
  hospital behavioral services, 156-157
  referral process, 165
  vulnerable populations, 162-165
Community-based infections, 133
Community-based support systems, 176
Competition, 85
Complementary and alternative
    approaches (CAAs), 102-104,
    165-169, 215. *See also*
    Chemical and dietary therapies
  educational outcomes, 223-224
  trends, 220-222, 364-365

Complementary and alternative
    medicine (CAM), 221
*Complementary and Alternative*
    *Medicine: A Research-Based*
    *Approach*, 221
Complete blood count (CBC), 125-126,
    133
Computer systems analysts, 18
Computers. *See also* Internet;
    Technology, impact on
    education; World Wide Web
  academic and training instruction,
    280-282
  occupational therapists, 69
  ordering laboratory tests, 123
  recording medical information, 278
  specimen record-keeping, 124
  teleconferencing, 169
  transmitting medical information,
    279-280, 354
Congress, role in education. *See also*
    Legislation
  legislation, 35-36
  lobbying, 33-34
  mandated reports, 34-35
  members of Congress, 33
  set-asides, 36
Congressional Research Service, 312
Congressional Review Act (1996), 305,
    307
Consent forms, laboratory test, 124,
    129
Consortium of Institutes of Higher
    Education in Health and
    Rehabilitation in Europe
    (COHEHRE), 230
Constitutional weaknesses, 166
Consumer needs, 85
Consumer organization interest groups,
    312
Content, professional alliance, 260
Continuing care retirement
    communities, 176
Continuity in health care, 47-48
Continuous improvement methods in
    control process, 93
Controlling function, management,
    91-94
Cooper, Ken, 227
Core competencies, 245

Core curriculum, technology, 276-277
Coryban-D caffeine content, 113
Costs
    access to technology, 274-275, 289
    accreditation, 196-197, 208-209
    complementary and alternative
        medicine, 221
    control of, and management, 76
    emphasis on cost-effective care, 322
    ergonomic legislation, 306, 307
    fixed costs (FC), in breakeven
        analysis, 93
    genetic testing, 241
    laboratory tests, 123
    long-term care, 177
    patient outcome and satisfaction, 59
    price (P), in breakeven analysis, 93
    variable (VC), in breakeven
        analysis, 93
COTA (Certified Occupational Therapy
        Assistant), 68, 69
Council for Higher Education
        Accreditation (CHEA), 193
Council on Academic Accreditation
        (CAA), 71
Council on Graduate Medical
        Education (COGME),
        339-340
Counseling, 229
CPU (central processing unit), 286
Cranberry, 107
Crick, Francis, 235
Crisis counseling, 165
Critical thinking, 145-146
Cross-disciplinary work
    case example, 254-255
    defined, 251
    gender issues, 256
*Cultural Competence: A Journey,*
        218-219
Cultural competency
    domains, 218-219
    education, 215-216
    interdisciplinary behavioral
        approach, 158
    sensitivity, 145, 178-179, 364
Cupping, 167
*Curanderismo,* 168
Cystic fibrosis, 240
Cytotechnology, 194, 324

Dalston, Jeptha, 342
Dance and movement therapy, 228
Daschle, Tom, 315
Davies, K., 239
Day treatment programs, 159
de Montesquieu, Baron, 308
de Secondat, Charles-Louis, 308-309
de Tocqueville, Alexis, 313
Death, leading causes, 240
Decentralization structure, 89, 91
Decision function, management, 94-97
DE/DL (distance education/learning).
        *See* Distance-based learning
        programs
Definition of allied health, 3-6
DeMarco, Rosanna, 249
*Democracy in America,* 313
Demographic trends, 171-172
    aging population, 173-177
    education, 216-218
    elderly population, 171
    family structure, 180-182
    impact on allied health professions,
        182-185
    population shifts, 172
    poverty and underserved
        populations, 179-180
    racial and ethnic diversity, 177-179
Demographics, defined, 84
Dental assistants
    employment opportunities, 355
    employment statistics, 18
    primary care, 53
Dental hygienists
    employment opportunities, 355
    employment statistics, 18
    occupational statistics, 77
    primary care, 53
Dentists
    employment opportunities, 355-356
    primary care, 53-54, 57
Deoxyribose nucleic acid (DNA),
        235-236, 237
Department of Defense, 292
Department of Education (USDE)
    accreditation recognition, 193
    financial aid eligibility, 189
    history, 27

Department of Education (USDE)
*(continued)*
professional association and
accrediting agencies
relationships, 200
Department of Energy, 245
Department of Health, Education and
Welfare (DHEW), 11, 12
Department of Health and Human
Services (DHHS)
allied health, defined, 3-4
CAHL grant, 343
history, 11
legionnaires, 312
Office of New Careers, 12-13
Department of Labor
Labor-HHS, 305
OSHA. *See* Occupational Safety and
Health Administration
Departmentalization, 79-80
Depression
primary care, 160-161
screening, 161
St. John's wort, 107, 108, 169
Designer foods, 103
Detoxification units, 157
DHEW (Department of Health,
Education and Welfare), 11,
12
DHHS. *See* Department of Health and
Human Services
Diabetic therapy, 108
Diagnosis, defined, 119
Diagnostic medial sonography, 194
Diagnostic services
case study, 120-121
discharge planning, 134
employment opportunities, 357
laboratory test, selection of, 121-125
multidisciplinary team, 119-120
procedures, 125-134
Diallyl sulfide, 108
Diet. *See also* Chemical and dietary
therapies
stress relievers, 149-150, 153
therapy, 102
Dietary supplements
defined, 102
flavonoids, 105-106
herbs, 106-109

Dietary supplements *(continued)*
phytosterols, 110
prebiotics and probiotics, 104-105
Dietary therapy. *See* Chemical and
dietary therapies
Dietitian
CAAHEP accreditation, 194
employment statistics, 18
genetics and, 245
occupational statistics, 77
roles, 17
Diffusion of innovation model, 274-275
Diffusion theory, 284-285
Digital divide, 274, 285, 289, 291
Digital Millennium Copyright Act of
1998, 272
Digital versatile disc (DVD), 286
Dip Tank Standard, 308
Disabled Veterans Service Dog and
Health Care Improvement Act
of 2001, 299
Distance learning, defined, 287
"Distance Learning" program, 292-293
Distance-based learning programs
accreditation, 195-196, 212
case studies, 287, 292-294
challenges, 288
features, 287-288
Internet, 280
program examples, 41-42
technology and online education,
287-290
trends, 289-290, 364
Diversity. *See* Cultural competency;
Minority groups
Division of labor, 89
DNA (deoxyribose nucleic acid),
235-236, 237
Doctor of audiology degree (AuD), 71
Doctor of occupational therapy (OTD),
68
Doctor of osteopathy (DO), 56. *See
also* Osteopathy
Dolan, Thomas, 342
Doll, R., 102
Domain expertise, 329
*Dorland's Illustrated Medical
Dictionary,* 142
Dossey, Larry, 229
Double helix, DNA, 237

Douglas, Harry E., III, 1, 363
Down syndrome, 240
DPT (doctor of physical therapy
    degree), 65, 66
Dream work, 228
Drucker, Peter, 75, 76, 83, 336
Dunton, William Rush, Jr., 67
DVD (digital versatile disc), 286
*Dying in the City of the Blues: Sickle
    Cell Anemia and the Politics
    of Race and Health,* 239


Early intervention program (EIP), 164
ECG (electrocardiogram), 132
Echinacea, 107, 108, 109
Echternach, John, 61, 364
Economic impact, 84
Economic Opportunity Act (1964), 12
Economic order quantity inventory
    systems, 93
Education. *See also* Accreditation
    achievement evaluation, 198
    certification, 16
    evolving role of, 13-16
    government role. *See* Government
        role in education
    historical overview, 7-9
    impact of technology. *See*
        Technology, impact on
        education
    institutional interest groups, 312
    interprofessional barriers, 257-258
    leadership, 339-340
    management, 77-78
    maximizing experience for future
        employment, 359-361
    medical technologies, 9
    nontraditional environments, 184
    occupational therapist, 9
    physical therapists, 9, 65
    recommended strategies, 23-24
    specialty medical, 10-11
    teaching assistantships, 361
Education, global community, 231
    complementary and alternative
        medicine trends, 220-222
    cultural competence. *See* Cultural
        competency
    cultural diversity, 222-223

Education, global community
    *(continued)*
    international study, 230-231
    medical philosophies summary,
        225-229
    outcomes, 223-224
    population demographics, 216-218
    recruitment, 223
    self-assessment checklist, 219-220
    strategies, 224, 229-231
EIP (early intervention program), 164
Eisenberg, David, 220
Elderly
    aging population trends, 173-175,
        353
    complementary and alternative
        medicine, 220
    demographic trends, 171-172
    health care trends, 174, 176-177
    independence, 176
    as vulnerable populations, 163
Electrocardiogram (ECG), 132
Electromagnetic therapy, 227
Electroneurodiagnostic technology, 194
Electronic classroom, 42
Electronic Patient Record, 42
Eligibility, training grant program, 40
ELSI (ethical, legal, and social
        implications of gene testing),
        242-244
Elwood, Thomas W., 23, 299, 365
Emergency medical technician (EMT),
        18, 120, 194
Emergency room
    functions, 54
    medical care for the poor, 180
    psychiatric, 156
    trauma patients and psychiatrists, 156
Empathy, 142-143
Employment, 353, 361
    allied health, 16-19, 365-366
    demand for workers, 353
    high-tech preparation, 353-354
    locations, 355-356
    maximizing experiences, 359-360
    occupational statistics, 77
    shortages, 361
    statistics, 17, 18, 353
    types of jobs, 356-358
    working conditions, 358-359

EMT (emergency medical technician), 18, 120, 194
End-of-life issues, 176
Energy drinks, 114
Energy medicine, 227
Engineers, employment statistics, 18
Enlightenment, 308
Environment, influence on health, 241
Environmental medicine, 225
Ephedra, 108
E-rate services, 285
Ergonomics
    chronology, 303
    congressional reaction to regulations, 305-306
    criticism of standards, 307-308
    dispute elements, 304-305
    history and, 310
    legislation, 300, 302
    litigation phase, 306-307
    risk factors, 302
*Espiritismo,* 168
Ethernet, 286
Ethical, legal, and social implications of gene testing (ELSI), 242-244
Ethnic population. *See* Minority groups
Ethnomedicine, 226
*Eupsychian Management,* 151
Evidence-based practice, 322
Excedrin caffeine content, 113
Executive branch, role in education, 36-41
Executive management, 77-79
Exercise
    aerobic, 227
    anaerobic, 227
    Chinese therapy, 3
    medical philosophy, 227
    stress reliever, 150, 153
Exons, 238
External analysis, 84

Fabricated foods, 103
Facility assets, in strategic planning, 86
Factor V Leiden allele, 241
Fair Use guidelines, 272
Faith-based health care organizations, 76

Families USA, 311
Family medicine, 50, 51
Family structure demographics, 180-182
Fat substitutes, 111-112
Fauser, J. E., 192
FCC (Federal Communications Commission), 291, 295
FDA (Food and Drug Administration), 103, 105
Federal Bureau of Prevention, 43
Federal Bureau of Primary Health Care, 52
Federal Commerce Department, 286
Federal Communications Commission (FCC), 291, 295
Federal Election Commission, 314
Federal government. *See also* Government; Legislation
    access to technology for everyone, 274
    access to technology policymaking, 286, 290, 295
    Department of Education, 189. *See also* Department of Education
    educational funding, 319, 364
    human genome issues, 243-244
    Internet funding, 292
    public policy roles, 310-312
    role in allied health advancement, 367
*Federal Register,* 36-37, 302, 305, 306
Federal Trade Commission, 294
*The Federalist,* 300-301
Feldenkrais method, 227-228
Feverfew, 107
File transfer protocol (FTP), 282
Finances, strategic planning, 86
Financial aid and accreditation, 189
First contact medicine, 49
Fitness/exercise medicine, 227
Fixed costs (FC) in breakeven analysis, 93
Flavonoids, 105-106
Flexner Report (1910), 7-9, 14, 26
Focusing, 228
Food
    alternative therapy, 102-104
    artificial sweeteners, 111-112
    caffeine, 112-114, 150, 153

Food *(continued)*
    fat substitutes, 111-112
    fermentation, 104-105
    fruit beverages, 114
    smoked and blackened, 110-111
    stress relievers, 149-150
    wines, 114-116
Food and Drug Administration (FDA),
    103, 105
Foot reflexology, 165
Fortune 500 companies survey, 252
Foster care parents and children as
    vulnerable populations, 163
Fragmentation, 25
French Philosophes, 308
Friends of HRSA, 314
Fruit beverages, 114
FTP (file transfer protocol), 282
Functional departmentalization, 79
Functional food, 102, 103-104
Functional medicine, 225
Funding factors, 38-39
Fuzzy medicine, 58


Gaby, Alan, 225
Gale, David D., 245
Gantt charts, 93
GAO (General Accounting Office),
    306, 312
Garlic, 107-109
Gatekeeper
    faculty, 280
    first contact function, 49, 56
Gatorade, 114
GDP (gross domestic product), 76
Gelsinger, Jesse, 236
Gender issues
    interprofessional work, 255-256
    postsecondary education, 290-291
Gene mapping, 235, 236
General Accounting Office (GAO),
    306, 312
General Health Questionnaire, 161
General medicine, 50, 52
General Notice, 37
Generally recognized as safe (GRAS),
    105
Genetic counseling, CAAHEP
    accreditation, 194

Genetics
    defined, 236-237
    disorders, 240-241
    ethical, legal, and social issues,
        242-244
    history, 235-236
    role in health care, 239-241
    testing, 240-241
Genistein, 106
Genome, defined, 237
Genomics, 237, 247
Geographical departmentalization, 80
Geriatric care. *See* Elderly
Gestalt therapy, 228
*Ginkgo biloba,* 107, 108, 169
Ginseng (Asian), 107, 108, 109
Given Diagnostic Imaging System, 279
Global community, education. *See*
    Education, global community
Glucosamine research, 169
GMENAC (Graduate Medical
    Education National Advisory
    Committee), 11, 26
Goldberg, Robert, 307
Goldstein, Harold, 5
Goode, T., 219
Gore, Albert, 310
Gould, K., 220
Governance, shared, 189
Government
    federal. *See* Federal government
    function in legislation, 308-310
    growing elderly health care,
        176-177
    historical overview of health care
        involvement, 7-9
    promotion of alternative treatment,
        168-169
    role in education. *See* Government
        role in education
Government role in education, 42-43
    executive branch, 36-41
    legislative branch, 33-36
    Nebraska story, 31-32
    program examples, 41-42
Graduate Medical Education National
    Advisory Committee
    (GMENAC), 11, 26
Grants, federal
    application process, 40-41

Grants, federal *(continued)*
  CAHL, 343
  distance education, 32
  eligibility, 40
  ergonomic studies, 303
  financial aid and accreditation, 189
  funding factors, 38-39
  program materials, 37-38
  promotion of alternative treatment,
    168-169
  rural community, 32
Grape skins, 110
GRAS (generally recognized as safe),
  105
Great Depression
  AMA and allied health partnership, 9
  development of physical therapy, 65
  occupational therapy, 67
Greater Media Cable, 292
Gross domestic product (GDP), 76
Guided imagery, 228
Guild system, 13-14, 21
Guttmacher, A., 239, 240
Gynecologists, 50, 51-53


Hall, Herbert, 67
Hamilton, Alexander, 300
*Handbook of Accreditation,* 190-191
Harland, Barbara F., 101, 364
Hawes, Bernadine, 293
Hayward, Lorna, 249
HCFA (Health Care Financing
    Administration), 76, 299
Head Start programs, 164
Healer interventions, 227
Healing arts, evolution of, 1-2
Health, defined, 140
Health and Human Services, 12
Health care, defined, 64
Health Care Financing Administration
    (HCFA), 76, 299
Health care management. *See*
    Management
*Health Groups in Washington,* 312
Health Information System Simulation
    (HISS) project, 42
Health maintenance organizations
    (HMOs), 138-139, 221

Health managers, employment
    opportunities, 358
Health Manpower Training Act of
    1985, 22
*Health Personnel: Meeting the
    Explosive Demand for
    Medical Care,* 5
Health Professions and Nursing
    Education Coalition
    (HPNEC), 314
Health Professions Education
    Extension Amendments, 3-4,
    34, 39, 337
*Health Professions Education for the
    Future: Schools in Service to
    the Nations,* 23-24
Health Professions Education
    Partnership Act of 1998, 35
Health Professions Extension
    Amendments of 1991, 24
Health Professions Network (HPN),
    339, 343, 348
Health promotion through technology,
    291-294
Health Resources and Services
    Administration (HRSA)
  Bureau of Health Professions. *See*
    Bureau of Health Professions
  Friends of HRSA, 314
  *Preview,* 37, 40
  program materials, 37
Health services managers, 18
Health Training Empowerment Act of
    1970, 20
Health Training Improvement Act of
    1970, 20
Health trends
  aging population, 174, 176-177
  family structure, 181-182
  impact on allied health professions,
    182-185
  racial and ethnic diversity, 177-179
Healthcare Insurance Portability and
    Accountability Act (HIPAA),
    76, 81
Healthy People 2010
  eliminating disparities in health
    care, 223
  improving quality of life, 163, 220
  public service, 229

Heart disease
  alcohol and, 114-115
  flavonoids and, 106
  lifestyle changes and, 220-221
Hellerwork, 227-228
Hematology laboratory procedures,
    125-126
Herbal medicine
  alternative therapy, 102-103
  herbs, 106-109, 229
  history, 17
  trends, 220
Herbology Chinese therapy, 3
Heteroglossia, 315
"The Hidden Health Care Workforce,"
    338-339
Hierarchy of needs, 151-152
HIPAA (Healthcare Insurance
    Portability and Accountability
    Act), 76, 81
Hippocrates, 17
HISS (Health Information System
    Simulation project), 42
Historical overview, 26-27
  accreditation, 191-192
  allied health, defined, 3-6
  early approach, 2-3
  education and standards roles, 13-16
  evolution of healing arts, 1-2
  modern approach, 3
  new majority, 16-19
  occupational therapy, 67
  recognition of professions, 19-26
  rehabilitative and restorative
    therapies, 64-72
  speech/language pathology, 70
  U.S. health care system, 6-13
HIV/AIDS, 159
HMOs (health maintenance
    organizations), 138-139, 221
Holistic health
  early medicine, 2-3
  education, 224
  nursing, 169
Home health care
  employment opportunities, 355
  speech/language pathology, 72
  for vulnerable populations, 164
Home modification programs, 176
Homeless populations, 162-163

Homeopathic medicine
  complementary and alternative
    medicine, 165
  energy medicine, 227
  medical philosophy, 227, 229
  trends, 220, 221
Honolulu heart study (1977), 115
Horowitz, Morris A., 5
Hospital Survey and Construction Act
    (1946), 10
Hospital-based education, 13-15
Hospital-borne infections, 133
Hospitals
  behavioral services, 156-157
  consultation and liaison units, 157
  employment opportunities, 355
  functions, 55
  medical care for the poor, 180
  satellite behavioral health clinics,
    159
  specialty, 76
Howard University iridology study, 166
HPN (Health Professions Network),
    339, 343, 348
HPNEC (Health Professions and
    Nursing Education Coalition),
    314
HRSA. *See* Health Resources and
    Services Administration
*HRSA Preview,* 37, 40
Human cloning, 243-244
Human Genome Research Project, 242
Human genome sequence, 236, 365
*Human Side of Enterprise* (1960), 152
Huntington's disease, 242
Hydrotherapy, 229
Hyper Studio, 288
Hypnotherapy, 228

*I Know Why the Caged Bird Sings,* 168
IAM. *See* Interprofessional Alliance
    Model
Iammarino, N. K., 230
ICM (intensive case management)
    workers, 160
Illusion of power, 256
Immigration Public Policy Center,
    217-218
Immune system and stress, 149-151

*The Impact of Diversity on Students,* 230
Implementation Task Force, 344
In vitro fertilization, 243
Indian Health Service, 43
Industrial police, 6
Infections
    community-based, 133
    nosocomial (hospital-borne), 133
Information technicians, 77, 194
Information technology, 195-196
Inhalation therapy, 11
Inoperability, computer, 285-286
Input accreditation standards, 201-202
Institute for Alternative Futures, 221,
    222
Institute for Healthcare Improvement,
    340
Institute of Medicine (IOM)
allied health, defined, 3, 5
    *Allied Health Services: Avoiding
        Crises* (1989), 22-23
    Committee on the Future of Primary
        Care, 46-47
    leadership education, 340
    OB/GYN recognition, 52
    primary care definition, 49
Insurance
    chiropractic coverage, 166
    drugs, government's role, 177
    employee-based, 180
    gene tests and, 242
    home health care coverage, 164
    interest groups, 312
    Medicaid. *See* Medicaid
    Medicare. *See* Medicare
    payment for complementary and
        alternative care, 102, 221
    pre-approval of claim, 119
    social experiments of the 1960s, 12
    training cost write-off, 15
    uninsured poor, 179-180, 364
Intensive case management (ICM)
    workers, 160
Interdisciplinary health care
    behavioral approaches, 156
    behavioral services, 156-157
    case study, 157-160
    depression in primary care, 160-161
    focus, 155-156
    Interprofessional Alliance Model,
        263

Interest groups, 312-315
Interim Final Rule, 37
Internal analysis, 84, 85
Internal medicine, 50, 51-52
International study, 230-231
Internet. *See also* Computers;
        Technology, impact on
        education; World Wide Web
    academic and training instruction.
        *See* Distance-based learning
        programs
    access to complementary medicines,
        365
    accreditation information, 206-207
    advertising for complementary
        medicines, 102
    distance-based learning programs,
        41-42, 195-196
    health information, 220
    history, 292
    patient health care involvement, 76
    patients' rights information, 138
    searching, 282-285
    technology for African-American
        women, 293
    virtual campus, 201, 212
Internet Service Provider (ISP), 282
Interprofessional Alliance Model
        (IAM), 251, 259
    basis of model, 260
    caring, social support, personal
        knowledge, 261-262
    case example, 263-268
    illustrated, 261
    phases, 262
    theory, 260-261
Interprofessional collaborative
        alliances, 249
    barriers, 255-259
    case study, 253-255
    defined, 250-251
    education to explore barriers,
        257-258
    gender issues, 255-256
    group goals, 258-259
    illustrated, 250
    model. *See* Interprofessional
        Alliance Model
    need for, 251-253
    power illusions, 256

Interprofessional collaborative alliances
  *(continued)*
  reducing barriers, 256-257
  work interpretations, 251
Introns, 238
Intuition, 144-145
IOM. *See* Institute of Medicine
Iridology, 165, 166
ISP (Internet Service Provider), 282
Issues, strategic planning, 84, 86-87

Jaklevic, Mary Chris, 342
Japanese versus American decision-
  making, 95-96
Jay, John, 300
JCAHO. *See* Joint Commission on the
  Accreditation of Healthcare
  Organizations
Jerman, Ed C., 14
Jesus Christ, 143
Jin Shin Jyutus, 167, 227
Job corps program, 12-13
Joint Commission on the Accreditation
  of Healthcare Organizations
  (JCAHO)
  importance of management, 76
  interest groups, 312
  management ensuring compliance,
    81
  mandated evaluation methods, 92
  standards regulation, 81
*The Journal of Speech Disorders,* 70
*Journal of Telemedicine and Telecare,*
  279
Journaling, 228
Judgment, superior, 145-146
Jungian analysis, 228

Kaiser Permanente, 115, 312
Kanter, Rosabeth Moss, 76
Kardec, Allan, 168
Kava, 107, 108, 114
Keyboarding training, 281-282
Khan, K. Habib, 137, 365
Kiel, Joan M., 75
Kinesiotherapy, 194
Kirkeeide, R., 220

Knowledge. *See* Research
Kotter, John P., 335, 336
Kraemer, L. G., 231

Laboratory employment opportunities,
  356
Laboratory science, 195, 324
Laboratory technicians, 77
Laboratory technologist, 77
Laboratory tests. *See also* Clinical
  laboratory technologists and
  technicians
  analytic factor, 121, 124
  arterial blood gases, 133
  blood bank, 129, 194
  chemistry studies, 126-129, 133
  coagulation studies, 130, 133
  diagnostic X rays, 131-132
  electrocardiogram (ECG), 132
  factors in selection of, 122-123
  hematology procedures, 125-126
  infections, 133
  Magnetic Resonance Image, 132
  microbiology procedures, 134
  point-of-care testing, 130
  postanalytic factor, 121, 124-125
  preanalytic factor, 121-124
  selection of, for diagnosis, 121-125
  specimen collection, 123-124, 125,
    126, 129, 134
  urinalysis, 126-127, 133
Labor-HHS, 305
*The Lancet,* 220
Language
  bilingual personnel. *See* Bilingual
    personnel
  pathologists. *See* Speech/language
    pathology
Last, J. M., 140
Latin American folk practices, 167-168
Law of Similars, 227
Law of the Infinitesimal Dose, 227
Leaders, 349-350
  acquiring skills, 360-361
  association outreach, 349
  CAHL. *See* Coalition for Allied
    Health Leadership
  case study, 333-336

Leaders *(continued)*
 Center for the Health Professions
  recommendations, 338-339
 collaboration across disciplines, 348
 collaborative education, 339-340
 Commission on Allied Health
  recommendations, 337-338
 health care administrator
  observations, 340-342
 Health Professions Network vision,
  339
 health workers, 151-153
 knowledge of leadership
  development, 349
 management versus, 335-336
 need for, 367
 Pew Health Professions
  Commission report, 338
 preparing for the future, 336-340
 recommendations for students,
  348-349
Lecca, Pedro J., 353
Lee, J. K., 244
Legal issues, gene testing, 242-244
Legionnaires, 312
Legislation. *See also* Congress, role in
  education; Public policy
 Economic Opportunity Act, 12
 food regulation, 103
 genetic discrimination bills, 243
 health policy formulation, 299
 Immigration Public Policy Center,
  217-218
 occupational therapy, 68
 physical therapy licensure law, 64
 purpose of, 39
 speech/language pathology, 71
 state, 91-94
 statutory authority, 35
 in strategic planning, 85
 technology, 286, 290, 295
Legislative branch role in education,
  33-36
"Lessons learned" guidelines, 145
Librarians' Index to the Internet, 284
Licorice, 108
Lifestyle modification, 229
Light and color techniques, 227
Listening skills, 141-142, 152
*Live Longer, Live Better,* 149

LiveTalk, 288
Lobbying, role in education, 33-34
Long-term care costs, 177
Lycopene, 105-106
Lyme disease, 243
Lynch, M. Marcia, 249
Lyons, Kevin J., 319, 366

M2A Ingestible Imaging Capsule, 279
Madison, James, 300-301, 309
Magnetic Resonance Image (MRI), 132
Malpractice lawsuits, 122-123
Managed care, 138
Management, 98
 controlling function, 91-94
 decision making, 94-97
 defined, 75
 education, 77-78
 example, 75
 functions, 82-83
 importance of, 76
 leadership versus, 336
 organizational structure, 79-82
 organizing, 89-91
 planning function, 83-89
 roles, 75-76
 three-legged stool, 77-79
Mandates, congressional, 34-35, 36
Manual medicine, 227-228
Marshall, E., 238
Maslow, Abraham H., 137-138,
  151-153
*Maslow on Management,* 151
Massage therapy, 227
Master of physical therapy (MPT), 65,
  66
Master of science in physical therapy
  (MSPT), 65
Master's degree, occupational therapy
  (MSOT), 68
Masters in business administration
  (MBA), 78
Masters in health management systems
  (MHMS), 78
Materials, program, 37-38
MBA (masters in business
  administration), 78
McGregor, Douglas, 152
McKusick, V., 236, 247

McLanahan, S., 220
McMillan, Mary, 64
Measurement science, 91
Medicaid
    children's health care, 182
    CMS program instructions, 311-312
    compensation for health
        professionals, 182
    history, 12
    HMOs for the underserved, 180
    implementation of laws, 299
    serving the poor, 179
    training cost write-off, 15
Medical assistants, 18, 194
Medical doctors (MD), training, 56
Medical illustrator, 194
Medical police, 7
Medical profession, 7-9
Medical records and health information
        technicians, 18, 77, 194
Medical supply company interest
        groups, 312
Medical technologists, 9, 324
Medicare
    aging population trends, 174
    CMS program instructions, 311-312
    elderly, failure to see doctors,
        163-164
    future adequate funding, 176-177
    history, 12
    implementation of laws, 299
    interest group influence on policy,
        314-315
    occupational therapy services, 69, 72
    physical therapy services, 65, 72
    speech/language pathology services,
        72
    training cost write-off, 15
Medicinals, caffeine content, 112, 113
MEDLINE, 283
Mehl, Lewis, 226
Mendel, Gregor, 235
*Mental Health and Mental Disorders,*
        160-161
Mental health care
    employment opportunities, 357
    primary care, 48, 53
Mental Illness Awareness Week, 161
Mercy Hospital, Des Moines, Iowa,
        303

Mergers, 76
Methadone maintenance clinics, 159
MHMS (masters in health management
        systems), 78
MICA day treatment programs, 159
Microbiology procedures, 134
Middle line, 81, 82, 83
Midol caffeine content, 113
Military health care services
    federal support, 43
    occupational therapy, 67
    physical therapy, 65
    speech/language pathology, 70-71
Milk thistle, 107
Mind/body medicine, 228
Minority groups
    allied health occupations, 22
    demographic trends, 177-179, 184
    education, 222, 290-291
    health care access, 363-364
    referral process, 165
    student applicants, 26
    as vulnerable populations, 162
Mintzberg, Henry, 82-83
Mission, strategic planning, 84, 87-88
Model. *See* Interprofessional Alliance
        Model
Moonlighting, 80
Mortality, leading causes, 240
Mouse genome, 238
Moxibustion, 167
MPT (master of physical therapy), 65,
        66
MRI (Magnetic Resonance Image), 132
MSDs (musculoskeletal disorders),
        302, 304, 307
MSOT ( master's degree, occupational
        therapy), 68
MSPT (master of science in physical
        therapy), 65
Multidisciplinary work
    case example, 254-255
    defined, 251
    gender issues, 256
Murray, Michael, 228-229
Musculoskeletal disorders (MSDs),
        302, 304, 307
Music therapy, CAAHEP accreditation,
        195
Mutations, 235, 239, 240

NACNAH (North American Consortium for Nursing and Allied Health), 230-231

NACNEP (National Advisory Council on Nurse Education and Practice), 339-340

NAFEO (National Association for Equal Opportunity in Higher Education), 293

National Academy of Sciences, 306

National Advisory Council on Nurse Education and Practice (NACNEP), 339-340

National Allied Health Week, 344

National Association for Equal Opportunity in Higher Education (NAFEO), 293

National Association of Manufacturers, 306

National Center for Complementary and Alternative Medicine (NCCAM), 102, 116, 169, 224

National Center for Education Statistics, 290

National Centers for Toxicogenomics, 243

National Coalition for Health Professional Education in Genetics (NCHPEG), 245, 246

National Coalition on Ergonomics, 306, 308

National Commission on Allied Health (NCAH)
 congressional establishment of, 34, 337
 employment, 17, 19
 future of allied health, 21-22, 222, 223
 Implementation Task Force, 338
 leadership training, 344
 review of health issues, 24-26

National Commission on Allied Health Education, 3

National Depression Screening Day, 161

National Institute of Environmental Health Sciences (NIEHS), 243

National Institute of Health, 169, 221

National Library of Medicine, 283

National Network of Health Career Programs in Two-Year Colleges (NN2), 343, 348

National Nursing Research Agenda (NNRA), 155

National Society for the Promotion of Occupational Therapy, 67

National Society of Allied Health, 367

Native American medicine, 167, 226

*Nature,* 235

Naturopathic medicine, 228-229

NCAH. *See* National Commission on Allied Health

NCCAM (National Institute of Health's National Center for Complementary and Alternative Medicine), 102, 116, 169, 224

NCHPEG (National Coalition for Health Professional Education in Genetics), 245, 246

Nebraska story, 31-32

Neel, James, 235

Neighborhood clinics, 162, 180

Neighborhood health centers (NHC), 253-254

Neita, Marguerite E., 119

Networking, 293-294

Neurolinguistic programming, 228

Neurology, 55

*New Careers for the Poor,* 12

*New England Journal of Medicine,* 220

New majority, health professions, 16-19

*A New Majority in the Health Profession,* 11

NHC (neighborhood health centers), 253-254

NIEHS (National Institute of Environmental Health Sciences), 243

Nielsen, Gail A., 333, 367

Nightingale, Florence, 155

NN2 (National Network of Health Career Programs in Two-Year Colleges), 343, 348

NNRA (National Nursing Research Agenda), 155

No-Doz caffeine content, 113
North American Consortium for Nursing and Allied Health (NACNAH), 230-231
North Central Association of Colleges and Schools, 190-191
North Central Association of Colleges and Secondary Schools, 192
Nosocomial (hospital-borne infections), 133
Notice of Proposed Rulemaking, 36, 308
Nuclear Medical Technology, 194, 195
Nuclear medicine technologists, 77
Nurse practitioners
    functions, 56
    holistic nursing, 169
    mental health care, 53
    primary care, 51, 52
    public health nursing, 155
    subspecialties, 55
    surgery, 54
Nursing facilities, employment opportunities, 355
Nuru-Jeter, Amani M., 271, 366
Nutraceuticals, 103
Nutrient supplement, 102. *See also* Dietary supplements
Nutrim, 112
Nutrition, Chinese therapy, 3
Nutritional medicine, 225, 229
Nutritionists, 18, 77


Oatrim, 112
Obesity, 111
OB/GYN, 50, 51, 52-53
Occupational Safety and Health Administration (OSHA)
    construction standards, 307
    Dip Tank Standard, 308
    economic-impact analysis, 306
    Ergonomic Program Standard, 302
    ergonomics costs, 306, 307
    ergonomics legislation, 300, 304, 308
    ergonomics standard, 306
    perspective on ergonomics legislation, 310

Occupational therapists
    AOTA. *See* American Occupational Therapy Association
    education standards, 9
    employment statistics, 18
    occupational statistics, 77
    secondary care, 48
Occupational therapy
    CAAHEP accreditation, 194
    education, 67-68, 319
    employment, 68-69
    genetics and, 246
    history, 67
    licensure, 68
    purpose, 69
    research, 324
    role of research, 73
    teamwork, 72-73
Occupations, employment statistics, 18
Office of Complementary and Alternative Medicine, 221
Office of New Careers, 12-13
Olestra, 111
Oliver, Richard E., 171, 363
Onions, 108
Operating core, 81, 82
Operational planning, 83
Ophthalmic medical technologist/technician, 194
Options, strategic planning, 84, 87
Optometrists, 57
Orderlies, 11
Oren, E., 244
Organizational structure, management departmentalization, 79-80
    parts of, 80-82
    in strategic planning, 86
Oriental medicines, 165, 166, 222
Ornish, D., 220
O'Rourke, T. W., 230
Orthodontics, 53
Orthomolecular medicine, 225
Orthopedics, 55
Orthoptist, CAAHEP accreditation, 194
Orthotic and prosthetic practitioner, 194
Orthotics, 14
OSHA. *See* Occupational Safety and Health Administration
Osler, William, 225

Osteopathy, 56, 228, 355
OTD (doctor of occupational therapy), 68
Outcomes
    accreditation standards, 198, 201-202
    educational, 223-224
    professional alliance, 260-261
Outsourcing information and public policy, 315-316
Overlap, practice, 58

PACs (political action committees), 314-315
Para-professionals, 12-13
Pareto charts, 93
Partial hospitalization programs (PHP), 159
Partial thromboplastin time (PTT), 130
Patient feedback, 59
Patients Are People Too, 138
Patients' Bill of Rights, 138
Pau d'Arco, 108
PDA (personal data assistants), 278, 354
Peanut butter, phytosterols, 110
Pearl, Arthur, 12, 24
Pediatrics, 50, 51, 52
Pennyroyal, 108
People skills versus technical competence, 138-139. See also Psychosocial interaction
Perfusion, 194
Personal care facilities, employment opportunities, 355
Personal data assistants (PDAs), 278, 354
Personal knowledge, 261
Personnel
    poorly defined roles, 58
    in strategic planning, 85, 86
Perspective variations, 58
PERT analysis, 93
Peto, R., 102
Pew Advisory Panel for Allied Health, 5
Pew Health Professions Commission
    background, 23
    disadvantaged students, 222

Pew Health Professions Commission (continued)
    education of health care providers, 224
    findings and recommendations, 338
    public service goals, 229
    skills of future workers, 27
    strategies for educators and schools, 24
Pharmaceutical company interest groups, 312
Pharmacist Workforce Study, 34
Pharmacogenomics, 244-246
Pharmacy assistants, 18
Pharmafoods, 103
Phillips, K., 244
Philosophies summary, 225-229
Phlebotomy, 121
PHO (physician hospital organization), 80
PHP (partial hospitalization program), 159
Physical education model, 8
Physical therapists. See also Rehabilitation
    access to patients, 66
    CAAHEP accreditation, 194
    demand for services, 65-66
    education, 9, 65
    employment statistics, 18
    genetics and, 246
    occupational statistics, 77
    secondary care, 48
    veterans' benefits, 299
Physical therapy
    educational requirements, 319
    occupational statistics, 77
    research, 324
    role of research, 73
    teamwork, 72-73
Physical therapy degree (DPT), 65, 66
Physician assistants (PA)
    CAAHEP accreditation, 194
    employment statistics, 18
    exclusion from allied health definition, 4
    genetics and, 246
    mental health care, 53
    occupational statistics, 77
    primary care, 51, 52

Physician assistants (PA) *(continued)*
  subspecialties, 55
  surgery, 54
  training, 56
Physician hospital organization (PHO), 80
Physician offices, employment opportunities, 355
Physicians
  management responsibilities, 77-79
  role in organizational structure, 80
Phytochemicals, 104
Phytosterols (PS), 110
Picture archiving, 354
Planning, management, 83-89
Play therapists, 158
Pliny, 108
POCT (point-of-care testing), 130
Podiatrists, 57
Point-of-care testing (POCT), 130
Police, industrial, sanitary and medical, 6-7
Policy. *See* Legislation; Public policy
Political action committees (PACs), 314-315
Polyphenols, 106
Population shifts, 172
Ports, T., 220
Postanalytic factors for laboratory tests, 121, 124-125
Postoperative diagnostic testing, 132-133
Postural integration, 228
Poverty and underserved populations, 179-180, 184, 364
Power illusions, 256
Power Point, 288
Practice overlap, 58
Prayer, complementary and alternative medicine, 168, 229
Preanalytic factors for laboratory tests, 121-124
Prebiotics, 104-105
Preservice technology recommendations, 275, 294-295
Preventive care, 48, 49-50, 149-150
Price in breakeven analysis, 93
Primary care, 59
  case study, 45-46

Primary care *(continued)*
  clinicians, 55, 56-57
  components flowchart, 50, 51
  continuity, 47-48
  controversies and conceptual flaws, 58
  defined, 45, 46-47, 48
  dentists, 53-54
  first contact, 49
  integration of services and care, 49-53
  levels of care, 48-49
  mental health, 53
  practice of, 57-58
  therapy, 228
Prison health services, 160
Probiotics, 104-105
Process, professional alliance, 260
Process accreditation standards, 202
Process departmentalization, 80
Product departmentalization, 79
Professional accreditation, 192-193
Professional organization interest groups, 312
Professional specialty, 356
Professionalism concept, 81
Professionals, defined, 40
Program examples, 41-42
Programmatic accreditation
  background of, 190-191
  costs, 196-197
  functions, 15-16
  process of, 193
Projection by health worker, 143-144
Prosthetics, 14
Proteomics, 237
Prothrombin time (PT), 130
Protocols, 81, 157
Provider organization interest groups, 312
Prudden, Bonnie, myotherapy, 227-228
Psychiatric
  emergency room, 156
  inpatient units, 157
  outpatient unit, 158-159
Psychiatrists, 53
Psychodrama, 228
Psychologists, 156
Psychoneuroimmunology, 228

Psychosocial interaction, 137-138
  empathy, 142-143
  health, defined, 140
  health worker leaders and managers,
    151-153
  health worker stress, 147-151,
    152-153
  intuition, 144-145
  listening skills, 141-142, 152
  patient expectations, 146-147
  reflection, projection, clarification,
    summarization, 143-144
  sensitivity, 145
  superior judgment skills, 145-146
  technical competence versus people
    skills, 138-139
  therapies, 140-141
  total acceptance, 143
Psychosocial therapies, 140
Psychosynthesis, 228
PT (prothrombin time), 130
PTT (partial thromboplastin time), 130
Public Health Service, 311, 367
Public Health Service Act, 3-4, 77, 314
Public Law 105-392, 35
Public policy, 315-316. *See also*
    Legislation
  determinants, 310-312
  ergonomics legislation. *See*
    Ergonomics
  government mechanism, 299-300,
    315
  interest groups, 312-313
  political action committees, 314-315
  separation of powers, 300-301
Public service, 224, 229-230
"Publius," 300
PubMed database, 224


Qigong, 167, 227
Quackwatch Web site, 294
Quality management, 91
Quantitative methodologies in control
    process, 93
Quervalu, Ivan, 155, 366


Radiation technologists, 48
Radiation therapy, 77, 195

Radiographer, 33
Radiologic technologists, 14, 18, 246
*Raising Standards in American
    Healthcare: Best Practices,
    Best People, Best Results,* 342
Random access memory (RAM), 286
Rapp, Doris, 225
Rational emotive therapy, 228
Reader's Digest, *Live Longer, Live
    Better,* 149
RealAudio, 288
Reality therapy, 228
Rebirthing, 228
Recognition, accreditation, 193
Recreation, therapeutic, CAAHEP
    accreditation, 195
Red wine, 110
Referral process, 165
Reflection by health worker, 143-144
*Reforming Health Care Workforce
    Regulation: Policy
    Consideration for the 21st
    Century,* 24
Regulations, federal
  cable television, 291
  executive branch, 36-41
Rehabilitation
  case study, 61-63
  counseling, 195
  defined, 63
  history of therapy, 64-72
  purpose, 64
Reichian analysis, 228
Reiki, 227
Reissman, Frank, 12, 24
Religious-based health care
    organizations, 76
"Report of the National Commission on
    Allied Health," 3-4, 25
Report of the Sanitary Commission of
    Massachusetts (1850), 6-7
Reports, mandated, 34-35
Research, 319-320, 331
  by allied health professionals,
    324-325
  applied, 324
  basic, 324
  case study, 320-322, 323
  graduate projects, 360-361
  importance of, 322-323

Research *(continued)*
   individual strategies, 326-330
   professionwide strategies, 325-326
   role in rehabilitative therapies, 73
Resident training programs, 14
Resources, accreditation standards, 189
Respect for patients, 142-143
Respiratory therapists
   CAAHEP accreditation, 194
   employment statistics, 18
   genetics and, 246
   historical overview, 11
   occupational statistics, 77
Rest, stress reliever, 150, 153
Restorative therapies. *See*
   Rehabilitation
Resveratrol, 110
Retinoblastoma, 241
RHEN (Rural Health Education
   Network), 32, 42
Robert Wood Johnson Foundation, 245,
   342
Rogers, Carl, 141, 142, 143
Role-playing and Capitol Hill visits,
   343-344
Rolfing, 227-228
Rote learning, 14
Ruggiero, V. R., 146
Rural communities
   accessibility to health care, 182
   support of elderly populations, 176
Rural Health Education Network
   (RHEN), 32, 42

Sadee, W., 244
Safety issues, 333-334
Salaries and accreditation, 190
Samuels, Cheryl T., 215, 363-364
Sanitary police, 6
*Santeria,* 168
SASHEP (Study of Accreditation of
   Selected Health Education
   Programs), 20-21
Satellite
   behavioral health clinics, 159
   distance education, 287
   health clinics, 162
Saw palmetto, 107

Scherwitz, L., 220
Schloman, Barbara F., 4-5
School of Allied Health, 41
Scientists, 18
Screening, 161
Secondary care, defined, 48
SEIU (Service Employees International
   Union), 303
Self-actualization, 151, 152
Self-care tools, 221-222
Self-study, 195
Selye, Hans, 150
Senna, 108
Sensitivity, 145, 178, 364. *See also*
   Cultural competency
Separation of powers, 300-301
Service, R., 237
Service Employees International Union
   (SEIU), 303
Service occupations, 356
Set-asides, 36
Severely and persistently mentally ill
   (SPMI), 159
Shadowing a professional, 13-14, 359,
   361
Shamanic healing, 167
Shattuck, Lemuel, 6
Shattuck Report (1850), 6-7, 17, 26
Shealey, Norm, 227
Sherman, V. Clayton, 342
Shiatsu, 167
Sickle-cell anemia, 238, 239
Simplesse, 111
Site visits, accreditation, 195, 198-199,
   203-204, 210
Slagle, Eleanor Clark, 67
Smart cards, 354
Smith, Carole I., 271, 292-293, 366
Smith, D., 230
Smith, T., 140
SoBe drink, 114
Social
   experiments, 12-13
   gene testing implications, 242-244
   lag, 17
   responsibilities, 8
   well-being, 140
   workers, 18, 156
Software, 280, 286. *See also*
   Computers

Southwest Texas State University, training programs, 42
Soy, genistein, 106
Span of control, management organizing, 89, 90-91
Special consideration, funding factor, 38
Special Supplemental Nutrition Program for Women, Infants, and Children (WIC), 182
Specialized accreditation, 15-16, 190-191, 192-193
Specialty medicine
education programs, 10-11
functions, 55
management organizing, 89-90
speech/language pathology, 71-72. *See also* Speech/language pathology
Specimen collection, 123-124, 125, 126, 129, 134
Spectrometry, 241
Speech/language pathology
audiology and, 69-70
CAAHEP accreditation, 195
education, 71, 319
employment statistics, 18
function, 69
genetics and, 246
history, 70
home health care, 72
occupational statistics, 77
research, 324
role of research, 73
specialization, 71-72
teamwork, 72-73
*The Spirit of the Laws,* 308
Spiritual medicine, 168, 229
SPMI (severely and persistently mentally ill), 159
SportBrain First Step, 279-280
St. John's wort, 107, 108, 169
State government and public policy, 311
State laws. *See also* Legislation
lack of uniformity, 25
standards evaluation, 92
Statistics
aging population, 173-175
education, 290

Statistics *(continued)*
employment, 17, 18, 353
occupational, 77
racial and ethnic diversity, 177-179, 216-218
Stem cell research, 243-244
Straker, Howard, 45
Strategic apex, 80, 82, 83
Strategic planning
defined, 83
organizing, 89-91
steps, 84-86
Streaming technology, 292
Stress
depression and, 160-161
handling of, 148
health worker, 147-151, 152-153
immune system and, 149-151
relievers, 149-151, 152-153
Structure accreditation standards, 201
"A Structure for Deoxyribose Nucleic Acid," 235
Study of Accreditation of Selected Health Education Programs (SASHEP), 20-21
Sub-professional, 12-13
Subspecialties, 55
Substance abuse
CASAC counselor, 160
hospital detoxification units, 157
screening, 161
Summarization by health worker, 143-144
Supplements. *See* Dietary supplements
Support staff, 81, 82
Surgery
CAAHEP accreditation, 194
functions, 54-55
primary care, 51
Sweating and purging practice, 167


TAA marker, 239
Tai Chi, 167, 227
Tank jockey, 11
Tax entity considerations in strategic planning, 86
TCM (Traditional Chinese medicine), 3, 221, 226. *See also* Traditional Oriental medicine

Team care approach
  diagnostic services, 119-120
  interdisciplinary behavioral
    approach, 158
  occupational therapy, 69, 72-73
  physical therapy, 72-73
  in rehabilitation, 63
  relevance in health care, 153
  speech/language pathology, 72-73
Teas
  adverse effects, 108
  caffeine, 112
  polyphenol antioxidants, 106
Technical competence versus people
    skills, 138-139
Technicians, employment
    opportunities, 357
Technology, impact on education
  access to technology, 273-275, 285,
    286, 291, 295
  adult learning trends, 290-291
  case studies, 271-273, 276-279,
    292-294
  connecting theory and practice,
    277-280
  core curriculum, 276-277
  distance education, 287-290. *See
    also* Distance-based learning
    programs
  health promotion, 291-294
  inoperability, 285-286
  Internet searching, 282-285
  learning technology skills, 280-282,
    284-285
  policymaking, 286, 294-295
  preservice technology, 275, 294-295
  watchdog, 294
  well-trained providers, 274
"Technology and Sports" program,
    292-293
*Technology and You: Another Point of
    View,* 292-293
Technostructure, 81, 82
Telecommunications Act of 1996, 291
Teleconferencing, 169
Telemedicine, 354
Tertiary care, defined, 49
Tests. *See* Laboratory tests
Theory X, 152
Theory Y, 152

Therapeutic nursery services, 159-160
Therapeutic recreation, CAAHEP
    accreditation, 195
Therapeutic touch, 17, 165, 227
Three-legged stool of management,
    77-79
Time orientation, 321
Tomatoes and lycopene, 105
Touch, therapeutic, 17, 165, 227
*Toward a Psychology of Being,* 138
Traditional Chinese medicine (TCM),
    3, 221, 226
Traditional Oriental medicine, 165,
    166, 222
Trager approach, 227-228
Transactional analysis, 228
Transdisciplinary work
  case example, 255
  defined, 251
  gender issues, 256
  illustrated, 252
Trends
  adult learning, 290-291
  complementary and alternative
    medicine, 220-222, 364-365
  demographic. *See* Demographic
    trends
  distance education, 289-290, 364
  health. *See* Health trends
  strategic planning, 85
Triaminicin caffeine content, 113
Trufant, John E., 187, 365
Truth in Regulating Act of 2000, 306

UCSF (Center for the Health
    Professions), 338-339
Unconditional positive regard, 143
Underserved populations
  demographic trends, 179-180, 184
  Medicaid HMOs, 180
  setting up practices, 222
United States Distance Learning
    Association, 287
Unity of command, management
    organizing of, 89, 90
Universal access, 285
Universal Serial Bus (USB), 286
Universal service, 285

University of California
botanical research, 168-169
grants for preventing lifting injuries,
303
interest groups, 312
University of Illinois botanical
research, 168-169
University of Texas, HISS project, 42
University of Utah, osteoarthritis
research, 169
Upledger, John, 227-228
Urgent care clinics, 54
Urinalysis, 126-127, 133
U.S. Department of Education. *See*
Department of Education
U.S. Department of Health and Human
Services. *See* Department of
Health and Human Services
U.S. Division of Allied Health
Manpower, 4
U.S. Public Health Service, 311, 367
USB (Universal Serial Bus), 286
USDA, 112
USDE. *See* Department of Education
Utilization of services, 85-86


Valentine, Peggy, 353
Valerian, 107, 108, 114
Vanquish caffeine content, 113
Variable costs (VC) in breakeven
analysis, 93
Veenstra, D. L., 244
Venipuncture, 121
Venter, J. Craig, 236
Virtual campus, 201, 212
Visualization, 228
Vivarin caffeine content, 113
Voice recognition programs, 281-282
Voluntary organization interest groups,
312
Voodoo, 168


W. K. Kellogg Foundation, 21
Wallace, Narissa, 293
"Wanted: A Few Good Leaders," 342
Watchdog, technology, 294

Watson, James, 235
Web sites. *See also* Internet
"Ask Jeeves" search engine, 283
Digital Millennium Copyright Act
of 1998, 272
Fair Use guidelines, 272
Librarians' Index to the Internet,
284
MEDLINE, 283
NCCAM, 224
Quackwatch, 294
searching the Internet, 282-285
technology for African-American
women, 293
WebsMostLinked.com, 293
*Webster's Collegiate Dictionary,*
intuition, defined, 144
Weeks, John, 221
Weil, Andrew, 225
White, Ryan, programs, 159
WHO (World Health Organization),
140
WIC (Special Supplemental Nutrition
Program for Women, Infants,
and Children), 182
Williams Interoral Protective Sports
System (WIPSS), 292-293
Wilson, Stephen L., 171, 363
Wines, 114-116
WIPSS (Williams Interoral Protective
Sports System), 292-293
Wolf, L., 230
Women
aging and health care, 176
interprofessional barriers, 255-256
postsecondary education, 290-291
technology Web site, 293
trends in family structure, 180-182
"Women and Technology" program,
292-293
Word processing training, 281-282
Work projects for leadership training,
344-345
Workers' compensation and
ergonomics laws, 308
Workforce shrinkage, 176, 183, 184
Working conditions, 190
Workplace Preservation Act, 305
World Health Organization (WHO),
140

World War I
  hospital-based training programs, 14
  occupational therapy, 67
  physical therapy, 64
  speech/language pathology, 70
World War II
  consequences of, 10-11
  occupational therapy, 67
  physical therapy, 65
  speech/language pathology, 71
World Wide Web (WWW). *See also*
      Internet; Web sites
  application process, 40-41
  training programs, 41-42

X-ray technician
  diagnostic tests, 131-132
  training program, 14

Y Diagram, 84
Yoga, 220
Young, Wendy B., 315
Youtsey, John W., 11

Ziegler, J., 221
Zinc excretion and alcohol
      consumption, 115
Z-Trim, 112